introduction to

Blood Banking

THIRD EDITION

Robert M. Greendyke, M.D.

Former
Blood Bank Director
and
Clinical Associate Professor of Pathology
University of Rochester Medical Center
Rochester, New York

Medical Examination Publishing Co., Inc.
an Excerpta Medica company

Garden City, New York

SIMULTANEOUSLY PUBLISHED IN:

Europe   : HANS HUBER PUBLISHERS
                    Bern, Switzerland

United Kingdom : HENRY KIMPTON PUBLISHERS
                    London, England

PREFACE

This volume is an outgrowth of the Blood Bank training program for technologists and resident physicians formerly conducted by the author at the University of Rochester Medical Center. In the interest of brevity many subjects of considerable interest have been touched upon only fleetingly and others omitted altogether. The author admits to a measure of dogmatism in his approach and hopes that the student will pursue areas of interest by consulting the references listed at the end of each chapter. I have attempted to distinguish throughout these pages between speculation and what seems to be reasonably supported fact, but caution the reader that some of our current concepts of blood group immunology are more plausible theory than proven certainty. That there is still so much to be learned about immunohematology is one of its fascinations.

For the current edition of my work, as for its predecessors, I have drawn heavily upon Dr. P.L. Mollison's *Blood Transfusion in Clinical Medicine,* and wish to gratefully acknowledge the debt to Dr. Mollison which I share with Blood Bank workers everywhere.

Robert M. Greendyke, M.D.

CONTENTS

1 Introduction to Blood Banking 1

2 The Composition and Functions of Blood 3

3 Hematologic Diseases 21

4 Principles of Blood Transfusion Therapy 33

5 Characteristics of Antigens and
  Antibodies 39

6 Reactions Between Antigens and
  Antibodies 61

7 Antiglobulin Testing and Complement 75

8 Genetics in Blood Banking 91

9 The ABO System 98

10 The Lewis System 112

11 The Rh System 119

12 The Kell, Duffy and Kidd Systems 134

13 The MNSs, P, and Lutheran Systems 145

14 The I and Other Blood Group Systems 155

15 Autoimmune Acquired Hemolytic Disease 167

16 Practical Considerations in Blood
   Bank Methodology 181

17 Blood Grouping and Compatibility
   Testing 196

18 Detection and Identification of
   Alloantibodies 213

19 Immunologic Complications of Blood
    Transfusion 226

20 Nonimmunologic Complications of Blood
    Transfusion 245

21 Hemolytic Disease of the Newborn 259

22 Histocompatibility Testing Leukocyte and
    Platelet Antigens 274

23 Blood Collection, Processing and Storage 281

24 Blood and Red Blood Cell Transfusion 291

25 Platelet and Granulocyte Transfusion 298

26 Plasma Coagulation Factor Deficiencies 304

27 Administrative Regulations and Practices 315

28 Quality Assurance 320

    Index 330

notice

The editor(s) and/or author(s) and the publisher of this book have made every effort to ensure that all therapeutic modalities that are recommended are in accordance with accepted standards at the time of publication.

The drugs specified within this book may not have specific approval by the Food and Drug Administration in regard to the indications and dosages that are recommended by the editor(s) and/or author(s). The manufacturer's package insert is the best source of current prescribing information.

CHAPTER 1

Introduction to Blood Banking

Recent advances in medical knowledge have significantly increased the volume and complexity of the work of the hospital blood bank. Surgical techniques are becoming increasingly sophisticated and complex procedures more numerous. Cancer surgery, reconstructive operations, open-heart procedures, and organ transplantation all make special demands upon the blood bank. Greater clinical appreciation of hematologic physiology is reflected in requests for specific blood components, and the modern blood bank dispenses a wide variety of blood products tailored to specific patient needs. An array of techniques unknown to blood bank workers even a few years ago has come into routine use, ranging from radioimmunoassay to cytotoxicity testing.

Simultaneously with advances in clinical medicine has come an explosive increase in our knowledge of immunohematology, reflected by an almost threefold increase in the size of this book in three editions over the space of seven years. Whereas the ABO system and "Rh factor" were almost the only considerations of clinical significance a generation ago, we now recognize more than a dozen major blood group systems, each many times more complex than originally conceived, with some 400 blood group antigens defined as of this writing. Powerful new investigative techniques have been devised to extend our knowledge, some of which have been adapted to use in the blood bank. Immunoglobulin structure and the role of complement in red blood cell sensitization are now understood with considerable insight, and this knowledge has led to increased appreciation of the mechanisms of antibody-mediated red blood cell destruction. Increased understanding of the mechanisms of blood coagulation and clot lysis has resulted in major changes in the approach to the patient with a bleeding disorder.

1

This sophistication, however, has not been without its drawbacks. Burgeoning demands for blood products have posed problems in obtaining sufficient supplies. Transfusions of 20 pints of blood to a single patient are now commonplace, and 100 pints or more have been given in 24 hours to save a life. Awareness of the increased hazard of hepatitis transmission by blood obtained from paid donors has resulted in regulations requiring blood collection from a purely volunteer population, thus causing increased difficulty in procuring blood supplies in some areas. Widespread transfusion has caused widespread blood group sensitization, with resultant problems in antibody identification and procurement of blood of special types.

For the blood bank worker, these advances have special meaning. No longer is "blood banking" a casually acquired competence learned in a few hours' training on the job. Much highly specialized information is necessary for acceptable performance. For the blood bank director, the large amount of particular knowledge required almost precludes simultaneous competence in both immunohematology and the multiple other disciplines encompassed by the term "clinical pathology."

The amount of responsibility assumed by the blood bank technologist and its director has no parallel elsewhere in the clinical laboratory. There is no way for an attending physician to confirm through his own observation or judgement the adequacy of the testing performed in the blood bank until disaster occurs in the form of an untoward reaction. If the clinical chemistry laboratory reports a serum potassium level of 10 mEq/dl or the hematology laboratory says the hematocrit value is 5% and the patient is jogging about the solarium, his doctor may reasonably suspect a laboratory error. But there is no way that a physician can say, "I think you are an 'O', not an 'A' as the lab says," simply by examining his patient.

In the blood bank as in no other area of the clinical laboratory the patient's life may hinge upon a mistake, be it clerical, technical, or judgemental. Errors in other areas may be irritating, confusing, or embarrassing, but rarely are they immediately life-threatening. If someone errs in the blood bank, a patient may die. A standard of excellence that would be the envy of any hematology, chemistry, or microbiology laboratory is not satisfactory for a blood bank: "99 and 44/100% pure" is not good enough.

Challenge and responsibility are the daily substance of blood bank work; stimulation and gratification are the reward.

CHAPTER 2

The Composition and Functions of Blood

The blood circulatory system, as the main transport system of the body, is concerned with moving raw materials, finished products, and wastes from where they originate to where they are used, exert their effects, or are excreted. Blood is composed of an amazing variety of substances, including cells (red blood cells, white blood cells and platelets); gases (oxygen and carbon dioxide); mineral ions (Na^+, K^+, Ca^{++}, Mg^{++}, Cl^-, $H_2PO_4^-$, HCO_3^- to name just a few); metabolites of carbohydrates, proteins, and lipids (frequently in complex combinations); and specialized molecules such as vitamins, hormones, enzymes, antibodies, and complement components, all dissolved or suspended in water. The concentration of each component as well as total osmolality, oncotic pressure, pH, viscosity, and total volume of the blood are under rigid control, thought to be genetically determined but in general poorly understood. The measurement of deviations from the "normal," however defined, constitutes a major part of the work of the clinical laboratory, and a large though inexact body of knowledge has grown up about the diagnostic, therapeutic, and prognostic significance of these variations.

As in any transportation system, some of the components of blood are riders, simply going to a particular destination (e.g., blood glucose going from stores in the liver to muscle to be catabolized), while others are integral parts of blood, performing their function and spending their entire mature existence within it (e.g., red blood cells); and a few are stowaways, foreign elements that are not normal constituents of blood but which have managed to gain access to it (e.g., bacteria or foreign protein antigens). Particular attention will be paid in this chapter only to those elements in blood that are relevant to our understanding of immunohematology.

3

FORMED ELEMENTS

1. Red Blood Cells

Human red blood cells or erythrocytes (RBC) are normally bi-concave discs measuring 7 to 8μ microns in diameter, and in health compose approximately 40% to 50% of the total blood volume, or about 4×10^6 to 5×10^6 RBC/μl. Normal blood volume is 7% to 8% of body weight at maturity, so that a 70 kg adult has about five liters or roughly 10 pints of blood containing some 1.1×10^{13} (eleven tril-lion) RBC. A normal erythrocyte has a life span of 110 to 120 days, and thus the body's red blood cell population must be replaced by the bone marrow at a rate of about 0.9% per day (100 billion RBC or about 18 ml of cells per day).

The mature RBC has a very specialized role in the bodily econ-omy and as such has a limited array of metabolic capabilities. It lacks a nucleus, can synthesize no nucleoprotein and little lipid, and thus is unable to reproduce itself. The energy production of the red blood cell is dependent upon glucose metabolism to lactate via glycolysis (the nonoxidative, or Embden-Meyerhof pathway) and to a lesser extent through the hexose-monophosphate shunt (pentose-phosphate pathway). A constant source of energy is necessary to the red blood cell to enable it to carry out the reactions involved in gas exchange, defense of the integrity of the cell membrane, ion trans-port, and maintenance of its hemoglobin in the reduced state. (Ox-idized hemoglobin is incapable of gas transport. Note the distinc-tion between oxidized hemoglobin, the iron of which is in the ferric state, and oxygenated hemoglobin, or oxyhemoglobin, which is he-moglobin carrying oxygen and bearing its iron in the normal ferrous state.)

Red blood cells normally contain the series of enzymes neces-sary to produce adenosine triphosphate (ATP), the energy trans-ferring compound found in essentially all human cells. A fundamen-tal relationship has been shown to exist between glucose metabol-ism, ATP levels, and the energy required to keep RBC alive. With aging, gradual loss of certain enzymes involved in energy production and generation of ATP leads to loss of cell membrane integrity, RBC death, and breakdown. As will be discussed in greater detail in the section on blood preservative solutions, in vitro red blood cell storage requires provision of glucose to maintain cell viability.

Structurally the mature RBC is composed of a lipoprotein envelope (stroma) enclosing a red, iron-containing protein known as hemoglobin. Hemoglobin concentrations in adult males range from 14 to 17 gm/dl of blood and in adult females from 12 to 15 gm/dl. Because of its marked affinity for oxygen and carbon dioxide, hemoglobin is ideally suited for one of its major functions, the transport of oxygen to body tissues and of carbon dioxide to the lungs. Hemoglobin also plays a major role in the buffering capacity of blood, whereby major changes in pH are minimized as carbon dioxide enters and leaves. Normally RBC in the lungs are almost fully saturated with oxygen, giving up on average about one fourth of this oxygen in the peripheral tissues. Several factors affect the unloading of oxygen, including the blood pH, the partial pressure of carbon dioxide in the tissues (P_{CO_2}) the genetically determined structure of the hemoglobin in the RBC, and the concentration in the red blood cells of an intermediate substance in the glycolytic pathway known as 2,3-diphosphoglycerate (2,3-DPG). This compound interferes with the stable binding of oxygen to hemoglobin, and in normal concentrations facilitates the unloading of oxygen in the tissues. Depleted 2,3-DPG levels in RBC, though not damaging to the integrity or viability of the cells, increase their affinity for oxygen and thus interfere with their ability to function in a physiologically normal fashion. The theoretical desirability of maintaining normal 2,3-DPG levels in stored RBC is apparent.

Of significance to the understanding of some of the phenomena to be discussed in subsequent chapters are recent advances in our understanding of the molecular structure of the red blood cell membrane. See Figure 2-1. The membrane is thought to be composed of a double layer of phospholipid molecules with their hydrophilic ends oriented toward the surface or toward the cell interior. The hydrocarbon chains of the fatty acids of these phospholipids are in motion, continuously flexing. Moreover, these molecules are capable of moving rapidly along the lateral plane of the bilayer, i.e., over the surface. Cholesterol molecules form part of the membrane structure, apparently imparting chemical stability to it. Half of the mass of the red blood cell membrane in man is composed of proteins, with at least seven different polypeptide chains identified. These fall into two groups, one loosely attached to the outer surface and quite easily removed, the other inserted deeply into (or through) the bilayer and tightly fixed as an integral part of the membrane structure. One of the most characteristic of the intrinsic membrane proteins is known as spectrin. These molecules do not intercalate with the phospholipid bilayer but are held electrostatically to the other proteins of the membrane or to polar groups of the phospholipids. A major component of the intrinsic membrane protein is a sialoglycoprotein called glycophorin A. The polypeptide portion of this molecule consists of 131 amino acid residues and extends perpendicularly completely through the bilayer. Sixteen oligosaccharide chains are attached to the polypeptide near its outer end, some of which may well represent antigenic determinants, specifically receptor sites for antibodies and lectins in the ABO, Lewis, I, and other blood group systems. Glycophorin A may exist as a multimeric complex (several linked molecules forming a single large unit) in which association-dissociation reactions could theoretically play a role in regulating the functional capabilities of these molecules as antigenic determinants and antibody receptors. Though most of the RBC membrane proteins are probably fixed, it is possible that some are mobile. It is postulated that interactions between the buried part of glycophorin A and the spectrin polymers may have an effect on the stability of the red blood cell membrane.

The significance of these observations will become apparent in later chapters when we shall discuss the oligosaccharide nature of the ABO, Lewis, and I antigens, as opposed to the lipoprotein character of the Rh antigens, and contrast the lack of physiologic significance of absence of antigens of the former type, e.g., O or Le(a–b–) or i, versus the structural deformity and shortened life span of RBC lacking Rh or Kx antigens, e.g., Rh_{null} or McLeod types. The observations on the dynamic state of the red blood cell membrane are particularly interesting as a possible explanation for the effects of enzymes on RBC: the enhancement of certain serologic reactions involving red blood cells might be a result of aggregation of antigens normally dispersed evenly over the surface. The interested reader is referred to the recent review by Marchesi for a discussion of the subject.

2. White Blood Cells

Total peripheral blood white blood cell counts normally range between 4,500 and 12,000/μl. Five different varieties of white blood cells (WBC), or leukocytes, are normally found in peripheral blood: neutrophils (polymorphonuclear leukocytes) including both seg-

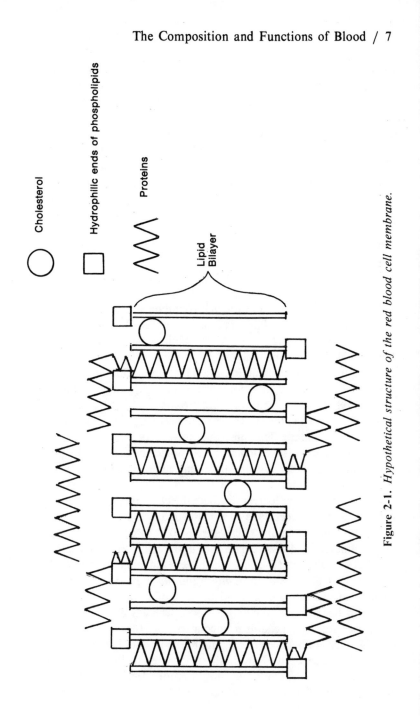

Figure 2-1. *Hypothetical structure of the red blood cell membrane.*

mented and band forms, lymphocytes, monocytes, eosinophils, and basophils. Neutrophils serve as a major body defense against invading organisms such as bacteria, which are ingested by the process of phagocytosis and usually destroyed by the digestive action of enzymes contained within the cytoplasmic granules (lysosomes) of the cells. Neutrophil maturation in the bone marrow requires about four days. After being released, neutrophils spend only a few hours in the peripheral blood. Because they are actively mobile and possess a "sticky" cell surface, neutrophils normally marginate in small vessels with sluggish blood flow, clinging to vessel linings. Thus their true numbers in the circulation are not fairly represented in a venous blood sample, the usual white bood cell count underestimating their true concentration by 50% or more.

Neutrophils may be thought of as circulating in the blood as cruising patrolmen, remaining only long enough to get where they are needed. The life span of the neutrophil once it has migrated into the tissues is unknown, but it is brief. A reserve of 20 to 30 times the circulating granulocyte pool (neutrophils, eosinophils, and basophils) exists in the bone marrow. In response to chemical mediators released from sites of tissue injury and inflammation (including portions of the third and fifth components of complement as discussed in Chapter 7) neutrophils migrate from the bloodstream through capillary walls to enter the tissues and become part of the acute inflammatory exudate. The anaerobic (glycolytic) metabolism of the neutrophil renders it particularly well suited to carry out its phagocytic function in the oxygen-poor environment of abscesses and similar such lesions.

Lymphocytes are currently the subject of intense interest, and major recent advances have been made in our understanding of their production and function. There appear to be two major populations of lymphocytes and their derivatives in the body: those participating in cellular immunity (T-cells) and those responsible for humoral immunity (B-cells). The term *humoral immunity* refers to immune responses mediated by cell-free solutions of immunoglobulins contained in body fluids, including blood, whereas *cellular immunity* comprises defense mechanisms mediated directly by lymphocytes. T-lymphocytes are believed to migrate to the thymus in embryonic life, where *thymosin* derived from the thymic epithelial cells exerts a humoral influence upon them, programming the T-cells to participate in cell-mediated immune reactions. The T-cells then migrate into the peripheral blood, where they constitute perhaps 85% of the lymphocytes, and to the lymph nodes and spleen. Here they play several major roles, including participating in delayed hypersensitivity reactions, functioning as "killer" cells in graft-versus-host reactions, protecting against facultative bacterial, viral, and fungal diseases, and serving as "helper" cells in the production by B-cells of antibody directed toward a particular group of antigens. It is also thought that certain groups of T-cells function in "turning off" antibody production by B-cells at the appropriate time, serving in a suppressor role. T-cells are involved in the switch from production of immunoglobulins of the M class (IgM) to those of the G class (IgG) during the immune response, and are also thought to influence production of antibodies of the IgA and IgE classes.

B-cells are lymphocytes that are potential plasma cell (immunocyte) precursors. Their site of origin is variously speculated to be the fetal gut, liver, or bone marrow. B-cells comprise 10% to 15% of the peripheral blood lymphocytes and populate the bone marrow and germinal centers of lymph nodes. Upon exposure to appropriate antigenic material, with or without the associated action of T-cells and macrophages (depending on the nature of the antigen), B-cells are transformed to cells of the plasma cell series and begin production of humoral antibody. Other B-cells do not make the transition to plasma cells with active antibody production but rather serve as "memory cells" capable of rapid proliferation and vigorous antibody production if re-exposed to the antigen at a later time. The antibodies produced by B cells include all immunoglobulin classes and are primarily involved in reactions with bacteria and a variety of foreign proteins, including antigenic determinants on RBC.

Although plasma cells are readily identified using conventional staining techniques, simple morphologic distinction between T- and B-cells cannot be made. Rather the use of special techniques using surface markers is required: T-cells form rosettes when incubated with sheep RBC, while B-cells have a surface coating of immunoglobulin that can be detected by fluorescence or other methods. Alternatively, histochemical staining for alpha-napthyl acetate esterase can be employed: T-cells yield positive results; B-cells do not. The surface immunoglobulin on B-cells probably acts as antigen receptor. As described in Chapter 4, antigen attached to this immunoglobulin is internalized by pinocytosis and concentrated to initiate humoral immune response. It should be noted that all lymphocytes are not classifiable as T- or B-cells. A third small population of "null" cells is presumed to represent precursor lymphocytes that have not yet acquired the identifying characteristics of mature T- or B-cells.

Monocytes are probably best thought of as peripheral blood macrophages and function as phagocytes or scavengers in the removal of tissue debris, damaged cells, and foreign material that has gained access to the body. They participate in bodily defenses against microorganisms, including phagocytosis of both facultative and obligate intracellular bacteria such as the tubercle bacillus. Macrophages possess surface receptors for the Fc portion of IgG molecules and for C3b (i.e., receptors for certain antibody molecules and for one of the members of the complement system), which facilitate this function. Macrophages kill ingested bacteria probably by two processes, one involving the formation of peroxides and similar compounds and the other related to the entry of microbiocidal substances into the phagocytic vacuole. Monocytes spend only a few hours in the peripheral blood, migrating into the tissues where they undergo a change into cells variously called histiocytes or macrophages. Under some circumstances macrophages are involved in altering ("processing") antigenic foreign materials and transporting and transmitting them to antibody-forming cells. It has been suggested that antigen molecules actually ingested by macrophages are generally destroyed and that only those retained on the surface membrane are presented to lymphocytes to initiate immune responses. Some macrophages apparently retain antigen molecules for protracted periods, serving as "immunologic islands" interacting with lymphocytes. Not only do macrophages affect lymphocytes, but the reverse also occurs: lymphocytes produce lymphokines, which activate macrophages to be more effective killer cells.

The functions of eosinophils and basophils are poorly understood. Eosinophils are involved in a number of allergic reactions. The granules of basophils are known to contain a variety of potent chemical principles, including histamine.

3. Platelets

Platelets are small (1 to 3μ in diameter) non-nucleated fragments of the cytoplasm of bone marrow megakaryocytes. Platelets are normally present in peripheral blood in concentrations of 150,000 to 450,000/μl. The spleen usually contains up to 20% of the circulating platelet pool, though in diseases in which the spleen is enlarged this figure may increase to as much as seven times the number of circulating platelets. The normal platelet life span in peripheral blood is eight to nine days. Metabolic activity in platelets is considerable, with a contractile protein and a variety of potent vasoactive substances (e.g., serotonin) contained within their cytoplasm. Platelets are structurally complex, containing an assortment of cytoplasmic granules, mitochondria, lysosomes, and a tubular system. They bear a peripheral coating of plasma proteins, including molecules participating in the coagulation and fibrinolytic systems (Factors II, V, VII, VIII, IX, and X). Seven platelet factors have been identified as participating in primary hemostasis and/or coagulation: Platelet factor 2 activates the clotting of fibrinogen by thrombin. Platelet factor 3 is required by the complex of Factor Xa, Factor V, and calcium to convert prothrombin to thrombin and is also necessary for the activation of Factors XII, XI, X, and IX. Platelet factor 4 enhances the polymerization of fibrin monomer and exhibits antiheparin activity, while platelet factor 6 is an antiplasmin. Energy for platelet function is derived in about equal amounts from glycolysis and the tricarboxylic acid cycle.

The chief functions of platelets are participation in 1) primary hemostasis or the formation of platelet plugs, and 2) the coagulation of blood (described below). These two processes, though intimately related, should be distinguished from each other for a clear understanding of the mechanisms involved in the control of hemorrhage due to trauma or that occurring in deficiency states. Primary hemostasis is effected solely by interaction between platelets and the walls of blood vessels and does not involve or require the remainder of the plasma proteins participating in the formation of a blood clot (thrombosis). The body defense against hemorrhage is a complex process in which three major components participate: platelets, arterial smooth muscle, and the plasma procoagulants, the last of which interact in delicate balance and are affected by both activators and inhibitors. Platelets function in this scheme by releasing platelet factors, by providing a surface upon which plasma procoagulants can react, by causing clot retraction, and by interacting with endothelial cells in a support function. Platelets also release vasoactive substances and chemotactic principles. When a small blood vessel is damaged, it contracts and retracts. Platelets immediately adhere to the exposed subendothelial collagen, changing their shape from discs to spheres with pseudopods, and undergo a "release reaction" with liberation of adenosine diphosphate (ADP), serotonin, epinephrine, calcium, and platelet factor 4. ADP and epinephrine cause platelet aggregation with formation of a plug that occludes the vessel or seals defects in its wall. An alternative explanation of this phenomenon assigns the major role in producing the plug to prostaglandins released from platelet cytoplasm instead of to ADP. In either scheme the process is self-amplifying. Thrombin formation causes irreversible platelet metamorphosis and secondary release of ADP, platelet factors, and a substance that activates Factor XIII. The release reaction occurs in two phases: the first is characterized by liberation of the content of the cytoplasmic dense bodies and does not interfere with platelet metabolism; the second involves disruption of the alpha granules and is irreversible. A Factor VIII constituent (von Willebrand Factor) is also required, and aspirin inhibits the reaction. The primary hemostatic platelet plug is not stable and if blood coagulation does not supervene with definitive fibrin clot production, bleeding may recur. During disc-to-sphere transformation the platelet surface is reorganized to provide a phospholipid matrix that accelerates the interaction of Factors VIII, IX, and X with prothrombin. Hereditary diseases of platelets are classified as a result of defects of adhesion of platelets to collagen, defects of adhesion of platelets to subendothelium, defects in the release reaction, and defects in ADP-induced aggregation.

PLASMA

Plasma contains a wide variety of protein constituents including hybrid molecules containing carbohydrate portions (glycoproteins) or fats (lipoproteins). Plasma proteins may be characterized by their electrophoretic mobility. Large complex molecules such as plasma proteins form charged groups in solution, for example by dissociating H^+ from $-COOH$ groups to form $-COO^-$ or adding H^+ to $-NH_2$ groups to form $-NH_3^+$. Depending on the pH of the solution, positively or negatively charged groups may predominate in the molecule, leaving it with a small net charge. If an electric current is passed through the solution, the molecule will migrate toward the pole opposite its electrostatic charge. At pH 8.6, most plasma proteins have a negative charge and will migrate in electrolyte solution toward the anode (positive pole) if a current is passed. The rates of migration of different types of proteins vary among other factors with the differences in electrostatic charge on various molecular species, permitting their separation. Electrophoresis, as this technique is called, can be carried out in electrolyte solution or more easily on various supporting media, including starch, agarose, cellulose acetate, or polyacrylamide gel, producing bands of proteins migrating at various speeds. Staining of the strips and their analysis in a densitometer converts the amount of protein in each band into a tracing with peaks representing major molecular types. The area under each peak is approximately proportional to the concentration of protein in the corresponding band. For serum proteins these bands correspond to albumin, alpha-1, alpha-2, beta and gamma globulins (see Figure 2-2). The quantitative distribution of each fraction is shown in Table 2-1, where it will be seen that albumin constitutes the largest component of serum total protein. The predominant components of alpha-1 globulin are alpha-1 antitrypsin orosomucoid or alpha-1 glycoprotein, thyroid binding globulin, and transcortin. The major contributors to alpha-2 globulin are alpha-2 macroglobulin, ceruloplasmin, and haptoglobin, whereas the principal constituents of the beta globulin fraction are the third component of complement (C3), beta lipoprotein, transferrin, and hemopexin. Immunoglobulins (i.e., antibody globulins) comprise almost all of the serum gamma globulin. Although not separately defined by serum protein electrophoresis, the contribution of each of the quantitatively major immunoglobulins to the serum protein electrophoretic pattern is shown in the shaded areas in Figure 2-2.

The technique of immunoelectrophoresis combines separation of

Table 2-1

Normal Ranges for Serum Protein Fractions in Adult White Subjects as Determined by Electrophoresis in Barbital Buffer at pH 8.6 on Cellulose Acetate

Protein Fraction	Concentration (gm/dl)	Relative Percent
Albumin	3.6–4.8	56–68
Alpha-1 globulin	0.013–0.30	2–5
Alpha-2 globulin	0.45–0.87	7–13
Beta globulin	0.51–0.99	8–15
Gamma globulin	0.55–1.30	9–19

proteins by electrophoresis with double-diffusion precipitin technique. Antisera capable of combining with a variety of plasma proteins to form visible precipitates are introduced into slots cut into thin agar plates on which serum proteins have already been separated by electrophoresis into bands. Identification and crude semiquantitation of specific proteins can be accomplished by noting the location of the arcs of precipitated antigen-antibody complexes deposited in the agar.

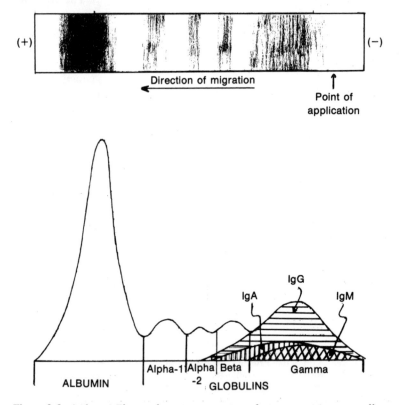

Figure 2-2. *(Above) Electrophoretic separation of serum proteins on a cellulose acetate strip after staining. Individual groups of proteins migrating at different speeds have traveled as discrete bands for varying distances. (Below) Densitometer analysis of the above pattern. The areas under each peak in the tracing are proportional to the amount of protein present in the corresponding band on the lectrophoretic pattern. The areas occupied by the major classes of immunoglobulins have been shaded in.*

Quantitation of individual serum proteins is usually accomplished by taking advantage of the fact that specific antisera can be made to most proteins (i.e., antisera that will react with a particular molecular species and no other). If a specific antiserum is mixed with agar and a serum sample introduced into a well in the agar plate, a precipitin ring will form about the well at the point where diffusing serum protein and agar-embedded antibody meet in optimal proportions to form insoluble antigen-antibody complexes. Measurement of the diameter of the precipitin ring provides quantitative information about the concentration of the serum protein under study. This methodology is widely used for the quantitation of the major serum immunoglobulins. A variant combining this technique with electrophoresis is the basis of so-called rocket electrophoresis.

Another popular means for quantifying individual serum proteins is nephelometry. In this procedure the combination of dilute solutions of specific antibodies and test serum proteins produces faintly turbid suspensions of antigen-antibody complexes whose light-scattering properties can be measured and related to a calibration curve.

A different means of characterizing serum proteins employs ultracentrifugation. Serum is layered over a sucrose solution and then subjected to great centrifugal forces. Larger, heavier molecules sediment more rapidly than smaller lighter molecules and are said to have a higher sedimentation coefficient (expressed in Svedberg units). Proteins such as IgM molecules with molecular weights approximating 1,000,000 have sedimentation coefficients of 19S, while smaller proteins such as IgG molecules whose molecular weights are about 160,000 have sedimentation coefficients near 7S.

BLOOD COAGULATION

Plasma is the fluid portion of unclotted blood, or blood free from formed elements. Untreated plasma, like untreated whole blood, will clot upon removal from the body. The fluid remaining after clotting of whole blood or plasma is called serum. Blood banking depends upon the ability to maintain blood in the fluid state for transfusion. Moreover, because treatment of coagulation disorders is one of the indications for transfusion of blood components, it is necessary for the blood bank worker to have some acquaintance with the blood coagulation scheme. The coagulation sequence as it is currently understood is represented in Figure 2-3. Note that clotting can be initiated either by tissue damage, with activation of the "extrinsic" system, or by contact of blood with an appropriate surface, activating the "intrinsic" system. Although this distinction is traditionally presented, in actuality it appears that both are simultaneously operative in most physiologic situations and may be synergistic. As seen in the diagram, the initial stages in the two differ, but both eventuate in the conversion of prothrombin to thrombin, which catalyzes the polymerization of fibrinogen to fibrin. The blood coagulation process is thought of first as a cascade, with each component in the reaction activated by its predecessor; second, as self-amplifying, with small amounts of initial products multiplying their effects to produce a large end result; and third, though not shown completely in Figure 2-3 in the interest of clarity, as exhibiting positive and negative feedback. As noted previously, many of the reactions in plasma coagulation at least initially appear to occur on the surfaces of platelets. Table 2-2 presents some pertinent data concerning plasma protein coagulation factors, or, as they are known, procoagulants.

The question as to why blood remains fluid and does not normally clot in the circulation has always attracted interest. Two areas require attention: first, the existence of naturally occurring inhibitors of coagulation, and second, the fibrinolytic system. It should be appreciated that the blood-clotting process is normally self-limited by the adsorption of thrombin by fibrin. Further, Factors V and VIII are unstable after thrombin exposure, making the effects of thrombin self-limiting. Finally, activated Stuart factor (Xa) is removed by the liver, possibly along with other activated clotting factors. In pathologic clotting (discussed in Chapter 26) depletion of coagulation factors also occurs.

A small amount of blood coagulation may normally be constantly in progress, counteracted by a small amount of thrombolysis (clot liquefaction) and fibrinolysis (fibrin liquefaction), the two coexisting in delicate balance. Tissue trauma may activate both mechanisms through the activation of Hageman factor or by other means, and in certain pathologic conditions, imbalance in the two systems may occur. The plasmin (fibrinolysin) system consists of four parts: plasmin, plasminogen, plasminogen activators, and a series of inhibitors. (See Figure 2-3.) Plasmin is an enzyme capable of degrading both fibrin and fibrinogen as well as other plasma procoagulants

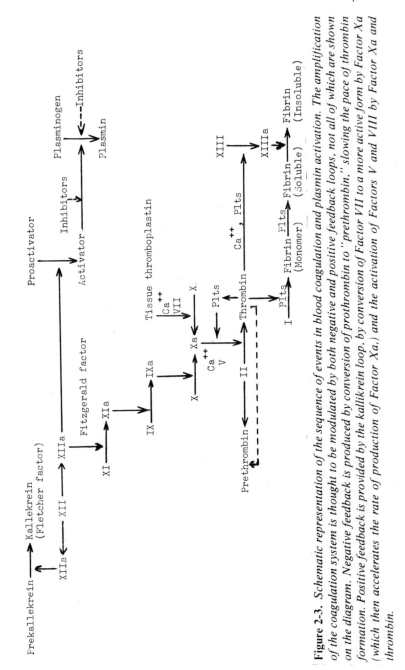

Figure 2-3. Schematic representation of the sequence of events in blood coagulation and plasmin activation. The amplification of the coagulation system is thought to be modulated by both negative and positive feedback loops, not all of which are shown on the diagram. Negative feedback is produced by conversion of prothrombin to "prethrombin," slowing the pace of thrombin formation. Positive feedback is provided by the kallikrein loop, by conversion of Factor VII to a more active form by Factor Xa (which then accelerates the rate of production of Factor Xa,) and the activation of Factors V and VIII by Factor Xa and thrombin.

Table 2-2

Nomenclature and Properties of Major Plasma Coagulation Factors

Factor	Name	Biologic Half-Life (hr)	Plasma Concentration Required for Hemostasis (% of normal)	Present in Serum	Present in Adsorbed Plasma	Stability in Stored Blood	Recovery in Blood (% of dose transfused)
I	Fibrinogen	96–120	10–25	No	Yes	Good	50
II	Prothrombin	60–72	40	No	No	Good	40–80
V	Proaccelerin	12–15	10–15	No	Yes	Fair	80
VII	Proconvertin	4–6	5–10	Yes	Yes	Good	70–80
VIII	Antihemophilic factor (AHF)	12–15	10–40	No	Yes	Poor	50–80
IX	Christmas factor (PTC)	20–30	10–40	Yes*	No	Good	25–50
X	Stuart factor	30–48	10–15	Yes	No	Good	50
XI	Plasma thromboplastin antecedent (PTA)	48–72	30	Yes	Yes**	Good	90–100
XII	Hageman factor	50	?	Yes**	Yes	Good	?
XIII	Fibrin stabilizing factor (FSF)	96–144	1–5	Yes**	Yes	Fair	?

* = increased; ** = decreased

(Factors V and VIII). In addition, plasmin can activate Hageman factor and complement and induce platelet aggregation. Degradation products of fibrinogen and fibrin exert anticoagulant effects by interfering with fibrin polymerization. Normally no free plasmin activity is demonstrable in blood, probably because its presence is masked by inhibitors. The precursor of plasmin is called plasminogen, a plasma beta globulin with a molecular weight of about 60,000, which is converted to plasmin by the proteolytic action of plasminogen activators. These activators occur naturally in the blood, other body fluids and tissues, and are found in the plasma in increased amounts after exercise, trauma, and in other stressful situations.

A series of inhibitors that affect not only plasma coagulation but plasmin, kallikrein (Fletcher factor) and the complement system as well is also present in the plasma. These inhibitors include alpha-1 antitrypsin, alpha-2 macroglobulin, antithrombin III, interalpha inhibitor, and C1 inhibitor. They act on thrombin, Fletcher factor, Factors Xa, XIa, and XIIa, plasmin, and the first component of complement. Of the naturally occurring inhibitors, alpha-2 macroglobulin and antithrombin III appear to be the most important. Alpha-2 macroglobulin is active as an inhibitor of fibrinolysis, but its main function in vivo may well be to preserve a portion of the activity of the plasmin molecule by reversibly binding it and allowing it to act in the presence of other inhibitors. Antithrombin III serves to inhibit thrombin, Factor Xa and plasmin, but again its biologic significance may be more complex. As a cofactor to heparin, a naturally occurring anticoagulant found in tissue mast cells and blood basophils, antithrombin III activity in neutralizing thrombin is increased by heparin release (or therapeutic administration). It has been postulated that heparin is normally bound to the surfaces of platelets and the endothelial cells lining blood vessels where it serves locally to increase the activity of antithrombin III, providing a barrier against the action of the hemostatic mechanism. The significance of antithrombin III is underlined by the major thrombotic episodes experienced by patients deficient in this inhibitor.

The requirement for ionized calcium for blood coagulation is the basis for the use of most of the anticoagulants employed in the clinical laboratory. Any compound that will complex or bind with calcium ions will render blood incoagulable. In practice, citrate and EDTA (salts of ethylenediamine tetra-acetic acid) are commonly used. Heparin is employed as an anticoagulant in vivo and in special circumstances in the laboratory. Heparin blocks the interaction between Factors XI and IX, interferes with the functions of thrombin, and prevents activation of Factor XIII.

RECOMMENDED READING

Biggs, R. (Ed): *Human Blood Coagulation, Hemostasis and Thrombosis*, 2nd ed. Blackwell, Oxford, 1976

Brozovic, M.: Physiological mechanisms in coagulation and fibrinolysis. *Br Med Bull* 3:231, 1977

Cline, M.J. (Mod): Monocytes and macrophages: functions and diseases. *Ann Intern Med* 88:78, 1978

Deykin, D.: Platelet physiology. In: *Human Hemostasis*. Am Assn Blood Banks. Washington, 1975, p. 5

Hardisty, R.M.: Disorders of platelet function. *Br Med Bull* 33:207, 1977

Henry, R.L.: Platelet function. *Semin Thrombosis and Hemostasis* 4:123, 1977

Hurtubise, P.E.: B and T lymphocytes: the cells of the immune response. In: *Blood Bank Immunology*. Am Assn Blood Banks. Washington, 1977, p. 1

Kernoff, P.B.A., McNichol, G.P.: Normal and abnormal fibrinolysis. *Br Med Bull* 3:239, 1977

Marchesi, V.T.: Structure of biological membranes. In: *Membrane Structure and Function of Human Blood Cells*. Am Assn Blood Banks. Washington, 1976, p. 1

Ratnoff, O.D.: Interaction of soluble procoagulants in blood clotting. In: *Human Hemostasis*. Am Assn Blood Banks. Washington, 1975, p. 15

Rosenberg, R.D.: Protease inhibitors of blood coagulation. In: *Human Hemostasis*. Am Assn of Blood Banks. Washington, 1975, p. 25

Williams, W.J. et al: *Hematology* 2nd ed. McGraw-Hill, New York, 1978

Wintrobe, M.W. et al: *Clinical Hematology*, 7th ed. Lea & Febiger, Philadelphia, 1974

cases there may be a decrease in the normal stimulus to red blood cell production (the renal hormone called erythropoietin), which may be deficient in patients with renal failure or chronic inflammatory disease. Other patients may be anemic because there is congenital or inherited abnormality in their red blood cell-producing mechanism resulting in delivery of biochemically or metabolically defective RBC that are destroyed in the bone marrow or bloodstream before they live out a normal life span. These anemias include 1) those associated with defects in the red blood cell membrane such as are found in hereditary spherocytosis; 2) those caused by abnormalities in the glycolytic metabolism of the RBC such as pyruvate kinase deficiency; 3) those due to defects in the pentose-phosphate metabolic pathway, such as glucose-6-phosphate dehydrogenase deficiency; 4) those occurring as a consequence of the production of structurally abnormal hemoglobins such as that found in sickle cell disease; 5) those resulting from quantitative defects in hemoglobin production, such as the thalassemias; 6) those due to blocks or defects in synthesis of the precursor substances of hemoglobin (the porphyrias); and 7) those caused by production of RBC with multiple or unknown defects such as occur in paroxysmal nocturnal hemoglobinuria. Acquired RBC metabolic defects include those due to abnormalities of iron metabolism (the sideroblastic anemias), those due to blockage of iron incorporation into hemoglobin ("simple chronic anemia" of chronic disease), and those due to the effects of toxins, such as lead poisoning or acquired methemoglobinemia.

The most common cause of anemia in the face of normal red blood cell production is, of course, blood loss (hemorrhage). A variety of extracorpuscular defects, however, can result in premature RBC destruction. Antibodies (immune globulins) attached to RBC, with or without interaction with complement can bring about untimely red blood cell destruction. Physical damage to erythrocytes as a consequence of burns or that which occurs during contact with prosthetic heart valves or heart-lung machines may result in their accelerated destruction. Red blood cell fragmentation may occur in certain small vessel diseases (microangiopathic hemolytic anemia), in march hemoglobinuria, and in some diseases of heart valves.

Other anemias are more complicated, for instance the anemia of the cancer patient. In such cases there may be a combination of inadequate dietary intake, insufficient bone marrow stimulation, defective iron incorporation into immature RBC, abnormal bleeding, shortened RBC life span, and other factors — some or all of which are operative at various times in different patients.

B. Polycythemia

This condition is characterized by overproduction of RBC, either as a response of the body to chronic hypoxia such as occurs in chronic lung disease, or as a primary, unexplained (idiopathic) condition. The patient with polycythemia has an excess of RBC; his blood is abnormally viscous and tends to clot abnormally. Therapeutic phlebotomy is frequently employed in treating patients with primary polycythemia.

C. Leukemia

Leukemias are malignant diseases of the blood-forming organs, characterized by blood and tissue infiltration by abnormal white blood cells. Leukemia is classified on the basis of cell type as myelocytic, lymphocytic, or monocytic, plus other rare variants, and further as acute, subacute, or chronic, based upon the morphologic maturity of the leukemic cells and the rapidity with which the disease progresses. Abnormalities of function such as impaired phagocytic ability or deficient response to antigenic stimulation are found in many leukemic leucocytes. The bone marrow of the patient is often replaced by leukemic cells so that normal RBC, WBC, and platelet precursors are crowded out. The treatment of leukemia often entails the use of toxic drugs, which may destroy remaining normal bone marrow elements as well as leukemic cells. As a result, the leukemic patient may become anemic, thrombocytopenic, and, in terms of normally functional leukocytes, leukopenic. Autoimmune hemolytic disease is sometimes found in patients with chronic lymphocytic leukemia.

D. Lymphoma

Lymphomas are malignant diseases of lymphatic tissues, including lymph nodes, spleen, and the reticuloendothelial portions of liver and bone marrow. Peripheral blood involvement, if it occurs, is a secondary phenomenon. Various categories of lymphoma are recognized, including Hodgkin's disease and the non-Hodgkin's lymph-

omas previously known as lymphosarcoma and reticulum cell sar-
coma. Anemia, sometimes autoimmune, is frequently encountered in
patients with lymphoma, and the occurrence of leukopenia and/or
thrombocytopenia is a common complication of treatment.

E. Infectious mononucleosis

This disease is a generally benign, self-limited viral infection
which occurs primarily in young adults, and is characterized by an
atypical lymphoid infiltration of the peripheral blood and lymphoid
organs. Autoimmune hemolytic disease or thrombocytopenia are
rare components of infectious mononucleosis.

F. Thrombocytopenia

Idiopathic thrombocytopenia is a moderately common condition
usually occurring after a viral illness in children, less often in adults,
and presumably is caused by autoimmune platelet destruction. In
children the disease generally is self-limited and responds to treatment; results in adults are not always satisfactory. A hemorrhagic
tendency may appear when the platelet count falls below $50,000/\mu l$,
and may eventuate in serious complications if not corrected.
Thrombocytopenia is frequently encountered in patients with acute
leukemia and after the use of antimetabolites in cancer chemotherapy. Thrombocytopenia due to abnormal platelet pooling may be
found in disease conditions causing marked splenomegaly. Decreased platelet counts are common in patients with bone marrow replacement. Mild thrombocytopenia is sometimes seen in cases of
megaloblastic anemia.

G. Thrombocytosis

Some elevation of the platelet count is frequently found in patients with malignant diseases or severe inflammation. Marked
thrombocytosis is common in patients with untreated chronic myelocytic leukemia or other myeloproliferative disease.

H. Functional platelet disorders

A number of rare hereditary disorders of platelet function have been defined, each characterized by biochemical abnormalities that render the platelets functionally defective though quantitatively normal. Much more common is acquired platelet dysfunction due to the administration of antiinflammatory drugs, of which the best example is aspirin. Aspirin has been shown to impair the platelet-release reaction and secondary platelet aggregation for several days after a single therapeutic dose. Platelet dysfunction is common in uremia, and hemorrhagic complications are frequently seen in patients in renal failure. A bleeding tendency may also be found in patients with paraproteinemia (see below), myeloproliferative disease, or disseminated intravascular coagulation. Platelet dysfunction is characteristic of patients with von Willebrand's disease, a hemophilia-like coagulation disorder caused by failure of production of a component of Factor VIII necessary to normal platelet function.

I. Pancytopenia

Aplastic anemia is characterized by loss of bone marrow precursors for granulocytes, erythrocytes, and platelets, although occasionally some progenitor cells of one or another cell line persist. Aplastic anemia may be idiopathic, in which case it may be a preleukemic state, or it may be the consequence of exposure to poisons or drugs. Rarely is the former condition reversible, but the bone marrow may recover in the latter if the patient survives the pancytopenia long enough. There are also rare congenital deficiencies of production of erythrocytes only.

Drug toxicity is frequently seen in modern medicine and may take the form of hematologic abnormality, either as an idiosyncrasy (abnormal sensitivity) or as a predictable consequence, particularly of antimetabolite therapy. Certain drugs may cause lowered neutrophil counts (neutropenia) or destruction of all peripheral blood granulocytes (agranulocytosis). Others may effect destruction of platelets or RBC, mediated in many cases by drug-induced antibodies (see Chapter 15). Chemotherapy or radiation therapy for malignant tumors or leukemia, if intense or prolonged, often destroys much of the bone marrow, sometimes with fatal consequences.

DISEASES AFFECTING PLASMA PROTEINS

A. Paraproteinemias

Of practical concern to the blood bank worker is a group of diseases characterized by over-production of qualitatively abnormal serum globulins. The best known of these conditions is multiple myeloma, a malignant disease of plasma cells (immunocytes) involving bone and ultimately other organs. Multiple myeloma is usually associated with high concentrations of a single species of abnormal immunoglobulin in the blood and often by the presence of unusual protein fragments (L-chains) in the urine and blood. A related disease, Waldenström's macroglobulinemia, is typified by the presence in the blood of large amounts of macroglobulins (giant proteins with molecular weights of 1,000,000 or more). Rarely patients with diseases known as monoclonal gammopathies exhibit abnormally large amounts of electrophoretically uniform globulins in the plasma as an isolated abnormality.

B. Hyperglobulinemias

In contrast to the increased numbers of a single species of abnormal globulin molecules characterizing the diseases described above, elevated blood concentrations of normal gamma globulins consisting of a wide spectrum of molecules of slightly differing composition and electrophoretic mobility are found in diverse disease states such as cirrhosis, sarcoidosis, and systemic lupus erythematosus. Interference with blood grouping and compatibility testing procedures is frequently caused by the presence in serum of increased concentrations of globulins.

C. Hypogammaglobulinemias

An array of immune deficiency states has been described, including rare primary or genetically determined abnormalities of immunologic development resulting in defective antibody production or cellular immune responses. There also exist acquired or secondary immune deficiencies superimposed on a previously normal immune system. In the first category are included congenital defects in T- and/or B-cell function or stem-cell development. Probably the most common of the congenital hypogammaglobulinemias is selective immunoglobulin deficiency, particularly of IgA, which occurs in about one in 700 blood donors. In addition, isolated deficiencies of production of single molecular species such as specific complement components also occur, though rarely.

Relative hypogammaglobulinemia is a normal occurrence in early infancy. At birth, human infants are endowed with passively acquired maternal gamma globulin that is mostly IgG. This immunoglobulin, with a half-life of 22 to 26 days, however, begins to disappear. The infant's immature immunologic system begins to function only slowly, with only small amounts of IgM produced at birth, and no IgG for a month or two thereafter. As a result, by age three to five months quite low immunoglobulin levels are reached, though concentrations approaching adult values are achieved by the age of one year.

Acquired immune deficiency states are found most commonly in patients with advanced lymphoproliferative malignancies (multiple myeloma, Hodgkin's disease and other lymphomas, and chronic lymphocytic leukemia).

PLASMA COAGULATION DEFECTS

A specialized category of plasma protein abnormality of particular concern to the blood bank worker is that involving deficiencies of plasma procoagulants. Congenital deficiency of each of the factors participating in the scheme of blood coagulation previously shown in Figure 2-3 has been found. The most common and clinically most significant of these diseases is hemophilia, a deficiency disease caused by absent or defective production of Factor VIII, or antihemophiliac factor (AHF). Hemophilia is characterized by major bleeding during surgery or other trauma, or it may occur spontaneously, especially into joints, with crippling aftereffects. Christmas disease is a somewhat similar condition, occurring as a consequence of Factor IX, or plasma thromboplastin component (PTC) deficiency. Von Willebrand's disease is caused by genetic absence of the stimulus to the production of Factor VIII, including a component necessary for normal platelet function.

The most frequently seen acquired abnormalities of coagulation are therapeutically induced by administration of the warfarin group of drugs or of heparin in an effort to prevent thrombosis in diseased blood vessels. Such treatment has been popular for patients with thrombophlebitis, and, more controversially, with coronary artery disease. Warfarin drugs depress hepatic production of Factors II, VII, IX, and X, while heparin, through the action of antithrombin III, interferes with blood coagulation at several stages, as discussed in the previous chapter.

Coagulation defects are occasionally encountered in patients undergoing open-heart surgery. Several abnormalities, not all of them defined, may be present, including a dilutional effect of aqueous solutions and stored blood deficient in platelets and Factor VIII, thrombocytopenia, the anticoagulant effect of split fibrin products, and the inadequate postoperative neutralization of heparin used for anticoagulation during surgery. Further treatment of the subject of specific congenital and acquired coagulation defects is presented in Chapter 26.

A clotting defect due to imbalanced activation of the coagulation and fibrinolytic systems can occur in a number of disease states, including certain obstetric conditions, sepsis, intravascular hemolysis (including hemolytic transfusion reactions), advanced malignancy, shock with hypoxia, and massive tissue injury. The condition is variously known as disseminated intravascular coagulation (DIC), the defibrination syndrome, or consumption coagulopathy. Mild forms of DIC not requiring treatment are frequently seen and major life-threatening episodes are fortunately rare. Initiation of the process is in most cases the result of entry of thromboplastic materials from damaged tissue (including RBC) into the bloodstream, with widespread activation of the coagulation mechanism and vascular occlusion. Consumption of coagulation factors (I, II, V, VIII, and platelets) may occur to the point where little or no further clotting can occur, and bleeding ensues. In the meantime, the plasmin system has been activated to dissolve clots already formed. If excessive, plasmin activity not only lyses clots but destroys procoagulants, thereby aggravating the bleeding diathesis. The fibrin split products formed are themselves anticoagulant and interfere with fibrin polymerization and platelet function, further increasing the problem. The reticuloendothelial system, which normally clears the blood of active procoagulants, fibrin split products, tissue breakdown products, endotoxin, and red blood cell stroma may be blocked by an excessive load of such debris, resulting in perpetuation of DIC.

HEMORRHAGE

The causes of hemorrhage are fundamentally three: blood vessel trauma, inadequate hemostasis, and defective blood coagulation. Blood will continue to leak from a damaged vessel as long as the defect remains patent and the pressure within exceeds the pressure without. Bleeding ceases when the defect in the vessel wall is sealed or the pressures inside and outside the vessel are equalized. The first objective is accomplished by formation of the hemostatic platelet plug discussed in the previous chapter and by contraction and retraction of the injured vessel. Equalization of pressure is effected by the lowering of pressure within the vessel because of arteriolar contraction proximal to the damage, by shunting of blood through alternative channels, or by a generalized decrease in blood pressure such as occurs in shock, plus increase in pressure outside the vessel produced by accumulation of blood and edema fluid in the tissues involved by the injury. Localized sludging of blood with increased viscosity may occur as the result of plasma loss. Increased vascular permeability occurs as part of the inflammatory reaction to injury, thereby helping to cause sludging and promoting clotting.

Abnormality in vascular reaction, platelet function, or formation of the definitive thrombus may result in bleeding from even inconsequential trauma. Decreased production of procoagulants, synthesis of defective factors or their dilution, consumption, or inhibition can result in inadequate thrombosis. Management of hemorrhage is directed at removing the cause and temporarily supplying any deficiency present. The latter properly requires a knowledge not only of what is deficient but what the appropriate product is for replacing the deficiency, how much is needed, and how long the product can be expected to survive. Implicit in this statement are two facts: Administration of "blood" as a transfusion of whole blood is not the optimal treatment for most such patients, a fact to which we will return in Chapter 24 when blood component therapy is discussed. Secondly, the nature of the patient's disease and his clinical condition have a profound effect on the efficacy of transfusion of blood products and specifically on how long their beneficial effects can be anticipated to last.

Hypovolemia, or inadequate circulating blood volume, with associated circulatory collapse is one cause of the clinical condition known as shock. Shock may occur solely as a consequence of severe blood loss, but more frequently it involves a complex mechanism involving biochemical and neuogenic reactions to injury. Shock may also occur during massive heart failure (cardiogenic shock) or overwhelming infection (septic shock), as part of anaphylaxis (anaphylactic shock), as a consequence of extreme pain (neurogenic shock), or on an endocrinologic basis (endocrine shock). Hypovolemic shock occurs as a result of massive blood loss or of vasodilation with pooling of blood in the extremities and splanchnic bed. Hypovolemia causes inadequate blood return to the heart and consequent inadequate cardiac output. Tissue anoxia leads to acidosis, deranged cellular metabolism, impairment of vital cellular functions, and ultimately to death of both cell and body. Massive replacement therapy is indicated in this situation, which constitutes a clinical emergency. Common causes of hypovolemic shock include hemorrhage, massive trauma, fractures, crushing injuries, burns, acute pancreatitis, peritonitis, intestinal obstruction, and severe diarrhea.

Normally blood comprises about 7% to 8% of body weight, or somewhat over five liters in a 70 kg adult. Loss of 500 ml, or 10% of circulating blood volume by a healthy adult rarely produces symptoms on a physiologic basis (though psychically induced reactions may occur in up to 3% of first-time blood donors). Vasovagal attacks, with pallor, clammy moist skin, faintness, and nausea may be accompanied by decreases in pulse rate and blood pressure. Vomiting, incontinence, convulsions, and loss of consciousness occur in extreme situations. Autonomic nervous system stimulation appears to account for most of this picture, triggered by emotional factors rather than physiologic consequences of blood loss.

Blood loss of 1,000 ml or more is not unusual in patients sustaining major fractures or tissue trauma. A fracture of the femur can result in blood loss of 1,500 ml, a fracture of the pelvis, 1,500 to 2,000 ml. The patient who has lost 1,000 ml of blood acutely may be comfortable while supine but may experience tachycardia, a decrease in blood presure, and loss of consciousness if he attempts to arise. With acute hemorrhages of 1,500 to 2,000 ml, the subject slips into incipient shock, with air hunger, impaired tissue oxygenation, decreased cardiac output, and decreased blood pressure, even while lying down. Such findings indicate that compensatory efforts by the body in the form of increased respiratory and heart rate, decreased circulation time, vasoconstriction, and shunting of blood from skin, muscle, kidney, and GI tract to vital organs such as the brain are failing. Acute hemorrhage in excess of 40% of blood volume (over 2,000 ml in a 70 kg adult) may lead to irreversible shock and death. The severity of hypovolemic shock in a given patient is influenced by such factors as age, general state of health, and the nature of the accompanying trauma.

Physiologic restoration of blood loss may be considered in two sections: volume replacement and RBC replacement. Fluid replacement occurs relatively rapidly, although after a loss of 10% of blood volume (approximately 500 ml) only half is replaced in most subjects within 24 hours. It is important to note that the extent of hemodilution, that is to say the decrease in packed cell volume (or hemoglobin concentration or RBC count) is *not* a reliable guide to the magnitude of acute blood loss and always initially underestimates the amount. Indeed, the packed cell volume may not reach its minimum value until three days after hemorrhage ceases.

The extent of blood loss from trauma is best estimated by measurements of systolic blood pressure. Pressures of 120 to 140 mm Hg in adults indicate blood volumes of at least 80% of normal; of 100 mm Hg at least 70% of normal; and below 100 mm Hg less than 70% of normal. Signs of vasoconstriction (skin temperature) are valid guides to shock, while pallor is unreliable. It may be noted that estimates of surgical blood loss made by weighing sponges usually underestimate blood loss by at least 25%.

The limiting factor in the rate of blood volume replacement is the rate of protein addition to the blood, which initially occurs by transfer from the extravascular pool, but ultimately requires resynthesis. Restoration of red blood cells is dependent upon increased erythropoietin stimulation and occurs at a much slower pace. Bone marrow erythroid hyperplasia may be seen within three to five days after acute hemorrhage, but maximum reticulocyte response does not occur for six to 11 days, and depending on the amount of blood loss and various patient factors, normal red blood cell counts may not be achieved for 30 to 60 days.

Certain types of injury and disease result in disproportionate plasma losses. The burned patient is the classic victim of this phenomenon, but crushing injuries, acute pancreatitis, peritonitis, profound diarrhea, and small intestinal obstruction cause a similar problem.

RECOMMENDED READING

Biggs, R. (Ed): *Human Blood Coagulation, Hemostasis and Thrombosis*, 2nd ed. Blackwell, Oxford, 1976

Mollison, P.L.: *Blood Transfusion in Clinical Medicine*, 5th ed. Blackwell, Oxford, 1972

Williams, W.J. et al: *Hematology*, 2nd ed. McGraw-Hill, New York, 1978

Wintrobe, M.W. et al: *Clinical Hematology*, 7th ed. Lea & Febiger, Philadelphia, 1974

CHAPTER 4

Principles of Blood Transfusion Therapy

The clinical indications for transfusion of blood and blood components can be summarized as follows:

1) To restore circulating blood volume
2) To increase blood oxygen-carrying capacity
3) To supply missing plasma coagulation or other factors
4) To supply platelets or granulocytes
5) To dilute or remove (by exchange transfusion) toxic substances

Clinical judgement must determine when blood transfusion is indicated. Laboratory studies are of value in supplementing and confirming this judgement, but it is the patient who must be treated, not the laboratory report. The practice of arbitrarily setting values at which a patient must be transfused constitutes poor medicine. Many patients are quite comfortable with degrees of anemia that would be poorly tolerated by others. Blood transfusions should not be given as a tonic, nor are they a practical way to increase serum total protein concentrations. Asymptomatic anemia is not an indication for transfusion, nor is wound healing speeded by raising hemoglobin values to some predetermined value.

So that these comments may not seem too arbitrary, an example by way of illustration may be in order. In the case of the bleeding patient on the operating table, the surgeon who cannot predict with confidence how much additional hemorrhage will occur may reasonably elect to stay ahead of his patient's blood loss rather than to delay blood transfusion until a major deficit has occurred. On the other hand, there is now conclusive evidence that most surgical patients fare better with appreciable hemodilution, in part because of improved flow characteristics of less viscous blood, than do patients with "normal" concentrations of RBC.

33

Efficient compensatory mechanisms exist in patients with chronic anemia, which often permit them to carry out adequate tissue oxygenation. Among these may be cited decreased overall physical activity, increased cardiac output (with increased heart rate, increased cardiac stroke volume, and decreased circulation time), increased respiratory rate, the shunting of blood to vital tissues, increased oxygen extraction from RBC by peripheral tissues, and a shift where possible to glycolysis as an energy source. Increased red blood cell concentrations of 2,3-DPG provide an important mechanism in this regard by effecting a shift in the oxygen dissociation curve to the right. (It will be recalled that the oxygen dissociation curve describes the relationship between the partial pressure of oxygen in the blood and the percentage oxygen saturation of its hemoglobin.) If the oxygen dissociation curve is shifted such that the P_{50} value (the partial pressure of oxygen at which the blood hemoglobin is half saturated) is 32 mm Hg, assuming normal oxygenation, blood with a hemoglobin concentration of 8.4 gm/dl can deliver as much oxygen as it can with a concentration of 14.0 gm/dl when the oxygen dissociation curve is normally placed, i.e., a P_{50} of 27 mm Hg.

One of the disadvantages of blood transfusion to the patient with chronic anemia characterized by premature RBC destruction (i.e., hemolytic anemia) is that transfusion may suppress erythropoiesis. If maximal red blood cell production is necessary to maintain even subnormal hemoglobin concentrations, transfusion may create a vicious cycle of ever-increasing need for additional transfusions, with their repeated risk of alloimmunization and hepatitis transmission. On the other hand, transfusion in such cases may be beneficial by allowing normal bone growth in children, permitting the birth of viable babies, permitting surgery, or aborting crises. Levels of 15% to 40% of normal type A hemoglobin are the goal, for example, in pregnant patients with sickle cell disease.

In the normal 70 kg adult, red blood cell production approximates 18 ml per day. If a hemoglobin concentration of 10 gm/dl is accepted, and normal cell survival is assumed, transfusion of 24 ml of RBC per day or about one unit per week (allowing for nonviable RBC) will maintain this hemoglobin concentration in the total absence of endogenous RBC production. Blood volume readjustment after transfusion of 500 ml to a normal recipient is usually complete within 24 hours, but in patients with chronic renal failure the increase in blood volume may be prolonged, and the expected rise in hemoglobin concentration may not become apparent for as long as 48 hours after transfusion. Patients with splenomegaly may also not exhibit the anticipated increase in hemoglobin concentration after transfusion as a result of splenic trapping of transfused RBC.

Blood can be safely administered to normal recipients who are not bleeding at the rate of one unit each 60 to 90 minutes. If the infusion set delivers 15 drops/ml, transfusion of one unit of blood at a rate of 40 drops per minute will require 3.3 hours; at 60 drops per minute, 2.3 hours, and at 200 drops per minute, 40 minutes. In the patient with severe anemia (hemoglobin concentration of less than 4 gm/dl) Mollison recommends a transfusion rate of not over 0.5 ml/lb of body weight per hour, or 75 ml per hour to a 70 kg adult. To minimize the very real hazard of circulatory overload when transfusing the severely anemic patient, the transfusion should be given as red blood cells and administered with the recipient in the sitting position. Warming the patient permits peripheral pooling of blood and minimizes the amount of blood in the pulmonary circulation. If transfusion is required by patients in congestive circulatory failure a rapidly acting diuretic may be administered before the transfusion is begun and/or a partial exchange transfusion carried out using red blood cells. In patients with severe anemia no more than one unit of red blood cells should be given over a period of four to six hours. Circulatory overload with acute pulmonary edema often occurs in such patients during transfusion or even hours later. Increased systemic venous pressure, pulmonary congestion and decreased vital capacity are reflected by complaints of a sensation of fullness in the head, dyspnea, tightness in the chest, and cough. The transfusion should be stopped at once if such symptoms occur, the patient propped up, and a venesection carried out.

Blood administration is conveniently performed using a Y-set with a saline drip connected initially. Glucose-containing solutions are not proper for this because of the damage done to RBC by even transient exposure to the sugar (which causes subsequent osmotic lysis). Red blood cells for transfusion usually have a hematocrit of about 70%, though this value may range from 65 to 90. Objections are often raised over the difficulty of rapidly transfusing red blood cells or transfusing them through small-bore needles because of their sluggish flow. Permitting a one third volume of saline to pass through the Y-set into the bag of red blood cells will decrease the viscosity of the suspension from five times to 1.3 times that of whole blood and eliminate the problem. No medications or other solutions should be added to blood, not only because of the hazard of contamination but principally because of the possibly deleterious effects of the concentrated drug on RBC. Optimal transfusion practice requires that during the first ten to 20 minutes the blood be administered slowly (about 5 ml per minute) while the patient is closely observed. If there is no reaction or evidence of circulatory overload, the transfusion can then be accelerated to permit its completion in about 90 minutes.

The use of blood components for transfusion is now widespread. Whereas most transfusions in the past were of whole blood, it is now recognized that more suitable and effective treatment requires that the patient be given the particular component that he requires. Impetus was given to this approach by the development of plastic collection and storage bags that permit sterile manipulation of the blood and its fractionation. Furthermore, growing demands, shortages, and economic considerations preclude the wasteful administration of a whole unit of blood to a single patient when two or three patients could be effectively treated with various portions of the same unit. The use of particular blood components will be returned to in Chapter 24.

MANAGEMENT OF HYPOVOLEMIC SHOCK

By definition, hypovolemic shock is not a result of anemia. Treatment is aimed at restoring circulating fluid volume, and to this end, although blood transfusion may be indicated, initial measures need not await the availability of blood. Indeed, many patients experiencing acute blood loss of less than two liters can be satisfactorily treated without administration of whole blood. Exceptions include patients with cerebrovascular or coronary artery disease, respiratory insufficiency, or the potential for further bleeding. Colloid solutions useful for immediate expansion of blood volume include plasma, albumin, and dextran. Dextran is not only effective but improves the flow characteristics of blood, although large amounts may cause abnormalities of clotting. No more than 10 ml/kg of body weight of dextran should be administered in 24 hours. Problems due to rouleaux formation may be encountered in compatiblity tests using serum samples from patients treated with dextran. Plasma carries the risk of hepatitis transmission, while albumin solutions are moderately costly.

Saline infusion in acute hemorrhagic shock can be effective in combatting hypovolemia until blood or colloid infusion can be accomplished. Administration of crystalloid solutions in volumes equivalent to the amount of blood loss, however, is not sufficient, although greater volumes are effective. It will be recalled that plasma sodium and water exchange freely with that in the extravascular space. In acute hemorrhage both are depleted. If sufficient crystalloid solution is administered to replenish both fully, even though no colloid solution is infused, plasma volume can be restored. There is danger of vascular overloading, however, if crystalloid solutions are used to excess, and if saline is given exclusively, chloride acidosis may occur. For this reason buffered solutions such as Ringer's lactate are generally preferred.

PEDIATRIC TRANSFUSIONS

Transfusion therapy in children and infants presents several special problems, particular among them the need for precise control of the volumes administered. As in adults, estimations of hemoglobin or hematocrit are not useful guides to the extent of acute hemorrhage: the systolic blood pressure provides a much better indicator. It may be useful to remember, however, that a fall in hemoglobin concentration within three to six hours of acute hemorrhage indicates a loss of over 20% of blood volume. Blood loss of at least 30% in children 13 to 16 years of age is suggested by a systolic blood pressure of less than 90 mm Hg. For children nine to 12 years a similar loss is heralded by systolic pressure below 85 mm Hg, while in the five-to-eight-year age bracket the value is 75 mm Hg, and at age four or less, 65 mm Hg. Although true for adults, the danger of cardiac decompensation due to increased blood volume from transfusion in cases of severe anemia is particularly acute in children.

Two formulas are given by Kevy for the calculation of the volume of RBC to be administered in pediatric transfusions:

1. Volume of RBC to administer (ml) =

Patient wt (kg) × 75 × (Hgb concentration
desired—Hgb concentration observed)

2. Volume of RBC to administer (ml) = Patient wt (kg) × increase in Hct desired

Pediatric transfusions should not exceed 5 ml/lb of body weight, and if anemia is severe (hemoglobin concentration less than 5 gm/dl) they should not exceed 3 ml/lb. If congestive heart failure is present or incipient, a partial exchange transfusion using red blood cells (not whole blood) should be carried out instead of a conventional transfusion.

Extended red blood cell typings should be conducted on the patient who is a candidate for chronic transfusion therapy to permit attempts to select blood negative for some of the potent red blood cell antigens other than D that the patient may also lack. Later identification of blood group antibodies may also be facilitated by this knowledge.

Walking donor and syringe transfusions for pediatric patients are not recommended. Donor testing and screening are subject to shortcuts with this practice, and anticoagulation of the transfused blood may be excessive. A better practice is the use of pediatric or quadruple blood packs. There is no need to cross-match these units again once the initial compatibility testing has been carried out, and in the case of neonates up to 16 transfusions over a space of days can be given from one blood pack with one cross-match, saving multiple blood-lettings for the child and minimizing the danger of alloimmunization and posttransfusion hepatitis. The same considerations (with even less danger of hepatitis transmission) apply to the use of multiple small units of frozen RBC from a single donor.

The recommended dosage for platelet transfusion to pediatric patients is 0.1 unit/lb of body weight.

RECOMMENDED READING

Bergentz, S.E. et al: What is the significance of blood sludge today—cause or effect of disease? *Vox Sang* 32:250, 1977

Greenwalt, T.J. et al (Eds): *General Principles of Blood Transfusion,* 2nd ed. Am Med Assn, Chicago, 1977

Huestis, D.W. et al: *Practical Blood Transfusion,* 2nd ed. Little, Brown and Co., Boston, 1976

Kevy, S.V.: *Pediatric Transfusion Therapy.* Technical Improvement Service, No. 29. Am Soc Clin Path, Chicago, n.d.

Mollison, P.L.: *Blood Transfusion in Clinical Medicine.* Blackwell, Oxford, 1972

CHAPTER 5

Characteristics of Antigens and Antibodies

Immunohematology is the branch of immunology devoted to the study of blood cell antigens, antibodies, and related factors and constitutes the discipline underlying the scientific aspects of blood banking. Like many other specialized areas of knowledge, immunology has a particular vocabulary that needs to be mastered in the process of comprehending its concepts. The term antigen is used to describe any substance that, when introduced into the tissues of an immunologically competent animal, is capable of eliciting an immune response resulting in the actual or potential production of antibody. An alternative definition proposed by Fox describes an antigen as a macromolecule with internal chemical complexity that is foreign to and easily solubilized in the body fluids. As discussed below, immune responses may be of several types, but the one of greatest significance to the blood bank worker is the production of immune globulin. Immune globulins or antibodies are produced only in response to antigenic stimuli and are recognized by their ability to react in some detectable way with the antigens that excited their production. It is immediately apparent that recognition of the existence of an antibody depends upon identification of a corresponding antigen, and vice versa. It should be pointed out that the terms "immunoglobulin" and "antibody" are not completely synonymous: use of the word "antibody" implies a known reactivity while the term "immunoglobulin" is a chemical description.

The term "immunologic competence" refers to the unique ability of the lymphoid system of vertebrate animals to respond to the presence of foreign, or "not-self" substances (antigens) by producing immunoglobulins (antibodies). The expression "naturally occurring" antibody is still occasionally used to indicate antibody made in response to an unidentified stimulus, although the contribution of bacterial antigens in such situations is becoming apparent. The antigenicity or immunogenicity of a substance refers to its potency in eliciting antibody formation and is a measure of its degree of foreignness to the host. The strength of the serologic reactivity of an antigen is not necessarily related to its antigenicity. A hapten is a substance that can react with an antibody but can provoke its formation only when attached to a macromolecular carrier substance. An antigenic determinant is a particular three-dimensional arrangement of chemical groups on an antigen against which antibody is directed and with which it reacts. An antigenic site is the area on an antigen molecule occupied by an antigenic determinant. Thus, an antigenic determinant is that small portion of an antigen molecule responsible for specificity, the remainder serving as a carrier substance and conferring antigenicity on the whole. An antigen often bears multiple determinant groups and thus may be multispecific, eliciting the formation of and reacting with more than one antibody. The term "specificity" when applied to an antigen refers to the characteristics that enable its corresponding antibody to recognize and react with it. Dramatic differences in antibody specificity may result from minimal changes in the structure of an antigen molecule. When the term "antibody specificity" is used, reference is made to the antigenic determinant with which the antibody reacts.

Antisera may possess more than one specificity. Even monospecific antisera are not composed of pure molecular species but rather are mixtures of immunoglobulins sharing the ability to react with a specific determinant. A given antiserum usually contains a wide array of molecules that may vary as to immunoglobulin class and subclass, binding constant, thermal optimum, ability to fix complement, type of serologic reactions participated in, and ability to cross-react with other determinants. The chemical term "valence" is sometimes used to refer to the number of antigenic sites with which a single antibody molecule can react. As will be apparent from the description of the structure of immunoglobulins, IgG molecules have two combining sites, or a valence of two, while IgM molecules have ten such sites (although only five may be functional) for a valence of ten (or five).

Antigenic determinants are usually small, and may be composed of as few as five amino acids or six sugar residues. There is room for many antigen sites on an antigen, and further, a given antigen need not be identical in all areas. Thus similar antigenic determinants may vary slightly in specificity and elicit the formation of antibodies of somewhat varying reactivity. Complex antigens may bear regions to which antibody is not formed either because they are normally inaccessible or because they resemble similar areas in host molecules. Part of the function of these carrier regions is to preserve the spatial configuration of individual antigen sites. Thus, all the antigenic determinants on a molecule are not normally available to elicit antibody formation, the configuration of the antigen determining which determinants shall be functional. Hidden determinants, nonfunctional in an intact, or "normal," molecule may be exposed if the molecule is structurally altered. Forces of attraction and repulsion between chemical groups on a molecule determine its three-dimensional shape or conformation. When two molecules interact, e.g., antigen and antibody, the normally stable state of each is unbalanced, and new attractions and repulsions are introduced. The resulting rearrangement of molecular shapes to achieve a new stable state is called a conformational shift and constitutes a major example of a way in which hidden reactive groups may be exposed. Molecular interactions that result in a conformational shift that exposes new reactive sites are called allosteric reactions.

To act as an antigen a substance must not normally come in contact with the body's immune system. This system is capable of distinguishing between substances that are normal components of the body and those that are not, that is to say substances that are "foreign" or "not-self." Substances provoking antibody formation contain chemical groupings the body does not make. Because animals are genetically different, each will bear chemical configurations that another may recognize as "not-self," while others common to both will elicit no recognition or response. Only under pathologic circumstances will the body produce antibodies reactive with its own tissues, i.e., autoantibodies. It is postulated that antibodies to foreign antigens may occasionally cross-react with self antigens or modified self antigens.

Most antigens are proteins, often in hybrid form with carbohydrates or lipids. A molecular weight of at least 10,000 is generally necessary for molecules to be antigenic, though carbohydrate substances of this size may not be effective antigens nor are substances achieving this size with a simply repeating structure antigenic. All other factors being equal, and assuming internal structural complexity, the greater the molecular weight of a substance the greater its antigenicity.

Glycosphingolipids comprise 5% to 10% of the mass of the human red blood cell membrane, possessing a nonpolar end associated with the lipid part of the cell membrane and a polar end projecting from the surface. A number of fatty acids, sphingosines and sugars are employed in their composition, resulting in many compounds on the cell surface. The sugar moieties control the physiochemical properties of these substances and often have a major role in determining their immunologic specificities. These glycosphingolipids are not only characteristic cell markers (antigens) but also recognition sites for cell-to-cell interactions, regulators for cell division, and carriage sites for ion and metabolic transfer. The antigens of the ABO, Lewis, and P blood group systems have been characterized as glycosphingolipids, the M and N antigens as sialoglycopeptides, the I and probably Duffy antigens as glycoproteins, the Kidd antigens as glycolipids, and the Rh antigens as polypeptides requiring glycolipid for expression. Not all blood group antigens found on the red blood cell surface are fully developed at birth. The RBC of newborn infants react weakly and sometimes not at all with anti−A, −B, −Le[a], −Le[b], −Sd[a], −P₁, −I, −Yt[a], −Xg[a], and −Ch[a].

ANTIBODY CLASSIFICATION

Antibodies may be categorized in a number of ways. One of these depends on the separation of immunoglobulin molecules into five classes: IgM, IgG, IgA, IgD, and IgE. Table 5-1 presents some of the characteristics of each class. IgG and IgM antibodies are present principally in blood and extracellular fluid, while IgA antibodies are characteristically found in body secretions. IgD molecules are fixed to lymphoid cells, while IgE antibodies (reagins) are bound to reactor cells throughout the body. Antibodies circulating in the bloodstream are called humoral antibodies, while those fixed in tissues are referred to as cellular antibodies. Humoral antibodies yield immediate reactions either in the body (in vivo) or in the laboratory (in vitro) and include the blood group antibodies. Cellular anti-

TABLE 5-1

Characteristics of the Immunoglobulins

Characteristic	IgG	IgM	IgA	IgD	IgE
Molecular weight (approximate)	160,000	900,000	170,000	180,000	200,000
Sedimentation coefficient	7S	19S	7S (10, 13, 15, 17)	7S	8S
Serum concentration (mg/dl)	800–1600	50–190	140–420	0.3–4.0	0.05
Percent of total IgG	70–80	5–10	10–15	< 1	≤ 0.01
Half-life (days)	25–35	6–8	9–11	2–3	2–3
Synthesis (mg/kg body weight/day)	20–40	3–17	3–55	0.4	?
Percent intravascular	45	76	42	75	51
Inactivation by -SH compounds	No	Yes	Partial	No	?
Heavy chains	Gamma	Mu	Alpha	Delta	Epsilon
Light chains	Kappa or lambda	Kappa or lambda	Kappa or lambda	Kappa or lambda	Kappa or lambda
Gm specificity	Yes	No	No	No	No
Inv specificity	Yes	Yes	Yes	?	?
Electrophoretic mobility	Gamma	Between beta and gamma	Slow beta	Between beta and gamma	Slow beta
Placental transfer	Yes	No	No	No	No
Usual serologic behavior as RBC antibody	Non-agglutinating	Saline agglutinating	Non-agglutinating	?	?
Complement fixation	Few	Many	None	None	None

bodies cause delayed or hypersensitivity reactions and, being fixed to tissue cells, are not readily susceptible to laboratory manipulation. The antibodies mediating various allergies and tuberculin sensitivity fall into this group.

Antibodies are recognized by various manifestations of their activity, and this fact has been used as the basis for another, rather artificial scheme of classification. Humoral antibodies may behave as precipitins, forming insoluble precipitates upon combining with antigens; as agglutinins, binding together antigen particles to form clumps; as hemolysins, fixing complement that effects red blood cell lysis; as blocking antibodies, sensitizing RBC but preventing their agglutination by saline agglutinins; as sensitizing antibodies for immune adherence, in which indicator particles attach to antigen-antibody complexes; as opsonins, enhancing phagocytosis; or as cytotoxins, bringing about cell death; and this is not a complete catalogue of antibody activities. Many of these serologic properties are manifestations of different reactivities of the same molecule under different test conditions so that a classification based on such distinctions is more a list of antibody-detection techniques than of antibody types.

STRUCTURE OF IMMUNOGLOBULINS

Chemical characterization of immunoglobulins has shown that the basic unit of structure of all classes is a symmetrical Y-shaped molecule composed of two heavy or H-chains, each with a molecular weight of 50,000 to 70,000 and two light or L-chains, each of a molecular weight of 20,000 to 25,000, bound together by disulfide (S-S) linkages and noncovalent bonds (see Figure 5-1). L-chains are composed of an estimated 214 amino acid residues while H-chains have 446. Each immunoglobulin class or subclass has a characteristic and different H-chain, designated gamma for IgG molecules, alpha for IgA, mu for IgM, delta for IgD, and epsilon for IgE. There are two types of L-chains, differing only in amino acid sequence, and these are common to all five classes of immunoglobulin molecules. A given immunoglobulin molecule will possess either two kappa or two lambda L-chains, molecules with kappa L-chains occurring about twice as frequently as those with lambda L-chains. Thus a typical IgG molecule is composed of two gamma H-chains and either two kappa or two lambda L-chains.

IgG molecules occur in monomeric form, as illustrated in Figure 5-1, whereas IgM molecules exist as pentamers, or combinations of five units similar in structure to the basic IgG molecule, and held together by J (joining) chains, each with a molecular weight of about 15,000. IgA molecules exist in two structural types, a serum form and a secretory type, and are found as monomers in serum but as dimers or trimers (composed of two or three units) in body secretions. J-chains serve the same function as in IgM molecules. A secretory component with a molecular weight of about 85,000 is also attached to the molecule when it is found in body secretions. The IgG molecule has approximate dimensions of 50 × 250 Angstrom units, while the maximum dimension of the IgM pentamer is about 350 Angstrom units.

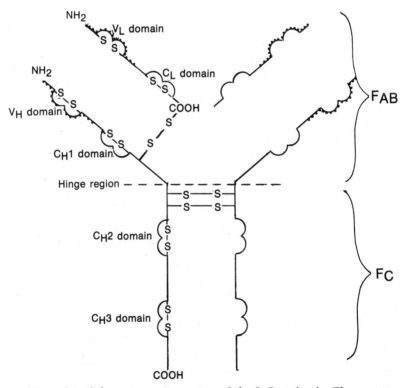

Figure 5-1. *Schematic representation of the IgG molecule. The constant regions of each chain are represented by solid lines and the variable regions by broken lines. A dotted line has been drawn through the hinge area.*

Whereas IgG and IgM molecules are found principally in blood and in the case of IgG in extracellular fluid, IgA molecules occur in such body fluids as tears, nasal secretions, saliva, milk, and urine and are thought to constitute a significant part of the local body defense mechanism. IgG molecules are characterized functionally as the only class of immunoglobulin capable of passage across the placenta to reach the fetus of a pregnant woman. This process is thought to require an active transport mechanism that will not accept IgM or IgA molecules. The significance of this observation will be returned to in the discussion of hemolytic disease of the newborn. IgG molecules of blood bank interest are characteristic of secondary immune responses, rarely behave as saline agglutinins, often do not fix complement (except for anti-A or anti-B), react optimally at 37 C, and are characteristically induced by exposure to foreign RBC. IgM molecules are typical of primary immune responses, are generally agglutinins in saline, fix complement, can cause hemolysis in vitro, and are usually non-RBC immune.

Four subclasses of IgG have been identified on the basis of differences in composition of their gamma chains and H-chain bonding. Table 5-2 presents some of their pertinent differences. Rh antibodies are usually IgG1 and less frequently IgG3 (which may be produced later). IgG anti-A is generally IgG1 or IgG2, while red blood cell autoantibodies are most frequently IgG1, either alone or mixed with other subclasses. As indicated in Table 5-2, IgG1 is transported preferentially across the placenta but is less effective in causing fetal red blood cell destruction than is IgG3. Recent observations also indicate the considerable importance of IgG subclass in autoimmune acquired hemolytic disease: marked shortening of red blood cell life span may occur if the RBC autoantibody is IgG3; IgG1 autoantibody may or may not cause premature cell destruction, and if the autoantibody is IgG2 and/or IgG4, red blood cell survival is said to be normal. Two subclasses each exist for IgA and IgM molecules, but little is currently known of their significance.

IgG and to a lesser extent IgA molecules are resistant to degradation by reducing agents such as 2-mercaptoethanol (2-ME) or dithiothreitol (DTT), whereas the agglutinating ability of IgM antibodies is destroyed by treatment with these compounds. Practical use of this observation is made in defining the IgG content of antisera.

The structure of a typical IgG molecule is represented diagrammatically in Figure 5-1. The molecule is conceived as a Y-shaped polypeptide composed of two outer, longer H-chains (gamma) and two shorter, inner L-chains (kappa or lambda) that form the inner portions of the arms of the Y. Interchain disulfide bonds formed by covalent linkage of cysteine residues join the two heavy chains and each heavy chain to its light chain partner to form a stable three-dimensional structure. The distal (amino) portion of each light chain and each heavy chain, comprising 108 to 125 amino acid residues, differs considerably in configuration and amino acid sequence among different antibodies. This variable region is responsible for the specificity of an antibody and differences in composition of these variable regions account for differences in specificities among different antibodies. The exact configuration of the antigen-binding site can vary from one molecule to another even if they have the same specificity. If an antigenic determinant fits into the binding site on an immunoglobulin molecule (i.e., if the two structures are complementary) the immunoglobulin will react as an antibody to that determinant. If the "fit" is good (that is to say, if the complementarity is high), binding between the two will be strong; if the fit is less good, binding will be weaker. This concept is shown schematically in Figure 5-2, where it will be seen that not only is complementarity of structure required for a good "fit" between antigenic determinant and antibody-combining site but complementarity of charge is necessary as well.

TABLE 5-2

Some Characteristics of the IgG Subclasses

Characteristic	IgG Subclass			
	IgG1	IgG2	IgG3	IgG4
Percent of total IgG	60–80	14–25	4–8	2–6
Half-life (days)	22	22	5–16	22
Complement-fixing ability	Fair	Poor	Good	Absent
Ability to cross placenta	Increased	Normal	Normal	Normal

The proximal (carboxyl) portions of both H and L-chains are quite constant in composition in the area of three loops, or "domains," in each H-chain and one in each L-chain. These loops are formed by disulfide bonding. The proximal portions of each chain are known as the constant regions. Even in the constant regions considerable variations in amino acid sequence occur in the areas between the loops. Slight differences in composition of the loops themselves are responsible for so-called allotypic variations or genetic polymorphisms such as the various Gm groups on gamma chains or Km groups on kappa chains. Cleavage by the enzyme papain splits the IgG molecule at the "hinge" region into two Fab fragments containing the antigen combining sites and each composed of the L-chain and the corresponding portion of an H-chain, plus an Fc (crystallizable) fragment composed of most of the two H-chains. At the point of juncture of the Fab and Fc fragments (the hinge region) the H-chains can bend from a T to a Y shape when the antibody

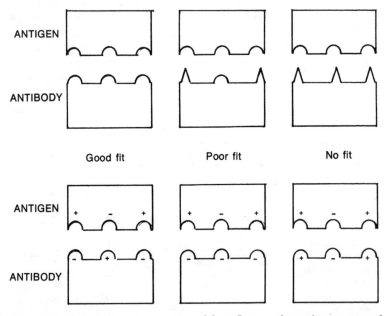

Figure 5-2. *Schematic representation of the influence of complementarity of structure and charge on the binding of antigen to antibody.*

molecule combines with its antigenic determinant. This change in shape of the molecule exposes previously hidden complement binding sites on the Fc portion of the molecule. Other biologic activities dependent on the Fc segment include placental transfer and, in the case of IgE molecules, cell fixation.

Recent work has shown that additional complexity exists in the composition of the immunoglobulin molecule beyond the description already given. Small areas in the variable regions of both heavy and light chains have been discovered to be hypervariable in terms of amino acid composition. Three such regions have been demonstrated in L-chains and four in H-chains, each composed of from five to 15 amino acid residues. It is now thought that antibody specificity is determined by these "hot spots" and that the remaining amino acids of the variable region of both H- and L-chains serve to fold the chains into a three-dimensional pattern that brings the hypervariable regions into optimal spatial relationship with their antigenic determinants.

The loops or domains within the H- and L-chains are each thought to participate in a different biologic activity. The light chains possess one domain each in the variable and constant regions (V_L and C_L) while the heavy chains of gamma type contain one domain in the variable region (V_H) and three in the constant region (C_H1, C_H2 and C_H3). IgA heavy chains also have three domains in the constant region and one in the variable region, while IgM and IgE H-chains each possess one additional domain in the constant region. The V_H and V_L domains determine the antigen-binding capabilities of the antibody molecule, and it is possible that the C_L and C_H1 domains assist in orienting antigen molecules toward the hypervariable foci of the variable regions. The C_H2 domain participates in binding the first component of complement (Clq), initiating complement activation by the classic pathway. The C_H3 domain is responsible for macrophage binding to the antibody molecule.

THE IMMUNE RESPONSE

Exposure of an immunologically competent host to an antigenic substance is necessary before an immune response can occur, but other factors are significant in determining whether actual antibody formation will ensue and what the amount and character of the response will be. All antigens are not equally effective in eliciting an immune response. Molecular size and internal chemical complexity, including such factors as variety and numbers of aromatic amino acid units and net molecular charges are important. With regard to immunization by red blood cell antigens, intact cells appear to be more antigenic than red blood cell stroma. The dose of antigen reaching the antibody-producing cells is generally important. For example, a 200 ml transfusion of Rh-positive RBC to an Rh-negative recipient is three or four times as likely to cause formation of detectable Rh antibody as is a 1 ml transfusion, although it is not true that more antigen is always more immunogenic. Other important factors include the number of times the antigen is introduced into the tissues, the length of time it persists before being destroyed or eliminated, the time intervals between exposures to the antigen, and the route by which the antigen is introduced.

Host factors are of major importance in determining whether an immune response will occur to a given antigen. Some persons produce antibodies readily in response to an antigenic stimulus while others may not respond to the same challenge. For example, about 30% of Rh-negative subjects do not respond in detectable fashion to the Rh blood group antigen no matter how often the stimulus is presented, yet these people respond normally to many other antigens. Immune response (Ir) genes are postulated to explain increased or decreased responses to particular antigens. There is no evidence that these genes are linked, although the possibility exists. At a practical level most blood transfusions do not cause blood group immunization either because the foreign red blood cell antigens are too weak (not sufficiently immunogenic) or because the recipient lacks the immune response genes necessary to react.

The ability of the host to respond to an antigenic stimulus may be reduced in congenital or acquired immune deficiency states, as discussed previously, or by certain drugs such as the antimetabolites or adrenal corticosteroids. On the other hand, patients with some diseases such as systemic lupus erythematosus appear to produce a variety of blood group antibodies in response to minimal provocation. It is a general observation that a patient who has made one blood group antibody is likely to form others. The reason for this however, may not be wholly genetic: antibody production in response to foreign antigens on RBC leads to the sequestration and presentation to the immunologic system of other foreign antigens in concentrated form.

The blood bank worker should appreciate that a number of statistical factors are at work in determining whether blood group immunization can take place in response to transfusion, based upon the frequency of occurrence of particular RBC antigens in donors and recipients. The considerable racial variation in occurrence of certain blood group antigens is illustrated in Table 5-3.

The speed with which antibody production is initiated after first exposure to a blood group antigen may vary widely. An induction period of seven to ten days is the minimum required for appearance of the first detectable antibody, although antibody in some patients may not appear for months if at all. In the latter situation, on subsequent re-exposure it may become apparent from the character of the response that the immunologic system was "primed" by the original contact. In the case of certain RBC antigens such as $Rh_O(D)$, it is traditionally taught that the first antibody molecules produced are 19S, IgM saline agglutinins, although it is apparent that IgG molecules are often made from the outset. If not restimulated, the immunologic system will produce antibody over the space of several weeks, with peak production occurring at about 30 days

TABLE 5-3

Percentage Frequencies of Occurrence of Selected RBC
Antigens in Various Races (after Mollison)

	Race		
Antigen	White	Black	Yellow
B	14	20	35
D	84	95	100
V (ce^s)	0	40	0
P	80	95	31
K	9	< 1	0
Fy^a	65	20	99
Js^a	0	20	0
Di^a	0	0	5

and a gradual decline in concentration thereafter, often to the point where the antibody can no longer be demonstrated.

Re-exposure to the antigen may provoke a response in as little as 24 to 48 hours. Clones of committed lymphocytes retaining the "memory" of the past antigenic exposure rapidly proliferate and differentiate into immunocytes with active antibody production. This secondary, or anamnestic, response is characterized by its short response time and production of large quantities of antibody molecules. Specifically in the case of blood group antibodies these molecules are usually of IgG class, and their production often persists for protracted periods, sometimes even for decades. IgG production tends to continue for longer periods than IgM production, though the specificity of the antibody influences the duration of its production.

Irrespective of how often an antigenic stimulus is repeated, there is always a point beyond which no increase in concentration occurs owing to a negative feedback effect, the amount of antibody formed controlling the subsequent rate of production. It is believed that there is competition for antigen between free antibody and receptor sites on antibody bound to the surface of immunocytes (see below), with the latter acquiring a progressively smaller share of antigen and consequently being stimulated less intensely. Actual prevention of primary immunologic sensitization can be accomplished by administering sufficient amounts of potent specific IgG antibody at the same time or shortly after antigen exposure. Clinical use of this observation is made in preventing sensitization of Rh-negative mothers who deliver Rh-positive babies.

If the receptor on an uncommitted lymphocyte (see below) fits an antigenic determinant closely, the final clones of immunocytes will produce antibody with binding sites highly complementary to it, and therefore will bind to the antigen strongly. Since the "fit" between antibody receptor and antigenic determinant does not have to be exact to stimulate cloning (the reproduction of identical cells), an antigenic determinant of a single specificity may stimulate lymphoid cells whose surface Ig molecules differ in their degree of complementarity to it. The result will be the production of antibodies with a range of binding strengths. This fact also explains why a secondary response may be caused by an antigen similar to, but not identical to, the one responsible for primary sensitization. The average binding strength of a population of antibody molecules is called the binding constant of an antiserum; the range of their binding strengths is the index of heterogeneity. Thus, the quantity of antibody molecules present plus their average binding constant and index of heterogeneity are the true measures of the potency of an antiserum. Repeated exposure to an antigen causes an increase in the average binding constant of the free antibody produced: immunocytes with surface antibody of high complementarity bind antigen more firmly and are more apt to be stimulated than those whose surface immunoglobulins fit poorly with the antigen.

The antibody molecules produced in response to an antigenic stimulus often represent a whole spectrum of types of serologic reactivity. Some of the molecules in an antiserum may react better by one method of testing, some by another. There may be wide ranges in their optimum temperature for reaction (thermal amplitude); some may fix complement while others fail to do so. Both increased thermal amplitude and acquisition of special abilities such as complement fixation are characteristic of some secondary responses to RBC immunization.

Another feature of repeated exposure to a complex antigen is increased breadth of response: determinants that did not stimulate antibody production originally may ultimately do so, and a previously monospecific antiserum may become multispecific. The complexity of the immune response, either initially or more typically on repeated exposure to the sorts of chemically complex antigens encountered by the host in nature may be illustrated by a hypothetical example. Consider an animal immunized with a human red blood cell antigen "XYZ." The resulting antiserum would be expected to have the specificity anti-XYZ. Some antibody molecules however might react only with determinant X, others only with Y, others only with Z, still others only with X in the presence of Y (anti-XY) or Z (anti-XZ) and so forth. If the antiserum is purified by absorption of all but anti-X activity, it may still be found that there are antibody molecules present that react with all of the X antigen plus others that combine with only a portion of it, so that "anti-X" may really be a mixture of anti-X plus anti-X_1, and sometimes of anti-X_2, -X_3, and more. Also present may be antibodies to other antigenic determinants on the immunizing RBC, so that, for example, the antiserum may exhibit "anti-human" activity, reacting with an antigen present on all human red blood cells. Further, if another antigen resembling XYZ is also found on human erythrocytes or RBC from other animals, or in bacteria or elsewhere, the antiserum may cross-react with it.

Three other immunologic phenomena should be noted. It was stated previously that prevention of immunologic sensitization can be accomplished if enough specific antibody is administered at the time of initial exposure to an antigen. If, however, only small amounts of antibody are given, particularly IgM antibody, host antibody production instead of being suppressed may be increased (immunologic enhancement). The administered antibody may act in this situation as an opsonin, increasing the likelihood of phagocytosis by macrophages, which, as will be discussed later, "process" certain antigens as the first step in the immune response to them. On the other hand, it should be appreciated that the administration of only very small amounts of antibody is required to suppress the immune response to RBC antigens. It has been shown that $25\mu g$ of a potent IgG anti-$Rh_0(D)$ prevents immunization of $Rh_0(D)$-negative adults by 1 ml of Rh-positive red blood cells. Even if every antibody molecule were attached to Rh-positive RBC there would only be enough antibody to combine with half of the D sites. In actuality, with the antigen distributed in a space equal to the blood volume, and the antibody in a space twice this (plasma volume plus extracellular fluid volume), at equilibrium only 5% of the D sites and 1% of the antibody are combined. It is speculated that antibody must be concentrated at the site of antigen processing to exert its effect.

Antibodies are normally made only to those antigens that the host is not genetically programmed to produce, a feature known as immunologic tolerance. It is postulated that in fetal life, immunologically competent cells, theoretically capable of making antibody against all possible antigenic determinants, meet their own complementary antigens and somehow are blocked. Escape from this block seems to be the cause of autoimmune diseases. Tolerance can also occur to foreign antigens introduced into the body during fetal life if these antigens persist. The best example of this is found in people who are red blood cell chimeras. Dizygotic (fraternal) twins may exchange hematopoietic tissue in utero with formation of two antigenically different RBC populations, each host accepting (tolerant to) the antigens of the other. A similar process characterizes the phenomenon of mosaicism, which is caused by the fertilization of two eggs by two spermatozoa, with formation of a single host with varying proportions of two cell lines throughout his tissues.

Massive exposure to a foreign antigen may fail to elicit antibody production, apparently by overwhelming the immunologic system, although the actual mechanism is unknown. This failure to respond is called immune paralysis and is most commonly induced by weak antigens that persist. The establishment of immune paralysis is facilitated by prior damage to the immunologic system, as, for example, by extensive host irradiation.

The distinction between "naturally occurring" and "immune" antibodies frequently made in the older literature is largely artificial but retains usefulness from a conceptual point of view. No antibody occurs naturally in the sense that it arises without antigenic stimulation, but the exact identification of the antigenic substances, and the means and occasion of exposure to them are often unknown, hence the term "naturally occurring." A better term for such antibodies is "non-red blood cell immune." As applied to blood grouping, these antibodies have generally common characteristics that usually distinguish them from red blood cell immune antibodies: they are usually saline agglutinins, of IgM class at least in part, are often complement fixing and potentially if not actually hemolytic, and react optimally at temperatures below 37 C. Antibodies in the ABO system fall into this category, as well as many antibodies in the MNSs, Lewis, P, I, and Wright systems plus some examples of anti-rh''(E). Some of the more common examples include anti-M^g (found in 3% of random blood donor sera), anti-Vw (2%), anti-Wr^a (1%) anti-Le^a (5% to 20% of Le(a–b–) and 0.3 to one percent of all persons), anti-P_1 (1% of P_1-negative or 0.2% of all persons) and anti-rh'' (E) (0.1%).

Antibody production occurs within the reticuloendothelial tissues or immunologic system of the body including lymphocytes, their precursors, and macrophages (both free and fixed) in the peripheral blood, lymph nodes, thymus, spleen, liver, bone marrow, gastrointestinal tract, and other tissues. As depicted in Figure 5-3, antigenic material introduced into the body may either be carried by the circulation to the lymphoid tissues or be ingested and carried there by macrophages (tissue histiocytes or blood monocytes). In some cases, depending on the antigen, fixed macrophages in the lymphoid tissues ingest or at least adsorb the antigenic material and "process" it, degrading or in other ways altering it. Messenger substances (mRNA) or the antigen itself are then transferred to inactive, "uncommitted" small lymphocytes. These cells then enlarge, morphologically coming to resemble "blasts," or primitive forms.

Cell multiplication occurs during this sequence. Depending on the nature of the antigen, the lymphoid cell, if a B-cell, is transformed into a plasma cell with concomitant humoral antibody production. If T-cells are involved in the process, no transformation by the T-cells to plasma cells occurs, but participation in the functional roles of T-cells does take place. Lymphocytes that have undergone functional transformation as a consequence of reaction to a specific antigen are called "committed." Their reaction is highly specific and can be elicited only by the particular antigenic determinant (or a closely similar chemical configuration) that originally induced it. In all cases some committed lymphocytes remain as "memory cells" — cells not functionally active but altered by exposure to antigen so that they will respond in accelerated fashion if re-exposed to it.

It is estimated that there exist in the body over 10,000 clones of lymphocytes, each committed to the production of a specific immunoglobulin. In the case of B-cells, during the process of commitment each has produced a small amount of immunoglobulin specifically reactive with a particular antigenic determinant, and never will that cell or any of its offspring for the entire life of the animal lose that capability or change it. Only one highly specific, unique immunoglobulin will or can ever be produced by that clone of lymphocytes. On first exposure to the antigen, the small amounts of immunoglobulin made in response to its presence by B-cells are transported to their surfaces and become fixed there, ready to interact with any antigen complementary to their receptors. Subsequent exposure to appropriate antigen plus receipt of an additional signal (from T-cells) leads to proliferation and differentiation into plasma cells that synthesize and excrete large amounts of immunoglobulin of the same specificity as that on the surfaces of their ancestral lymphocytes. The proliferative response to continuing or repeat antigenic exposure increases the number of "primed" precursor cells and results in an antibody response of increased effectiveness.

Both T- and B-lymphocytes require stimulation for formation of humoral antibody to most antigens. The antigen-specific receptor on the T-cell surface has not been identified. The B-cell apparently bears a receptor for a T-cell signal as well as its surface antigen receptor, and it is postulated that both must be occupied for stimulation to occur, thus placing humoral antibody production by B-cells under T-cell control. Although little is known about the subject, genes in the major histocompatibility (HLA) locus antigen appear to control formation of cell surface antigens (Ia genes) critical to T-B—cell interaction. As indicated in Figure 5-3 macrophages are also necessary to the immune reaction to most antigens, in some way presenting modified antigen to T-cells. Less than 10% of antigen molecules escape catabolism by the macrophages that ingest them. Possibly it is those only bound to the surface membrane of the macrophage that are effective in interacting with T-cells.

Recent work has filled some of the gaps in our knowledge of T-cell development and function. T-cells are thought to develop from bone marrow stem cells that migrate in early life to the thymus where they acquire their surface markers before migrating again, this time to the spleen, lymph nodes, and circulation. T-cell function appears to be dual: to regulate the immune response by helper or suppressor effects on B-cells and to serve as effector cells in cell-mediated immune responses, including delayed hypersensitivity and cytotoxic effects on foreign cells, tumor cells, and virus-infected host cells.

The origin of B-cells in man is not known, being variously cited as the fetal gastrointestinal tract, liver, or bone marrow. The model offered by Uhr and Vitetta proposes that in the bone marrow or fetal liver, stem cells develop a surface coating of IgM and later migrate to the spleen, where their offspring are found as lymphocytes bearing both IgM and IgD. These cells are thought to seed the peripheral tissues, including the lymphoid areas in the gastrointestinal tract, the lymph nodes, and other parts of the spleen. The theory holds that interaction of antigen with IgM-coated blasts in the spleen results in tolerance. Interaction of antigen however, with blasts bearing IgD as well as IgM, with the assistance of T-cell signals, causes proliferation of more precursors (memory cells coated with IgD and IgM) or differentiation into IgM-secreting plasma cells. Interaction of antigen with B-cells bearing IgD and IgM in nonsplenic lymphoid tissue results in differentiation of lymphocytes coated with IgD but not IgM. These IgD-bearing cells are the precursors of plasma cells that, after additional antigenic stimulation, produce IgA if situated in gastrointestinal lymphoid tissue or IgG if located in lymph nodes. This concept is diagrammatically summarized in Figure 5-4.

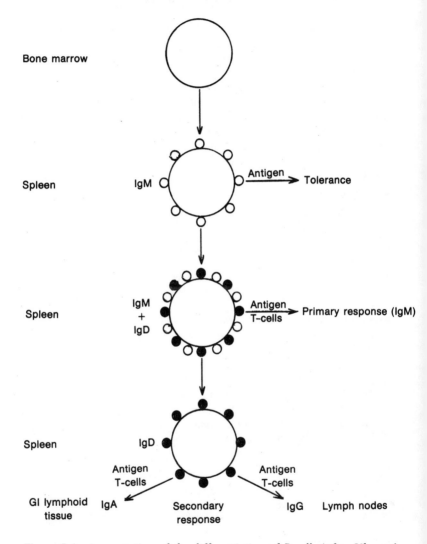

Figure 5-4. *A conception of the differentiation of B-cells (after Uhr and Vitetta).*

RECOMMENDED READING

Case, J.: The immune response. In: *Blood Bank Immunology.* Am Assn of Blood Banks. Washington, 1977. p.87

Dodd, B.E. and Lincoln, P.J.: *Blood Group Topics.* Williams & Wilkins. Baltimore, 1975

Fox, A.E.: The nature of antigen-antibody reactions. In: *Blood Group Immunology: Theoretical and Practical Concepts.* Dade. Miami, 1976. p.1

Huestis, D.W. et al: *Practical Blood Transfusion,* 2nd ed. Little, Brown & Co. Boston, 1976

Issitt, P.D.: The structure and function of antigens and antibodies. In: *Blood Bank Immunology.* Am Assn of Blood Banks. Washington, 1977. p.17

Issitt, P.D. and Issitt, C.H.: *Applied Blood Group Serology,* 2nd ed. Spectra. Oxnard, Calif., 1975

Kuhns, W.J.: Naturally occurring agglutinins in health and disease. In: *A Seminar on Polymorphisms in Human Blood.* Am Assn of Blood Banks. Washington, 1975. p.83

Mollison, P.L.: *Blood Transfusion in Clinical Medicine,* 5th ed. Blackwell. Oxford, 1972

Moore, B.P.L. et al: Serological and technical methods: *The Technical Manual of the Canadian Red Cross Blood Transfusion Service,* 7th ed. Canadian Red Cross. Toronto, 1972

Schanfield, M.S.: Human immunoglobulin (Ig) subclasses and their biological properties. In: *Blood Bank Immunology.* Am Assn of Blood Banks. Washington, 1977. p.97

Shohet, S.B. and Klock, J.C.: Red cell glycolipids and phospholipids: composition and metabolism. In: *Membrane Structure and Function of Human Blood Cells.* Am Assn of Blood Banks. Washington, 1976. p.15

Uhr, J.W. and Vitetta, E.S.: Receptors on lymphocytes. In: *Membrane Structure and Function of Human Blood Cells.* Am Assn of Blood Banks. Washington, 1976. p.81

CHAPTER 6

Reactions Between Antigens and Antibodies

Antigen-antibody reactions are specific, i.e., an antibody molecule reacts with only a single or a few closely related antigenic determinants. Reactions between antigens and antibodies are surface phenomena that do not alter the primary structure of either, although configurational changes may occur. Finally, as will be seen in the ensuing discussion, their reactions are reversible. The reaction conditions under which antigen and antibody meet in the laboratory are of major importance to their interaction and will be discussed in both their quantitative and qualitative aspects.

We have already noted the considerable variability encountered in the antibody molecules comprising an antiserum with regard to differences in specificity, immunoglobulin class, serologic detection methods, thermal amplitude, average binding constant, heterogeneity index, and other factors. At a practical level, blood group antibodies can be separated into two broad groups, saline agglutinins and "incomplete" antibodies. Saline agglutinins are capable of clumping or agglutinating suspensions of appropriate RBC suspended in saline (0.9% or 0.15 M aqueous NaCl), while incomplete or nonagglutinating antibodies are not and must be demonstrated by other means. Incomplete antibodies were first detected by virtue of their ability to "block" or prevent agglutination by saline agglutinins of the same specificity. Subsequently, it was shown that the addition of colloid materials such as bovine serum albumin to the suspending medium would permit agglutination by some incomplete antibodies. We now know, however, that many clinically significant antibodies are not detected by this technique either. Discovery of most of the complexity of modern blood group immunology awaited the introduction of the antiglobulin test by Coombs and his associates (see Chapter 7).

Once the specificity and qualitative reaction characteristics of an antiserum are known, its potency remains to be determined. The strength of an antiserum is traditionally indicated in terms of its titer, or the reciprocal of the greatest dilution of the antiserum that will yield a positive test result. Thus, an antiserum that can produce agglutination at a dilution of 1:256 is said to have a titer of 256 and is stronger than an antiserum with a titer of, for instance, 8. Table 6-1 shows results of a typical titration study. Note that antiserum #3 produced no or weak agglutination until it was diluted. This is an example of the prozone phenomenon: under conditions of marked antibody excess all antibody combining sites are occupied, leaving no free sites for formation of bridges between cells by molecules already attached to one cell. The result is little or no agglutination. Stated differently, we may consider the situation in which all antigen and antibody react and are consumed as a "zone of equivalence." If antibody is present in excess (prozone) agglutination does not occur, because when an antibody molecule dissociates from its antigen, there is a better chance for it to combine with a free molecule of antigen than for an antibody molecule already attached to antigen to combine with the same free molecule. The result of this situation is the formation of many but small agglutinates. Similarly, if antigen is present in excess (postzone) there is a better chance for a free antigen molecule to combine with antibody than for an antigen-anti-

---

TABLE 6-1

Results of typical titration studies using three different anti-A sera versus a suspension of group A_1 RBC. Agglutination is graded from 1+ (weak) to 4+ (strongest). The agglutinin titer of the antiserum is the highest dilution that gives a 1+ reaction. Thus antisera #1 and #3 have a titer of 256, while antiserum #2 has a titer of 8. Antiserum #3 demonstrates a prozone (see text).

Anti-serum	Antiserum Dilution									Control (saline only)
	2	4	8	16	32	64	128	256	512	
1	++++	++++	++++	+++	+++	++	+	+	−	−
2	++	++	+	±	−	−	−	−	−	−
3	−	−	++	++++	++++	+++	++	+	−	−

body complex to meet free antigen. The result is the formation of few, though large, agglutinates.

A property of importance in characterizing an antiserum is its affinity, or combining power, a term related to the binding constant. The term affinity refers to the ability of an antiserum to produce large, tightly adherent agglutinates, a property that correlates with the strength of the bond between antigen and antibody. The term avidity is frequently misused in this connection. Strictly speaking, avidity refers to the speed with which agglutinates of a specified size are produced by an antiserum. The distinction is trivial at a practical level, since avid antisera almost always exhibit high affinity. Correlation between titer and combining power, however, though frequent, is not absolute, and two antisera of equal titer may differ appreciably in the strength of agglutination produced by comparable dilutions.

The usage of titer as a measure of antibody concentration is conceptually invalid in that a titer estimates the amount of antibody attached to RBC, not the total amount in the antiserum. Thus, the proportion of high-affinity antibody molecules exerts an undue influence on titers. If two antisera contain the same number of antibody molecules, the antiserum with the higher average antibody affinity will have the higher titer. Another problem arises from the fact that the relationship between percent RBC agglutination and antibody concentration is not a simple straight line function but rather an S-shaped curve on a semilogarithmic plot. Thus, a large amount of antibody is required to change agglutination strength from 3+ to 4+ but relatively little to change it from trace to 1+. Attempts have been made to overcome some of these objections by using a scoring system in the grading of agglutination reactions, assigning a value of 10 for 4+ agglutination, 7 to 9 for 3+, 4 to 6 for 2+, 2 or 3 for 1+, and 1 for trace or ± reactions. The results of titration reactions are then added to produce a titration "score." The titration score for antiserum #2 in the example in Table 6-1 would be 55, while for antiserum #3, despite its identical titer, the score would be only 41.

Precise measurements of antiserum potency require estimates of the number of micrograms of antibody nitrogen per ml of antiserum plus a measurement of average binding constant and its dispersion or range (heterogeneity index). It is convenient to view the reaction between antigen and antibody as an example of the law of mass action:

antigen + antibody $\xrightarrow{\quad k_1 \quad}$ antigen-antibody complex

with the rate of complex formation governed by the association constant k_1. But antigen-antibody complexes also dissociate:

antigen-antibody complex $\xrightarrow{\quad k_2 \quad}$ antigen + antibody

with the rate of complex dissolution governed by the dissociation constant k_2. Combining these two expressions, we derive:

antigen + antibody $\xrightleftharpoons[k_2]{k_1}$ antigen-antibody complex

Because k_1 and k_2 are constant for a given system, we may divide k_1 by k_2, deriving the binding constant K. If the antigen and antibody are initially present in equivalent amounts, in systems in which this expression is shifted far to the right, there will be little free antibody, most being complexed with antigen. In this situation K will be high, which is a more precise way of saying that the antibody has a high affinity for its antigen. Conversely, a system employing an antiserum with a low value for K will contain few antigen-antibody complexes and much free antibody, which will be said to possess low affinity. K as thus defined is a quantitative measure of the complementarity between an antigenic determinant and an antibody binding site. The use of radioisotope labeling methods has made it possible to measure mean values for K.

The number of antibody molecules in a given system bound to RBC antigens is also dependent upon the total number, configuration or accessibility, and density of antigen sites per cell. These factors vary with the blood group system under consideration, the number of antigen sites per cell ranging from a few thousand for some of the Rh antigens to as many as a million for the A_1 antigen. Other influences also affect the number of antigen sites on the red blood cell. The term dosage refers to quantitative differences in antigenic strength of RBC in persons heterozygous and homozygous (see Chapter 8) for the genes determining a given antigen; the cells from homozygotes are the more reactive. This phenomenon is not seen in all blood group systems nor do all examples of antisera of a given specificity exhibit it. Dosage effects are commonly seen with antisera to the antigens M, N, hr'(c), rh''(E), hr'(e), Jk^a and Jk^b. Antigen expression on the red blood cell surface, and therefore cell reactivity, are also affected by the genotype (see Chapter 8) of the subject apart from considerations of dosage. Thus R^2r (CDE/cde) RBC have more D antigen sites than do R^1r (CDe/cde) cells. Or again, so-called "position effects" (see Chapter 11) may also exert an influence, e.g., expression of the D antigen is suppressed on RBC from persons with genotypes having C on a gene complex opposite (trans) to D, as in $R'R^2$ (Cde/cDE) subjects.

Whether or not the antigen is accessible to its antibody is of controlling importance, for reactions will not occur if antigenic determinant and antibody binding site cannot come into apposition. For instance almost all adult human sera contain anti-T and all human RBC bear the T antigen, but reactions do not normally occur because the T antigen is spatially masked on the normal red blood cell surface and inaccessible to anti-T. Antigen density is also important in some connections, particularly where the binding constant is low. IgM molecules possess ten potential binding sites and may attach by more than one site to the cell surface if such sites are close enough to be spanned by the size of the molecule. The importance of this occurrence will be returned to in the discussion of complement fixation. It should be recalled in this connection that the fluid mosaic model of the RBC membrane postulates a solution of integral proteins dispersed in a fluid lipid matrix in which both can be redistributed. The mobility of the components of the membrane bearing blood group antigens may be important in agglutination reactions, or even necessary to them. It has been speculated that the effects of enzyme treatment in enhancing red blood cell antigen-antibody reactions may be caused by inducement of increased antigen mobility.

Other factors affecting antigen reactivity of red blood cells include cell storage age and storage conditions. Certain RBC antigens such as those of the Lewis, MN, and P systems slowly deteriorate in vitro with loss of cell agglutinability. This effect is accelerated by storage of blood in clotted form or at temperatures above 4 C.

The relative concentrations of antigen and antibody are major factors in their interaction. The reaction of antigen with antibody is a random pairing, i.e., a chance meeting of complementary structures. The bonding between the two (see p. 66) is relatively weak, and as already discussed, reversible. The rate of random pairing or association of antigen and antibody and of bond cleavage or dissociation ultimately reaches a state of equilibrium expressed by rearranging the equation given earlier:

$$K = \frac{[\text{Antigen}]\ [\text{Antibody}]}{[\text{Antigen-Antibody complex}]}$$

From the expression it is obvious that increasing the concentration of one reactant (antibody) while holding a second constant (antigen) will increase the concentration of the third (antigen-antibody complexes). Thus, an increase in the proportion of antibody to antigen in a system will increase the number of complexes formed (assuming no prozone) and therefore will increase the likelihood of detecting the reaction. This fact can be stated in a different way: as shown in Figure 6-1, when antibody concentration is low, there is little free antibody, most being bound randomly to RBC, but the chance of two sensitized RBC colliding is low. With addition of more antibody, most RBC become sensitized and more numerous random collisions occur, leading to agglutination. Adding still more antibody does not proportionately further increase agglutination, because most cells are already maximally sensitized. On the other hand, increasing the concentration of antigen while holding antibody concentration constant, though increasing the number of antigen-antibody complexes formed, decreases the number of antibody molecules attached to each red blood cell. Increasing antibody concentration increases the number of complexes and increases the amount of bound antibody per cell. Since the sensitivity of agglutination reactions depends on the latter, the sensitivity of blood bank testing procedures can be increased by increasing the serum/cell ratio employed.

The binding forces involved in holding antigen-antibody complexes together are of four types: 1) Ionic or electrostatic attraction (the interaction between ionized groups); 2) Hydrogen bonding (an implied electrostatic interaction between a neutral and an ionic group, e.g., between amine or amide and carboxyl groups, or between neutral groups bonded to water). In hydrogen bonding, a hydrogen atom (proton) is shared between a proton donor or acceptor on an antigen molecule and its opposite member on an antibody molecule; 3) Van der Waal's forces (attractions between atoms and molecules). If we consider the electron cloud of an atom whirling about its nucleus, at any one moment it will be predominantly on one side of the nucleus, imparting a slight positive charge to the other side. This attracts the negative side of the electron cloud on an adjacent atom in which the same process is occurring. The process reverses itself rapidly and continuously. 4) Hydrophobic bonds. Molecules tend to exist in nature in their lowest energy state. To suspend hydrophobic (literally, "water-hating") molecules in water requires energy expenditure. To conserve energy, hydrophobic surfaces (e.g., antigenic determinants, antibody-binding sites) are drawn together. It is thought that hydrogen bonding and van der Waal's forces are important in antigen-antibody binding, with hydrophobic bonds less so, and ionic attraction of little significance.

"Environmental" factors or reaction conditions have a major impact on antigen-antibody reactions. The antigen-antibody reaction occurs in two stages, which will be considered in turn. Antibody binding to a complementary determinant occurs first, with associated conformational shifts, changes in intermolecular repulsions and attractions, and formation of intermolecular bonds. Then, antigen-antibody complexes may or may not form a lattice; whether

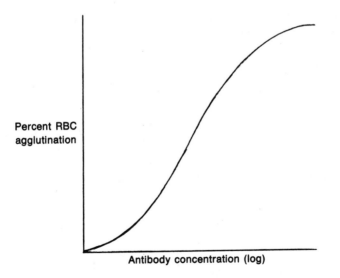

Figure 6-1. *The relationship between red blood cell agglutination and antibody concentration.*

agglutination occurs depends on some of the factors already noted plus others described below.

Reaction conditions in the suspending medium affecting the first stage of agglutination (formation of antigen-antibody complexes) and the binding constant (K) include:

1) *Temperature*. Increased temperature supplies heat energy that may increase complex formation by facilitating the reaction, or decrease it by increasing molecular motion and disrupting bonding, especially if K is low and complementarity is poor. The binding constant is not influenced by temperature in the case of 37 C-reactive antibodies, although the rate of association is slowed at low temperatures. On the other hand, the K value of cold agglutinins is markedly altered by changes in temperature.

2) *Ionic strength*. Decreased ionic strength increases antibody uptake by antigen, probably because the distortion of antibody structure by ionic attraction is decreased. Increased ionic strength results in interactions with small ions that can cause conformational shifts in antibody molecules and increase dissociation of antigen-antibody complexes. Decreased ionic strength also leads to exposure of oppositely charged groups on antigen and antibody molecules partially neutralized at higher ionic strengths, thus enhancing the association reaction. The rate of association between antigen and antibody as well as the strength of the binding is increased in many cases by the use of low-ionic strength solutions. The practical limit of their usefulness in the nonspecific binding of complement components to the cell membrane by immunoglobulins aggregated in low-ionic strength solutions.

3) *pH*. At ideal pH values, antigen and antibody molecules are stabilized in optimal configurations. At a pH in excess of 8 or below 6 RBC antigen-antibody reactions are inhibited, although those of anti-M may be enhanced at pH 6.5, as may agglutination of RBC from patients with paroxsymal nocturnal hemoglobinuria, reactions of enzyme-treated cells and cold agglutination. As noted below, the red blood cell surface bears a negative charge, while most antibody molecules carry a weakly positive charge at pH 7.0 to 7.5.

4) *Presence of albumin*. The effect of albumin in the suspending medium is similar to that of decreasing ionic strength in that albumin "absorbs" or neutralizes ion effects.

5) *Enzymes*. RBC treatment with enzymes causes release of surface sialic acid and enhancement of antibody uptake (unless the en-

zyme has destroyed antibody-combining sites, e.g., M or N determinants).

Practical use is made of our knowledge of the factors increasing the dissociation of antigen-antibody complexes in selecting the conditions for eluting (dissociating) antibodies from red blood cells. Heat, decreased pH, and increased ionic strength solutions are employed to break antigen-antibody bonds and release free antibody.

Before discussing the factors influencing the second stage of RBC agglutination, we must appreciate an important point about the size relationships between RBC and immunoglobulin molecules: namely, the RBC has a diameter of 7 to 8μ, the immunoglobulin molecule a maximum dimension of 250 (IgG) to 350 (IgM) Anström units. In more familiar terms, we are comparing a three-inch IgG molecule to a 50-yard red blood cell. It is immediately apparent that a bound IgG molecule could readily disappear into even minor irregularities in the RBC surface and thus be prevented from reaching a second combining site on another cell. The IgM molecule is only slightly larger, so that it shares this problem, but has an advantage over the IgG molecule in that it possesses five times as many combining sites. Moreover it is possible that in the case of an IgG molecule, both combining sites might attach to antigenic determinants on the same cell, whereas though two or even more sites on an IgM molecule might also attach to one cell, other sites would remain free to participate in reactions with another cell. It is possible that changes in location and/or distribution of antigenic determinants on the red blood cell surface may occur in RBC undergoing agglutination.

Environmental factors or reaction conditions affecting the second phase of RBC agglutination (lattice formation) include:

1) *Temperature*. Increased temperature increases the likelihood of cell collision, but also of separation. Different antisera are affected to various degrees in different ways.

2) *Enzymes*. The exact mechanism by which enzymes enhance RBC agglutination is unknown. Possible actions include reduction in steric hindrance, clustering of antigen sites, and changes in the hydration of cell surfaces as well as a decrease in cell surface charge.

3) *Albumin and ionic strength*. The effects of albumin or other large asymmetrical molecular species as well as the effects of ionic strength of the suspending medium on the second stage of agglu-

tination have been traditionally explained in terms of the zeta potential theory of Pollock and his colleagues. As shown in Figure 6-2, the
red blood cell surface carries a net negative charge when suspended
in electrolyte solution at neutral pH, owing to ionization of carboxyl
groups of surface sialic acid residues. When suspended in saline,
RBC are surrounded by a cloud of positively and negatively charged
ions about 1 nm thick, or 1/7000 the cell diameter, oriented as suggested in the diagram and partially neutralizing the negative charge
on the surface of the cell membrane. The electrical potential between the cell surface and the slipping plane or plane of shear of the
surrounding ion cloud is called the zeta potential. The mutual repulsion by the negatively charged cell surfaces prevents RBC from

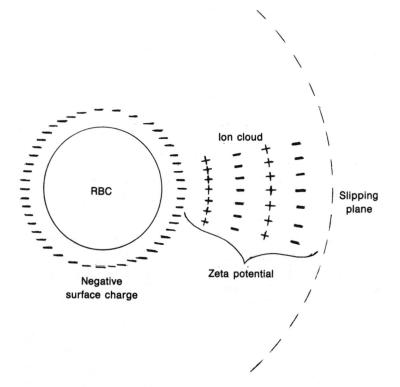

Figure 6-2. *Schematic representation of the concept of zeta potential.*

spontaneously agglutinating in vitro, or theoretically from normally approaching one another closer than 1,000 Angström units. In attaching to the red blood cell surface, antibodies reduce its negative charge, reduce the zeta potential, and allow the cells more closely to approach one another. If the cells approach sufficiently closely, antibody molecules may be able to span the gap between them, form a bridge, and produce agglutination. Differences in molecular size based upon immunoglobulin class play little part in determining whether agglutination will occur. IgG molecules are T- or Y-shaped, with the two combining sites a maximum of 140 Angström units apart, while pentagonal IgM molecules, with ten combining sites, have no two separated by more than 300 Angström units. The process of agglutination is probably best viewed in terms of random RBC collision with the cells prevented from separating if a sufficient number of strong enough antibody links are formed between them. The most probable reason for the failure of most IgG antibodies to produce agglutination in saline is that there are too few specific antigen sites on the RBC membranes to permit enough antibody molecules to form bridges and bind the RBC together. The lack of agglutinating capability of most IgG antibodies relates in this view to their specificity, not their immunoglobulin class, and explains why IgG anti-A is a saline agglutinin, A sites being very numerous on the red blood cell membrane. The existence of occasional IgG saline agglutinins of other specificities and of rare IgM incomplete antibodies might be explained by postulating unusual binding constants for these antisera.

According to the zeta potential theory, the enhancing effect of albumin in RBC reactions with certain incomplete antibodies (primarily in the Rh system) is explained by observing that albumin alters the dielectric constant of the suspending medium. In doing so, it neutralizes a portion of the ion cloud surrounding red blood cells suspended in electrolyte solutions, decreasing the zeta potential and permitting the cells to approach one another more closely and thus be agglutinated more readily. Decreasing the ionic strength of the suspending medium would have a similar effect in this view. Enzyme treatment of the red blood cell membrane, by decreasing its negative charge, also reduces the zeta potential.

Exception has been taken to the theory and significance of zeta potential by Steane. This author proposes an alternative explanation for the observed effects of various changes in reaction conditions on the second phase of red blood cell agglutination based on changes in water of hydration. According to this theory, it is the glycoprotein portion of the RBC membrane and its associated water molecules that prevent autoagglutination. The sialic acid residues on the cell surface bind water molecules as part of the membrane. The negative charge of the sialic acid residues and the steric hindrance of the bound water oppose cell cohesion. Any disruption will enhance the likelihood of antibody-mediated agglutination. Antigen-antibody reactions are seen as competition between the complex and the cell surface for bound membrane water, with antibody binding to cell surfaces releasing water and predisposing the cells to agglutination. If many antigen sites are involved, IgG molecules can effect agglutination; if not, additional measures must be taken to remove bound cell surface water before agglutination can occur.

As noted above, the dielectric constant of a solution is a measure of the ability of its molecules to dissipate charge. Dipolar molecules such as water orient themselves in electric fields and compete with oppositely charged groups attempting to interact. Water orients itself in such a way that it can react with either positively or negatively charged groups and decrease the interaction between the two, essentially getting in the way. The same argument holds in the case of hydrogen bonding. Addition of any molecule (e.g., albumin) that structures water so that water forms hydrogen bonds with it renders the water molecules less polarizable, thereby decreasing the dielectric constant of the medium and permitting hydrogen bonding and hydrophobic interaction between other molecules (such as antigens and antibodies) to increase. The role of the ionic strength of the suspending medium is viewed from the position that ions "shield" interacting molecules. Ions added to a solution must be hydrated to be soluble, thereby decreasing the amount of water available to protein molecules. Thus as ionic strength is reduced shielding decreases and the hydrogen bonding potential of antigens and antibodies increases, favoring agglutination. Hydrophobic bonding is affected similarly. The fundamental difference between the concepts of the zeta and the hydration theories is seen in their explanations of the mechanisms whereby RBC in suspension are prevented from approaching too closely: the zeta theory holds cell membrane surface charge responsible; the hydration theory maintains that the effect is a result of a tightly bound layer of water molecules.

Finally there remains to be discussed the effect of time on antigen-antibody reactions. The incubation time required for complete equilibrium to be reached between antibody association and dissociation, even at optimum temperature, may be several hours. Antibody binding occurs relatively rapidly, however, so that in practice it is not necessary to achieve a state of equilibrium before interpretation of serologic reactions is carried out. When discussing the effects of reaction conditions on antigen-antibody interaction, careful distinction should be made between factors actually altering the binding constant (such as pH and ionic strength) and those that do not affect the binding constant but alter the time required to reach conditions of equilibrium (such as temperature in the case of 37 C-reactive antibodies).

Time is also a factor in the second phase of the agglutination reaction. Normal centrifugation only speeds the rate of development of agglutination but does not produce agglutination which would not occur without it. As an exception to this generality, however, it has been observed that prolonged, very high speed centrifugation will produce agglutination by incomplete antibodies.

RECOMMENDED READING

Fox, A.E.: The nature of antigen-antibody reactions. In: *Blood Group Immunology: Theoretical and Practical Aspects.* Dade, Miami, 1976. p. 1

Huestis, D.W. et al: *Practical Blood Transfusion,* 2nd ed. Little, Brown and Co. Boston, 1976

Issitt, C.H.: Antigen-antibody reactions. In: *Advances in Immunohematology*, Vol. 1, No. 4, Spectra, Oxnard, Calif., 1971

Issitt, P.D. and Issitt, C.H.: *Applied Blood Group Serology*, 2nd ed. Spectra, Oxnard, Calif., 1975

Masouredis, S.P.: Red cell membrane blood group antigens. In: *Membrane Structure and Function of Human Blood Cells.* Am Assn of Blood Banks. Washington, 1976. p. 37

Mollison, P.L.: *Blood Transfusion in Clinical Medicine,* 5th ed. Blackwell, Oxford, 1972

Moore, B.P.L.: Antibody quantification, old and new. In: *A Seminar on Performance Evaluation.* Am Assn of Blood Banks. Washington, 1976. p. 75

Moore, B.P.L. et al: Serological and technical methods: *The Technical*

CHAPTER 7

Antiglobulin Testing and Complement

The coating of red blood cells by antibody molecules not capable of causing agglutination represents sensitization by incomplete antibody. If a bridge were to be constructed, reacting at either end with immunoglobulin or other molecules already fixed to the RBC, agglutination would occur. Antiglobulin serum serves as that bridge (Figure 7-1).

The reagents used for antiglobulin testing are sera of animal origin (usually from rabbits or goats) that react with human globulin. Such sera are produced by injecting human globulin, which acts as an antigen, into animal tissues to evoke formation of antibody directed against it. The use of such serum to detect globulin bound to red blood cell surfaces requires that unbound or free globulin first be excluded from the test system by washing the RBC suspension. The technique of the test involves incubation of the test cells with antiserum, washing three or four times with large volumes of saline to remove unbound globulin, addition of antiglobulin serum, centrifugation, and reading for agglutination. A positive test result indicates that incomplete antibody or other globulin attached to the RBC in the first step.

The direct antiglobulin test is performed on a washed suspension of RBC and does not entail prior incubation with serum. This test is carried out to detect whether red blood cells have been coated with globulin components in vivo and may be positive in instances of hemolytic disease of the newborn, autoimmune acquired hemolytic disease, hemolytic transfusion reaction, and drug-induced RBC sensitization. The direct antiglobulin test is occasionally positive on blood from patients exhibiting brisk reticulocytosis.

The indirect antiglobulin test consists of the incubation of a serum with red blood cells and their subsequent treatment with anti-

75

globulin serum to determine if sensitization of the cells by incomplete antibody in the test serum has taken place. A source of complement, either the test serum or added fresh normal serum without antibodies, should be present in the incubation mixture to permit detection of weak, complement-fixing antibodies. The indirect antiglobulin test can be used to detect blood group antigens using an incomplete antiserum of known specificity (typing), to detect antibody using a red blood cell suspension of known antigenic composition (screening), or to detect serum-RBC incompatibility (crossmatching).

The sensitivity of the antiglobulin test is considerable, manual

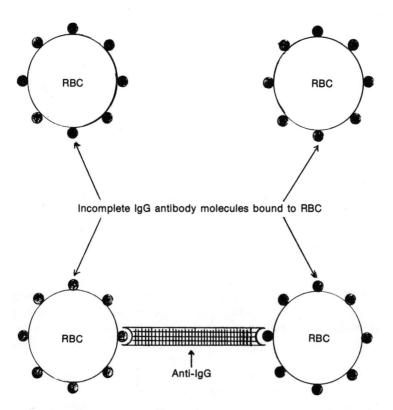

Figure 7-1. *Schematic representation of RBC sensitized by incomplete IgG antibody and agglutinated by anti-IgG.*

testing with a potent serum permitting detection of as few as 500 globulin molecules per RBC. The smallest amount of bound IgG demonstrable by antiglobulin testing varies with antibody specificity: one study showed minimal detectable antiserum levels of 65 ng/ml for anti-rh''(E), 24 ng/ml for anti-hr''(e), 65 to 90 ng/ml for anti-rh'(c), and 20 to 40 ng/ml for anti-Rh_O(D). Such sensitivity requires that after cell sensitization has occurred, extraneous unbound globulin be rigidly excluded from the test system by the washing step. As little as $2\mu g$/ml of residual globulin after washing can neutralize the conventional antiglobulin test. Issitt has calculated that, starting with a concentration of 15,000 μg of IgG per ml of test serum, the use of 2 ml wash volumes and the decanting of residual serum-saline to an 0.1 ml volume after each wash, the residual IgG after one, two, and three washings is 750, 37.5 and 1.8 μg/ml, respectively. If the decanting is more complete, leaving only a 0.05 ml residual volume, the respective values fall to 375, 9.4, and 0.2 μg/ml.

The amino acid sequence in the constant regions of an IgG molecule is important to its reactivity in the antiglobulin test. Anti-IgG is mostly anti-gamma (H-chain) and complexes primarily with Fc regions. It will be recalled that IgG subclasses are based on amino acid substitutions in the constant regions of the gamma heavy chains. Thus the Fc portions of the four IgG subclasses are not identical even for antibody molecules of the same specificity. It is not surprising that different anti-IgG sera vary in their ability to react with IgG antibodies of different subclasses. The ability of anti-IgG sera to detect antibodies of different specificities varies, particularly with regard to antibodies in the Duffy and Kidd systems, possibly because of differences in their IgG subclasses. IgG1 and IgG3 antibodies are the most common in nature though IgG2 and IgG4 also occur.

It should be recalled that, although most anti-IgG sera are directed against gamma heavy chains, antibodies to kappa and lambda light chains also may be present and react with the L-chains of IgM or IgA on RBC coated with antibodies of these classes. Thus, reaction with an anti-IgG serum does not guarantee IgG class specificity in the sensitizing antibody.

Some antigen-antibody reactions fix complement components to the red blood cell surface, and the antiglobulin test can also be used for their detection. This subject will be returned to at the end of the discussion of complement.

ENZYME TESTS

A sensitive technique to potentiate agglutination of red blood cells by certain incomplete antibodies is "enzyme testing." Red blood cells exposed to the action of a proteolytic enzyme, such as trypsin, ficin, papain or bromelin, lose part of their surface sialic acid as well as possibly undergoing other membrane alterations such as configurational changes and/or redistribution of antigenic determinants with resultant increased agglutinability by many antibodies. Excessive enzyme treatment may result in spontaneous agglutination of red blood cell suspensions in the absence of antibodies. Certain antigens are partially or completely destroyed by enzyme treatment, including M, N, S, Fy^a, Fy^b, Ch^a, Yt^a, Tn, and Pr (Sp).

COMPLEMENT

Originally thought to be a single substance, complement is now recognized to be a complex system of serum globulins interacting to play a large part in body defenses and involved in many serologic reactions. A major role of complement is the destruction of foreign cells, but this cannot be accomplished until they have been labeled as foreign by antibody attachment or other means. Whereas an antibody can react with only a specific or closely related antigenic determinant, complement is activated by a wide assortment of antigen-antibody reactions as well as by bacterial endotoxins, proteolytic enzymes, and other biologically active substances. The complement system is present in all animals and is nonspecific in that complement from one species is effective in serologic reactions in vitro with the cells of others. The blood bank is principally concerned with antigen-antibody reactions that fix complement to the surface of the red blood cell, where it may cause focal destruction of the surface membrane, producing defects through which ions, water, and ultimately hemoglobin can leak. This, of course, is the phenomenon known as hemolysis. Another effect of complement is the formation of reactive sites on cell membranes, which may then attach to specialized receptors for C3b on the surfaces of macrophages. Cleavage products of complement components also stimulate "effector functions" in other cells, such as histamine release and leukocyte migration.

The complement system consists of 11 glycoprotein components with molecular weights ranging from 80,000 to 400,000 and electrophoretic mobilities of alpha to gamma globulins. Their combined concentration in serum is about 300 mg/dl or about 10% of total serum globulins. Of this amount, about half is C3 and another 15% is C4. C2 is the component present in lowest concentration (25 μg/ml). Table 7-1 summarizes some of the known information about the components of complement.

Before proceeding to a description of the classic complement pathway, we should point out several features worth noting. Just as in the blood coagulation scheme, certain activated complement components exhibit enzymatic activity (i.e., are esterases), divalent cations (Ca^{++} and Mg^{++}) are required in certain phases of the complement-activation process, the reaction is self-amplifying as it proceeds, and the sequence occurs as a cascade, each step involving conversion of an inactive precursor to an active form that, either alone or more usually by forming a complex, activates its successor. Some of the components are fixed to the cell membrane, others (activated or inactive) are released. The system is held in check by the instability of the activated components and complexes and by the existence of C1 inhibitor and C3b and C4b inactivators in the serum. C1 inhibitor has already been met in the discussion of blood coagula-

TABLE 7-1

Complement Components in Human Serum (after Garratty)

Component	Molecular Weight (Daltons)	Electrophoretic Mobility	Serum Concentration (μg/ml)
C1q	400,000	Gamma	180
C1r	190,000	Beta	100
C1s	85,000	Alpha	80
C4	206,000	Beta	450
C2	115,000	Beta	25
C3	180,000	Beta	1500
C5	180,000	Beta	75
C6	128,000	Beta	60
C7	121,000	Beta	60
C8	154,000	Gamma	80
C9	80,000	Alpha	150

tion as an inhibitor of coagulation, fibrinolysis, and the kallikrein system. Another link between coagulation and complement activation exists in the ability of plasmin to activate C1 and to cleave C3 directly.

The notation employed in the following scheme of complement activation follows a convention now universally employed: the components are numbered, and a bar is placed over the number to indicate an activated form. Small letters denote fragments of the component.

Activation of the classic complement sequence on the red blood cell surface is accomplished by antibody attachment, with a resultant change in antibody configuration exposing an estimated six combining sites for Clq. Not all antibodies are capable of complement activation. IgM molecules are quite efficient at doing so, although only a portion of the IgM molecules in an antiserum may be active in this regard. Only some IgG molecules can activate complement, principally those of subclass IgG3 and to a lesser extent IgG1. IgG molecules of some specificities (e.g., antibodies in the Kidd system) regularly fix complement, while others (e.g., Rh antibodies) hardly ever do so. It has been estimated that the duration of the bond between Clq and IgG molecules may be critical, lasting less than 0.1 seconds. It is possible that the time required for activation of C1 may be greater than the duration of the bond between most IgG molecules and Clq.

Complement activation occurs with the attachment to the RBC surface of a single IgM pentamer or of two IgG molecules within a distance of 250 to 400 Angström units. Few of the antigens exciting the production of IgG molecules are sufficiently numerous on the red blood cell surface to fill this requirement (A and B are exceptions), and thus complement fixation by most IgG molecules is precluded. This is not the whole explanation, however, because some examples of IgG anti-K, anti-Fy[a], and a few antisera of other specificities bind complement despite the fact that the numbers of their combining sites on the RBC suface are smaller than those of Rh antigens. If antigen site distribution were uneven, this observation might be explained.

The classic complement sequence consists of the recognition unit (C1), the activation unit (C4, C2, and C3), and the membrane attack unit (C5–9) (Figure 7-2, A,B,C). C1 is a macromolecular complex, probably composed of one molecule of Clq, two molecules of Clr,

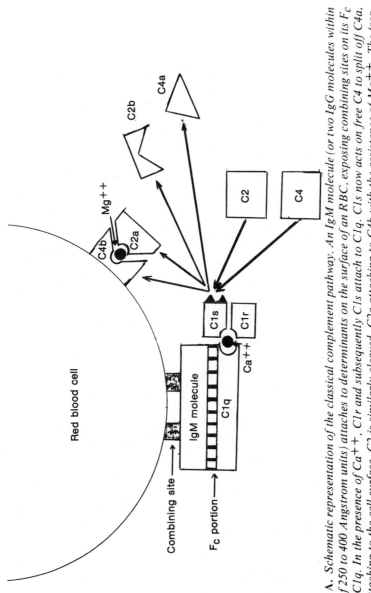

Figure 7-2. A. *Schematic representation of the classical complement pathway. An IgM molecule (or two IgG molecules within a distance of 250 to 400 Angstrom units) attaches to determinants on the surface of an RBC, exposing combining sites on its F_c portion for C1q. In the presence of Ca^{++}, C1r and subsequently C1s attach to C1q. C1s now acts on free C4 to split off C4a, with C4b attaching to the cell surface. C2 is similarly cleaved, C2a attaching to C4b with the assistance of Mg^{++}. The fragments C4a and C2b remain free.*

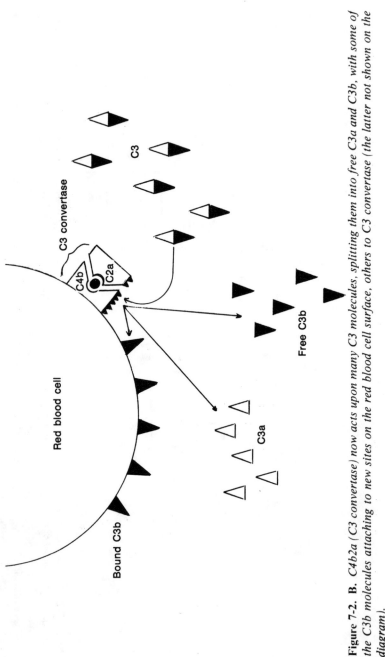

Figure 7-2. B. C4b2a (C3 convertase) now acts upon many C3 molecules, splitting them into free C3a and C3b, with some of the C3b molecules attaching to new sites on the red blood cell surface, others to C3 convertase (the latter not shown on the diagram).

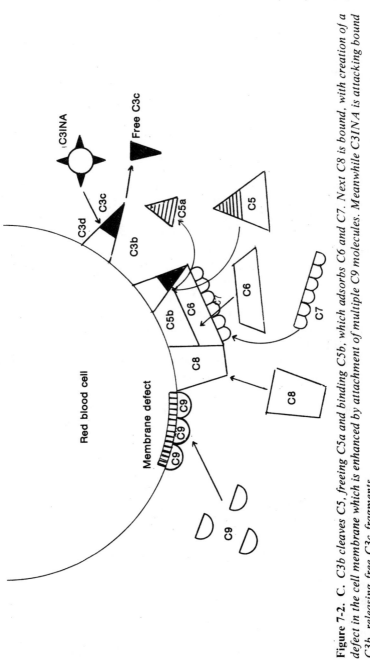

Figure 7-2. C. *C3b cleaves C5, freeing C5a and binding C5b, which adsorbs C6 and C7. Next C8 is bound, with creation of a defect in the cell membrane which is enhanced by attachment of multiple C9 molecules. Meanwhile C3INA is attacking bound C3b, releasing free C3c fragments.*

and four molecules of Cls, all held together by ionized calcium. Clq is a collagen-like globulin that is bound to receptor sites on the Fc portions of cell-bound IgM and IgG molecules to initiate the complement sequence. Clr appears to be a proenzyme that activates Cls. $C\overline{ls}$ splits C4 to release C4a and fix C4b to the Cl site by hydrophobic bonding. $C\overline{ls}$ activates hundreds of molecules of C4, but only 5% of these fix to the cell, and of these, only 5% produce a functional site. $C\overline{l}$ also cleaves C2, releasing C2b and binding C2a to C4b to form the activated complex $C\overline{4b2a}$, also known as C3 convertase. C3 convertase is unstable and must be continually regenerated by new C2. Because of its low concentration and the constant requirement for renewal, C2 concentration is the rate-limiting factor in the complement pathway. Mg^{++} is required at this step. C3 is attacked by the C3 convertase, which splits off C3a (anaphylotoxin I). Several thousand C3b molecules are produced, but only approximately 10% are cell bound and participate in the formation of the membrane attack unit. C3b molecules attach either to a nonspecific site on the cell membrane or to C3 convertase. It may be noted that after this step the presence of the antigen-antibody complex is no longer necessary for the remainder of the complement sequence to occur.

The complex $C\overline{4a2b3b}$ cleaves C5 to bind C5b and release free C5a (anaphylotoxin II). C5b adsorbs C6 and C7 to form a complex that attaches to the cell membrane. C8 is bound, with creation of a defect in the cell wall. The process is amplified by the attachment of six molecules of C9, resulting in the formation of a hole in the cell membrane measuring about 100 Angstrom units in diameter. Through this defect ions and water enter until the cell bursts with release of its hemoglobin.

It is emphasized that the "b" fragments released from C4, C3, and C5 have only transient capability (probably less than 0.1 seconds) to bind to the cell surface, and that there exists a second category of stable surface binding sites that are involved in immune adherence and phagocytosis.

There is present in the serum an inactivator of C3b (C3bINA) that attacks cell-bound C3b, releasing C3c, and leaving behind cell-bound C3d. C4bINA has also been discovered and functions in a similar way, inactivating C4b. A point of significance is the fact that complement activation does not necessarily progress to completion with cell lysis in every case: Inactivation of C3b or C4b by C3bINA or C4bINA or depletion of C2 may stop the sequence before progression occurs beyond the C1,4,2,3 stage. Even if terminated at this juncture, C3d remains on the cell surface. In addition, some antibodies appear able to fix only sublytic amounts of complement. The union between RBC and complement components is considerably stronger than that between RBC and antibody as evidenced by the elution of antibody in many situations, leaving behind fixed complement.

It has been shown that there exists an alternate pathway of complement activation involving direct C3 activation by such substances as aggregated immunoglobulins, immune complexes, bacterial endotoxin and plasmin. Four components are required, known as IF, properdin, and proactivators B and D. All are globulins of molecular weights ranging from 24,000 to 170,000 and exhibit electrophoretic mobilities of alpha to gamma globulins. A greatly simplified scheme depicting the alternative pathway is presented in Figure 7-3. In the presence of an activating substance, Factor D and Mg^{++} ions, IF and Factor B combine with C3 to form P-receptor forming enzyme, which then converts C3 to C3b. C3b combines with Factor B, again in the presence of Factor D and Mg^{++} ions to form properdin-activating principle, a labile C5 convertase, which is stabilized by interacting with properdin. The C5 convertase splits C5 to C5a and C5b, with the remainder of the scheme following the classic pathway. Thus antigen-antibody interactions and the recognition and activation units of the classic pathway are bypassed.

Among the biologic activities of complement, only cytolysis requires that the full sequence through C9 occur. Fragments C3a and C5a are anaphylotoxins, low molecular weight substances that cause smooth muscle contraction, increase vascular permeability and initiate anaphylaxis by causing histamine release from mast cells and platelets. Complement activation with release of anaphylotoxins is thought to be the cause of most of the symptoms of hemolytic transfusion reactions and may initiate disseminated intravascular coagulation. C3a, C5a, and $C\overline{5,6,7}$ are active chemotaxins, inducing neutrophil migration into the sites of their formation. C3b is bound during immune adherence, the process by which antigen-antibody complexes adhere nonspecifically to unsensitized particles such as RBC, WBC, platelets, bacteria or starch granules. Immune adherence may well be the precursor step to phagocytosis, which also requires C3b binding to occur. It will be recalled that macrophages possess C3b binding sites. Hence opsonization or antibody-mediated sensitization to phagocytosis is made possible by C3b. It has been reasoned that immune adherence greatly facilitates antibody-mediated destruction of bacteria and viruses by immobilizing them on various particles and rendering them more susceptible to ingestion by phagocytes. It may be speculated that immune adherence is also the process whereby antigens are localized and concentrated on the surface of B lymphocytes: it is known that B-cells have surface receptors for C3b/C4b and for C3d.

Complement concentrations in serum are generally increased in inflammatory conditions. They may be decreased in diseases associated with increased consumption caused by fixation to antigen-antibody complexes or to cells (e.g., systemic lupus erythematosus, acute glomerulonephritis, subacute bacterial endocarditis, autoimmune acquired hemolytic disease) or in diseases associated with decreased synthesis (e.g., cirrhosis of the liver). Congenital defects of synthesis of complement components occur, though rarely.

Certain of the components of the complement system are heat labile. C1 and C2 and to a lesser extent C4 are inactivated in sera heated to 56 C for 30 minutes. Slower deterioration occurs at 37 C or room temperature, but even on storage at 4 C or −20 C complement activity is slowly lost. It has been estimated that the presence of 60% of normal complement activity is necessary for detection of weak complement-binding antibodies. In a study by Garratty, serum complement activity was found to decrease to 30% of the original value after 24 hours at 37 C. After room temperature storage, complement levels were 80% at 24 hours and 40% after 48 hours. With 4 C storage, 90% of activity remained at 72 hours and 50% after two weeks. After −20 C, storage levels were 60% at two months. If storage was at −55 C, full activity remained after three months.

Bacterial contamination of stored sera may render them anti-complementary by altering Cls so that it is inactive. Altered Cls attaches to the cell surface but fails to cleave C4 and C2, thus preventing progression of the complement sequence past the detection unit. Because free Ca^{++} and Mg^{++} ions are necessary to the function of the recognition and activation units, anticoagulants such as EDTA or citrate, which act by complexing divalent cations, also prevent complement activity. Plasma is thus unacceptable for use in blood bank serologic studies. Antibodies that cause hemolysis in the presence of complement are usually saline agglutinins in its absence.

THE ANTICOMPLEMENT ANTIGLOBULIN TEST

In the discussion of the antiglobulin test it was stated that antiglobulin sera are used to detect the presence of globulin molecules attached to the surfaces of RBC. Antiglobulin serum may react not only with immunoglobulins but with nonantibody globulins as well. Depending on the purity of the globulin antigens used to immunize the animal in which the reagent is raised, an antiglobulin serum may be specific, for example, for IgG or may react with several different globulin determinants, all of which need not be gamma globulins. Antiglobulin sera prepared by injecting animals with whole human serum contain chiefly antibodies directed against gamma globulins, these being the most antigenic of the serum proteins. However, antibodies directed against other, nongamma (chiefly beta) globulins are also produced, though generally in lower concentrations. Among these beta globulins are complement components, and therefore anticomplement activity is also present in the antiglobulin serum. Such an antiglobulin serum, containing both anti-IgG and anticomplement activity, constitutes a "broad-spectrum" reagent. Monospecific antiglobulin sera are also commercially available.

Commercial broad-spectrum antiglobulin serum is capable of detecting either bound IgG and/or bound complement on the red blood cell membrane, but it does not differentiate between the two. It is held by many blood bank workers that both activities are essential in an antiglobulin serum to be used for compatibility testing. The antibody molecules of occasional antisera may be bound to the RBC surface in such small numbers (i.e., have such a low binding constant) that anti-IgG reactions may be weak, but because of the amplification occurring during complement activation, large numbers of readily detectable complement molecules may be bound. Anticomplement titration scores correlate well with the number of C3 molecules fixed to the red blood cell surface.

Today our sophistication has passed beyond the point of merely requiring "anticomplement" activity in an antiglobulin serum. All complement components are antigenic to varying degrees, and an anticomplement serum will contain a mixture of antibodies against individual components. Of greatest usefulness and desirability for detection of in vitro complement binding of potential clinical significance is activity against C3b. As described previously $C\overline{4b2a}$ (C3 convertase) cleaves C3 into C3a and C3b, with perhaps 10% of the C3b molecules attaching to the red blood cell membrane. About 100 times as many C3b as C4b molecules fix to the surface after sensitization with clinically significant complement-fixing antibodies, so that from a quantitative point of view it is much easier to detect cell-bound C3b than C4b. Additionally, as will be discussed in connection with compatibility testing problems (Chapter 17) difficulty in crossmatching is often encountered in the blood bank because of low-titered, clinically unimportant cold autoagglutinins that fix much C4b but little C3b. Minimizing the content of anti-C4b in antiglobulin sera to be used in compatibility testing is thus desirable. As will be discussed in Chapter 28, quality assessment of broad-spectrum antiglobulin sera should be conducted with tests that individually and specifically assess their anti-C3b and anti-C4b content.

As illustrated in Figure 7-2, C3b bound to the red blood cell surface is attacked slowly in vitro, and in time often completely destroyed in vivo by C3INA, with cleavage of C3b into two subcomponents, C3c and C3d. Only C3d remains fixed to the cell surface. C3 contains three antigenic determinants that elicit antibody formation to whole C3, to C3a, and to C3d. All three antibodies react with C3, which contains determinants called A, B, and D. (These bear no relationship to blood group antigens A, B or D.) Splitting off C3a removes the B antigen, leaving A and D. Splitting off C3c removes the A antigen, leaving D. Thus, anti-C3d reacts with the D antigen of C3. It is essential to the detection of in vivo complement binding, where, of the C3 components, only C3d remains attached to the cell surface, to have anti-C3d activity in any antiglobulin reagent used for direct antiglobulin testing. For testing of in vitro reactions where complement may have been bound, anti-C3b activity is needed inasmuch as the activity of C3bINA is relatively slow and may not be present in sufficient concentration or be permitted sufficient time in laboratory tests to split C3c from C3b.

A type of naturally occurring anticomplement called immunoconglutinin is found in the serum of man and most other mammals. Though normally low in human sera, immunoconglutinin activity increases in conditions in which complement fixation occurs, such as autoimmune diseases. Immunoconglutinins are usually IgM antibodies that react with bound complement components, predominantly C3b and to a lesser extent C4b. This reaction initiates further complement fixation and thus constitutes a positive feedback mechanism, but also inhibits C3b, thus resembling an inactivator. The biologic significance of immunoconglutinin is unclear.

CHAPTER 8

Genetics in Blood Banking

Genetics is the study of heredity, the transmission of bodily characteristics from generation to generation. Because red blood cell types can be determined with relative ease and certainty and because inheritance of these types behaves in accordance with the principles of heredity, blood grouping studies continue to contribute to our knowledge of genetics as a science. Conversely, the application of the general laws of inheritance to the field of blood grouping has permitted fuller understanding of otherwise puzzling observations.

Inheritance of bodily and cellular features is under the control of chromosomes, a specific number of which characterizes each kind of plant and animal. Each body cell in man contains 22 pairs of autosomal chromosomes plus two sex chromosomes for a total of 46. One chromosome of each pair plus one sex chromosome is contributed by each parent, and each of the multitude of cells in the body normally contains a perfect replica of the original set of chromosomes. Each chromosome contains thousands of bits of genetic information borne on units of inheritance called genes. Genes are composed of complex, coiled molecules of deoxyribonucleic acid (DNA). Genetic information is encoded into the DNA molecule by the sequences in which basic chemical building blocks called nucleotides are arranged within it. So coded, the DNA molecule controls the amino acid sequence of the protein synthesized under its control.

The term locus is used to describe the site of a gene on a chromosome. Alleles are alternative forms of a gene at a given locus. A subject is called homozygous for a given gene if identical alleles occupy a locus on each of a pair of chromosomes. If the alleles are different, the subject is heterozygous for that gene. Linked genes are located on the same chromosome within a measurable distance and behave as a set. Separated linked genes from a pair of chromosomes may be

91

interchanged during meiosis by the process known as crossing over, implying exchange of portions of homologous chromosomes. The further apart two genes are on a chromosome, the greater is the chance of crossing over. Loci are said to be syngeneic if they are located on the same chromosome. Genes on different chromosomes are said to segregate independently. The term genotype is used to indicate the sum total of the chromosomal makeup of a subject, while the phenotype refers to those characteristics which are apparent or manifest. A system of antigens is a group of associated antigens inherited independently from all other systems of antigens.

Obviously, genes cannot be tested for, but their products or expression frequently can be. If a gene produces a detectable result, it is said to be expressed. If a gene is expressed only when homozygous and produces no effect when heterozygous, we say that it is recessive. A dominant gene is the gene of a heterozygous pair of alleles that is expressed while the other is not. If both genes of a heterozygous pair are expressed (the usual situation in blood group genetics), they are said to be codominant. A gene without an observable effect is an amorph. In cases in which one of the allelic forms of a gene is an amorph, a given phenotype may be the consequence of two different genotypes, one homozygous and the other heterozygous for an expressed gene. Figure 8-1 illustrates this concept.

Structural genes actually construct a gene product, which is always a protein. This protein may, in the case of blood group systems, be an antigen and thus a direct gene product. In other cases in which a blood group antigen is at least in part carbohydrate or lipid, the antigen is an indirect gene product, produced by enzymatic activity of the protein coded by the gene. Thus, for example, the gene determining blood group A causes production of a transferase enzyme, which acts on a substrate preformed by other gene actions to add the sugar residue which determines group A specificity. Said in a different way, the nucleotide sequence that controls the production of N-acetyl-D-galactosamine transferase constitutes the A gene. An amorph may be the consequence of loss of DNA or of DNA that causes the production of inactive material. In the ABO system, for instance, the presence of the genes A, B, and H causes production of functional transferases, while the O and h genes produce no recognizable product.

In the Rh blood group system and probably in others, the situation is considerably more complex. Rh genes code for multiple products (e.g., R^1 codes for at least 15 products, R^2 for 13, r for nine) probably by producing a molecule with multiple determinants. To explain the existence of amorphs in such situations on the basis of loss by mutation of multiple different determinants is unreasonable. Hence, there was introduced the concept of operator genes, i.e., genes that activate or regulate the activity of structural genes. We

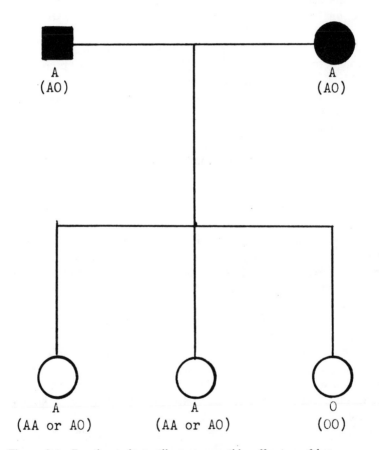

Figure 8-1. *Family study to illustrate possible offspring of heterozygous mating. Both father and mother are of phenotype A. The first two children are also of phenotype A, but the third is group O. If legitimacy is assumed, both parents must be of genotype AO: Each contributed a chromosome to their third child which lacked A, to produce the genotype OO. The other two children, of phenotype A, could be of either genotype AO or AA.*

now use the concept of the operon: a structural region on a chromo-some bearing the gene(s) that orders antigen synthesis, and an operator region containing the gene(s) that regulates it. It is seen that a single alteration in an operator region could switch off the entire operon, even though all of the structural genes were intact and poten-tially functional. With regard to many blood group systems, we now postulate genetically controlled production of precursor substances acted on by other gene products to produce a series of inter-mediates. These are in turn altered by the products of still other genes before the final antigenic form is achieved. Each of these steps is thought to be under the control of operator genes. Thus production of a blood group antigen frequently entails the activity of more than one structural gene and more than one operator gene operating in se-quential fashion. Nor is this the entire story, because in some systems, including Rh, we also recognize evidence for regulator loci, not linked to the operon, and producing mRNA, which influences the operator gene. Mutation can occur at regulator, operator, or structural loci. It is thought that the common type of Rh_{null} (RBC lacking common Rh antigens) is a result of supressor effects originating in a regulator locus.

Certain genes are known to compete for a common substrate upon which they exert their action (e.g., ABO and Lewis genes). Other antigens are recognized as different steps in a pathway (e.g., Rh and LW, T, and Tn, N and M). Still other antigens have the same immunodominant terminal group (e.g., A, Tn, Cad.) In light of the limited number of building blocks used, it is not surprising that structural relationships and serologic cross-reactivities exist among blood group antigens.

The term gene interaction refers to the modification of expres-sion of one gene by another gene and is best illustrated in the Rh system as discussed in Chapter 11. Dosage effect refers to the ability of certain antisera to react more strongly with RBC from homo-zygous subjects than with those from heterozygous donors. Rarely is the phenomenon of gene deletion encountered, wherein a gene ap-pears to have been lost, resulting in formation of an amorph. The phenomena of blood group chimerism and mosaicism were described in Chapter 5 in conjunction with the discussion of immunologic tolerance.

The subject of gene frequency is of considerable interest in blood group work from the viewpoints both of the anthropologist and the investigator elucidating new blood group systems. The frequency distribution of two allelic genes X and Y is given by the Hardy-Weinberg equation:

$$X^2 + 2XY + Y^2 = 1$$

Homozygotes for X and Y are represented by X^2 and Y^2, heterozygotes by XY. If a large population is screened with anti-X serum and the frequency of X-reactors determined, substitution of the value for X in the equation permits solution for Y. The expression $1 - Y$ then gives the frequency of occurrence of the X gene.

A number of practical considerations arise from the genetic data, which can be derived from the study of blood groups. We now recognize about 400 blood group antigens. If sufficiently numerous and reliable typing sera were available, it would be theoretically possible to type a donor's red blood cells for so many factors that the statistical likelihood of finding random persons of identical type would be almost nil. Use of such data is occasionally made in medicolegal work, for instance to identify a blood stain as having possibly originated (or not originated) from a victim or accused defendant. These observations also point up the impossiblity of obtaining a perfect match between blood donor and recipient unless they are identical twins.

Disputed paternity cases are also usefully studied from the viewpoint of inheritance of blood groups, not only of RBC antigens but also of red blood cell isoenzymes, lymphocyte HLA antigens, and serum protein groups. Paternity cannot be proved by such studies, but it can be excluded. A typical example of findings in RBC typings in such a case is illustrated in Table 8-1. To be of use in blood grouping studies for exclusion of paternity, the RBC antigens tested for must be stable and intrinsic portions of the cell (thereby excluding the use of Lewis groupings). Their gene frequencies must not be excessively low or high, the genetics of the system must be well established, and potent typing sera must be available. The red blood cell groups fit these criteria, are presently confined to the ABO, Rh, MNSs, Kell, Duffy, and Kidd systems, with rare additions of others. Proper testing procedures require foolproof identification of the concerned parties and their blood samples, duplicate testing and the use of adequate negative and positive controls.

Myhre cites four rules for exclusion of paternity:

1) A child cannot bear a gene absent from both parents. For exam-

ple, a K-positive child cannot be born of homozygous k-positive parents.

2) One or the other allele present in a heterozygous parent must be present in the child. For example, the child of a Cc parent must carry either a C or c antigen on his RBC.

3) Both parents must carry a gene for which a child is homozygous. For example, if a child is of genotype cc, each parent must be c-positive.

4) A gene for which a parent is homozygous must be present in his child. For example, a parent who is of genotype kk must have k-positive offspring.

If ABO red blood cell grouping alone is used, less than 20% of falsely accused men can be excluded in cases of disputed paternity. Further use of MNSs typing raises this figure to somewhat under 40%, while addition of Rh typing (C, c, D, E, and e) changes the value to over 50%. Inclusion of Kell, Duffy, and Kidd typings increases the chance of legitimate exclusion to about 70%. HLA typing or a combination of RBC isoenzyme and serum protein groupings can achieve exclusion rates of over 90% of theoretically true figures. Paternity testing is not a matter for the unsophisticated: even if technical errors and reagent failures are excluded, a whole host of genetic pitfalls exist to trap the unwary, including occurrence of genetic variables such as linked phenotypes (e.g., cis-AB), suppressor genes (e.g., O_h), silent alleles (e.g., Fy), gene deletions (e.g., some

---

TABLE 8-1

Results of blood grouping tests in a case of disputed paternity. The child of two group A people can be of group O if both are of genotype AO. The baby's D, C, e, M, s, k, and Fy^a genes could have come from either the mother or the putative father, while the Jk^a gene was of paternal origin. The Jk^b gene could have been from the mother. The N gene must have been of paternal origin inasmuch as the mother lacks N, but so does the accused man. Thus, the testing excludes him as a possible father of the child.

	A	B	D	C	c	E	e	M	N	S	s	K	k	Fy^a	Fy^b	Jk^a	Jk^b
Putative father	+	−	+	+	+	+	+	+	−	+	+	+	+	−	−	+	−
Mother	+	−	+	+	+	−	+	+	−	+	+	−	+	+	−	−	+
Child	−	−	+	+	+	−	−	+	+	+	−	+	+	+	−	+	+

Rh$_{nulls}$), rare variants (e.g., M^g), or decreased antigen strength (e.g., weak variants of A).

RECOMMENDED READING

Greenwalt, T.J. and Steane, E.A. (Eds): *CRC Handbook Series in Clinical Laboratory Science. Section D: Blood Banking*, Vol. 1. CRC Press. Cleveland, 1977

Huestis, D.W. et al: *Practical Blood Transfusion*, 2nd ed. Little, Brown and Co. Boston, 1976

Issitt, P.D. and Issitt, C.H.: *Applied Blood Group Serology*, 2nd ed. Spectra. Oxnard, Calif., 1975

Joint AMA-ABA guideline: Present status of serologic testing in problems of disputed parentage. *Family Law Court.* 10:247, 1976

Mollison, P.L.: *Blood Transfusion in Clinical Medicine,* 5th ed. Blackwell. Oxford, 1972

Myhre, B.A.: The use of red cell antigens for the determination of disputed parentage. In: *A Seminar on Polymorphisms in Human Blood*. Am Assn of Blood Banks. Washington, 1975. p.13

Race, R.R. and Sanger, R.: *Blood Groups in Man,* 6th ed. Blackwell. Oxford, 1975

CHAPTER 9

The ABO System

The discovery of the ABO system of blood group antigens and antibodies by Landsteiner and his colleagues in 1900 represented the beginning of modern blood group immunology. The ABO group is the most important of those dealt with in the blood bank. ABO antibodies universally occur when their reciprocal antigen is absent, and the biologic consequences of ABO-incompatible blood transfusion are generally serious and occasionally fatal. Red blood cells which contain a major ABO blood group antigen absent in the recipient should never be transfused. All human RBC belong to group A, group B, neither (group O) or both (group AB). An adult of group A has anti-B in his serum, while one of group B carries anti-A. Serum from a group O subject possesses both antibodies; that from a group AB subject, normally has neither. These relationships are shown in Table 9-1.

The antigens of the ABO system appear early in intrauterine life, having been demonstrated in a fetus of five and one half weeks but are not fully developed at birth. Combining sites for antigens of the ABO system continue to increase in numbers on RBC during the first months of life, approximating adult values by the age of a year. Table 9-2 lists the reported numbers of ABO antigen combining sites on newborn and adult RBC.

The ABO antigens are not confined to red blood cells but are found in the form of alcohol-soluble glycolipids on the cells of all body tissues except brain. ABO substances also occur in a water soluble glycoprotein form in body fluids and secretions, such as saliva in about 77% of white people. Such persons are called secretors. The remaining 23% of nonsecretors exhibit ABO antigens only on their

TABLE 9-1

Relationship Between Major ABO Red Blood Cell Antigens and Reciprocal Serum Antibodies

Blood Group	Antigen(s) on RBC	Antibodies in Serum
A	A	Anti-B
B	B	Anti-A
AB	A and B	Neither anti-A nor anti-B
O	Neither A nor B	Both anti-A and anti-B

tissue cells, including RBC. Depending on their ABO blood group, ABO substances are present in the plasma of all persons, irrespective of secretor status, but are present in larger amounts in the plasma of secretors. Note that the term secretor refers only to the ability to secrete water-soluble ABO substances into body fluids and has no connection with the presence of other blood group substances such as Lewis or Sid, which may also be present in such fluids. Depending on the genotype of the subject, the amounts of A, B and/or H substance secreted into body fluids vary as shown in Table 9-3. Secretor status

TABLE 9-2

ABO Antigen Site Density on Newborn and Adult RBC

RBC Group	Antigen Sites per RBC ($\times 10^5$)		
	A	B	H
A₁ (newborn)	2.5–3.7	—	—
A₁ (adult)	8.1–11.7	—	—
A₁B (newborn)	2.2	—	—
A₁B (adult)	4.6–8.5	3.1–5.6	6
A₂ (newborn)	1.4	—	—
A₂ (adult)	2.4–2.9	—	11
A₂B (adult)	1.2	6.1–8.5	—
B (adult)	—	6.1–8.3	9
O	—	—	19–20

TABLE 9-3

Relative Amounts of A, B, and H Substances Found in Secretions of Subjects of Various Phenotypes

Substance Secreted	Relative Amounts Secreted
H	$O > A_2 > A_1 > B \cong A_2 B \cong A_1 B$
A	$A_1 > A_1 B > A_2 > A_2 B$
B	$B > A_2 B > A_1 B$

Note that the relative amounts of H substance found in secretions differ from the amounts found on RBC from subjects of the same phenotype.

is determined by the presence of a dominant gene Se. Nonsecretors are of the genotype sese, while secretors are genotype Sese or SeSe.

Inheritance of the ABO genes follows the rules outlined in Chapter 8. Recall that the phenotype O represents the absence of A and B antigens. The RBC and (in secretors) the body fluids of people of group O, however, do carry the antigen H, which also occurs, though in smaller amounts, in subjects of other ABO groups. The amount of H substance is greatest on RBC of group O, followed by group A_2, A_2B, B, A_1, and A_1B cells in order of decreasing H content. H substance is significant as the precursor from which the A and B antigens are made, and will be returned to in conjunction with the discussion of the biochemistry of the ABO and Lewis systems. An instructive family tree illustrating possibilities of inheritance in the ABO system is shown in Figure 9-1. The distributions of ABO phenotypes and genotypes are given in Tables 9-4 and 9-5.

Attention has recently been paid to the relationship between ABO blood groups and the occurrence of certain diseases. Statistically significant increases in the ratios of subjects of group A to those of group O have been found in patients with carcinomas of the gastrointestinal tract, salivary glands, and uterus, and in people with pernicious anemia, chronic cholecystitis, rheumatic disease, and thromboembolic disease. In contrast, peptic ulcers are more prevalent in patients of group O than in those of group A.

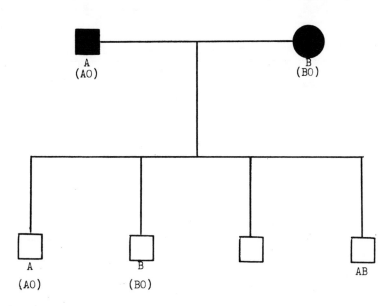

Figure 9-1. *Possible offspring of heterozygous group A and group B parents. The father may supply either A or O genes, the mother either B or O. Four different phenotypes may appear in their children.*

TABLE 9-4

Frequency of Occurrence of ABO Phenotypes

Phenotype	Approximate Frequency (%)	
	Whites	Blacks
O	44	49
A	45	27
B	8	20
AB	3	4

TABLE 9-5

Frequency Distribution of ABO Genotypes in Caucasians (after Race and Sanger)

Genotype	Frequency (%)
OO	43.6
A_1A_1	4.3
A_1O	27.6
A_1A_2	2.9
A_2A_2	0.5
A_2O	9.2
BB	0.4
BO	8.1
A_1B	2.6
A_2B	0.9

A number of variants of the A and B antigens have been discovered, of which the subgroups of A are the most important. Weak forms of A or B may be due to the presence of allelic genes, modifying genes, mosaicism, decreased antigen strength due to disease, or acquired reactivity. They are important to detect because RBC mistyped as group O but actually bearing weak A or B antigens may cause hemolytic transfusion reactions if administered to group O recipients. The most important of these subgroups are those designated A_2 and A_2B. About 20% to 25% of all group A RBC are A_2, and an equal proportion of group AB RBC are A_2B. A_2 and A_2B cells are more weakly reactive than A_1 or A_1B cells, possessing fewer antigenic sites. All group A and AB red blood cells are thought to possess A determinants, but in addition A_1 and A_1B cells bear a second determinant group called A_1. Anti-A serum from a group B donor is a mixture of anti-A and anti-A_1. If such a serum is suitably absorbed with group A_2 RBC, the remaining antibody will have anti-A_1 specificity, and be capable of reacting with group A_1 or A_1B red blood cells but not group A_2 or A_2B cells. Anti-A_1, in the form of a saline agglutinin rarely reactive above room temperature, is found in the serum of about 2% of subjects of group A_2 and at least a fourth of those of group A_2B depending on the test conditions. An extract of the seeds of the plant *Dolichos biflorus* has been shown to possess anti-A_1 reactivity and is used as an anti-A_1 reagent. Seed extracts exhibiting antibody-like agglutinating ability for RBC are known as lectins.

Rare examples of other genetically determined weak variants of group A are also found. A_3 red blood cells yield very weak reactions with anti-A sera; the pattern of agglutination is typically composed of small aggregates amidst large numbers of free cells (so-called mixed-field agglutination). Group A_x (A_o) RBC are also poorly agglutinated by anti-A sera but generally react well with serum from a group O donor (containing anti-A plus anti-B). Group A_{end} cells are similar in their reactions to group A_3 RBC, but A substance is absent from the body fluids of secretors. Group A_m cells are not agglutinated by anti-A or by O serum but can be shown to possess A sites by absorption-elution techniques, and A substance is found in the body fluids of group A_m secretors. Subjects with other very rare variants of A lack soluble A substance and can be detected only by absorption-elution methods. It has been suggested that the A receptors on some types of group A red blood cells may not be randomly distributed. It is thought that RBC antigens are mobile and able to cluster, a fact influencing the reactivity of cells with few antigen sites. Whereas the number of A combining sites on red blood cells from a single donor is quite uniform in the case of group A_1 subjects, individual cells from group A_2 persons vary somewhat in their numbers of combining sites, and RBC from A_3, A_m, and A_{el} donors appear highly heterogeneous. Cells of group A_{end} appear to be a true mixture of group A and non-A RBC.

Anti-A is found in the sera of subjects with several of the weak variants of A as shown in Table 9-6. Weak genetically determined phenotypes of B corresponding to their A counterparts exist, including B_3, B_m, B_x, and B_{el}, but save for B_3, which is missed in usual testing, are vanishingly rare. It will be appreciated that genetically determined weak forms of A and B as described above and due principally to the presence of allelic genes at the A and B loci (A_2, A_3, etc.) will not be apparent in tests on RBC from heterozygous subjects with a second, stronger group A allele.

A rare but very informative variant in the ABO system is the "Bombay" or O_h type. Group O_h RBC are not agglutinated by anti-

TABLE 9-6

Subgroups of A

Phenotype	RBC Agglutination with Anti-A	RBC Agglutination with Anti-B	Serum Agglutination of A_1 RBC	Soluble Substance	Frequency	No. of A Combining Sites per RBC
A_1	++++	++++	−	A, (H)	.80	810,000–1,170,000
A_2	+++	+++	−	A, H	.20	240,000–290,000
A_3	MF	MF	+ or −	A, H	.006	7,000–100,000
A_x	w	++	+	A, H	.002	1,400–10,300
A_{end}	MF	MF	+ or −	H	.001	0–200,000
A_m	−	−	−	A, H	.0007	200–1,900
A_y	−	−	−	(A), H	very rare	200–700
A_{el}	−	−	++	H	very rare	100–1,400

MF = mixed-field agglutination; w = weak agglutination. Parentheses indicate weak reactions in secretion tests.

RBC from subjects with weak variants of A have a generally heterogeneous distribution of the A antigen, with differing numbers of combining sites on different cells. Elution studies using anti-A are positive to varying degrees with all weak variants of A.

A, anti-B, or anti-H, and the serum of a Bombay subject contains agglutinins of all three specificities. A, B, and H substance are absent from the saliva. The parents and children of Bombay persons usually have normally expressed ABO genes. An explanation of this phenomenon is presented in Figure 9-2. In contrast to earlier concepts, it is now appreciated that individual, single genes do not always cause production of identifiable end products. Rather it is known that many genes act by preparing substrates for modification by other genes. The production of A and/or B antigens on the red blood cell surface begins with glycolipid precursor substance, which is acted upon by a product of an H gene to form H substance. In subjects with A and/or B genes, some or most of the H substance is then converted to A and/or B substance. If neither A nor B genes are pre-

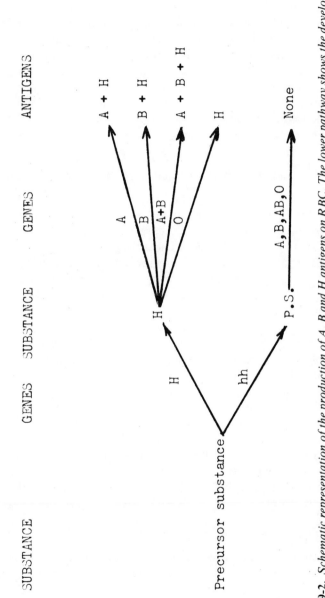

Figure 9-2. Schematic representation of the production of A, B and H antigens on RBC. The lower pathway shows the development of the "Bombay" or Oh type. Absence of an H gene prevents conversion of precursor substance (P.S.) to H substance. The A or B genes can exert their effect only on H substance and not on P.S.; therefore they cannot express themselves, and the A and B antigens do not appear.

sent (group O), only H substance will appear on the red blood cells. If no H gene is present (genotype hh), precursor substance cannot be converted to H substance, and consequently even if they are present, A and/or B genes cannot cause formation of A and/or B antigenic determinants on the cell surface. Discussion of the biochemical transformations involved in this sequence is presented in Chapter 10. It is apparent that offspring of a group O_h parent may express A or B genes derived from such a parent if they have received an H gene from the other parent. By convention the genetic but not-expressed type of a Bombay subject, if known, is written as a superscript, thus: O_h^A or O_h^B. Indeed, sophisticated absorption-elution techniques demonstrate that minute amounts of anti-A or anti-B are taken up by such cells. It should be noted in passing that a homozygous inhibitor gene (theoretical xx) could have the same effect in preventing formation of H substance as does the absence of an H gene.

Para-Bombay types are exceedingly rare but theoretically important in extending our appreciation of the complex genetic mechanisms involved in the production of ABO antigens:

1) A postulated third allele at the H locus may result in production of very small amounts of H substance, all of which is converted to A or B, resulting in very weakly reactive A or B antigenic determinants on RBC, development of anti-H in the serum, and absence of A, B, and H in the saliva of secretors. Such cells are designated by the symbols A_h and B_h.

2) A locus Zz has been proposed that controls ABO antigen production only on cells and not in secretions. In a subject homozygous for z, his RBC react weakly in agglutination tests, but anti-H is absent from his serum. ABH substances are normally present in the saliva (assuming he is Se positive). Hence Z is viewed as opposite in its effect to Se. Such RBC are designated by the symbols O_{Hm}, O_{Hm}^A, etc. It may be that the type A_h is sometimes (or always) an O_{Hm}^A nonsecretor. A related phenomenon is the postulated existence of an inhibitor gene y, which, if homozygous, suppresses the full expression of the A gene, though not B or H. Current theory explains the development of the group A_m variant in this fashion.

Although production of blood group antigens is typically under genetic control, it has become apparent that modification of ABO antigens may occur in certain diseases. ABH antigens are frequently lost from malignant cells and from tissues involved in wound healing. Weakened expressions of A, B, and H and increased or decreased expression of I antigens on RBC may occur in patients with acute leukemia, refractory anemia or other preleukemic states. Acquisition of weak B-like agglutinability may rarely occur with RBC of patients suffering from gastrointestinal disease or sepsis. This phenomenon occurs only in group A_1 patients and appears to be related to bacterial action on the red blood cell surface. Substances similar to the B antigen are elaborated by certain gram-negative bacilli and may be adsorbed to the RBC membrane, but a more likely explanation is that bacterial enzymes chemically alter some of the sugar residues on the cell surface, rendering them reactive with anti-B. The acquired B antigen will not react with the subject's own anti-B, suggesting that this phenomenon occurs only in people whose anti-B lacks a specific fraction, and that only a part of the B antigen is acquired. Anti-B from group A_2 and O serum reacts with RBC bearing acquired B antigens, but anti-B from A_1 subjects reacts poorly or not at all. The acquisition of B antigens is a transient phenomenon, disappearing with the recovery of the patient. Polyagglutinability occasionally occurs with RBC bearing acquired B antigens.

Rare examples have been reported of "*cis*-AB," a single gene determining the production of both A and B antigens. Group A reactivity of the red blood cells of such subjects is similar to that of A_2 cells, and the expression of B is also weak, while H is present in excess. The patient's serum usually contains weak anti-B. The saliva of secretors contains easily detectable A substance, but B substance is demonstrated with more difficulty. Differentiation from acquired B is accomplished by the tests summarized in Table 9-7.

A close relationship exists between the genes of the ABO, Lewis and I blood group systems, which will be explored in succeeding chapters. The genes of the ABO system may interact with those of the I system to produce compound antigens such as IH and IA. Antibodies formed in response to such antigens will react only when both parts are present, e.g., anti-IH will not react with H in the absence of the I antigen.

TABLE 9-7

Test Reactions Useful in Distinguishing *cis*-AB from Acquired B Blood Groups

Test	*Cis*-AB	Acquired B
Agglutination by anti-B at pH 4.5	+	−
Agglutination by *Dolichos biflorus* extract	−	±
Agglutination by *Ulex europeaeus* extract	+	−
B substance in saliva (secretors)	+	−

ABO Antibodies

The occurrence of anti-A and/or anti-B (the so-called isoantibodies) in the serum of persons lacking the corresponding antigens is such a constant and reliable finding that serum grouping or "backtyping" is conducted routinely in blood banks to confirm the accuracy of ABO red blood cell grouping. Unexpected findings require elucidation, and their explanation may range from a finding as simple as the occurrence of anti-A₁ in a patient of group A₂ to a rare weak variant of A, a Bombay patient, a blood group chimera, or a case of hypogammaglobulinemia.

Human infants are not capable of making appreciable quantities of blood group antibody until maturation of their immunologic system advances sufficiently. This does not generally occur until after the third month of life. Antibodies found in the serum of a newborn infant are of maternal origin, having crossed the placenta. For this reason, ABO blood grouping studies on infants less than three months of age are confined to testing their RBC, and serum groupings are omitted. The expected anti-A and/or anti-B are present by six months of age, reach adult potency by 20 to 30 months, and peak in concentration by age five to ten years, with a slow decline thereafter, though the decrease with age is less in group O people.

Classically ABO isoantibodies have been regarded as "naturally occurring," principally because of their universal occurrence and the absence of any obvious stimulus to their production. We now know that substances identical with or closely resembling the chemically rather simple ABH antigenic determinants are widespread in nature, being found in dust, bacteria, and plant and animal tissues, and are so ubiquitous that anti-A and anti-B surely occur as the result of antigenic stimulus. Non-red blood cell immune anti-A and anti-B are cold agglutinins, generally present in low concentration in human serum. They react in saline and their reactivity is not enhanced by the use of albumin or antiglobulin testing. Anti-A and anti-B from group B or A subjects are usually IgM antibodies. The isoantibodies of group O persons are often partially IgG and occasionally IgA also.

Exposure to incompatible A and/or B substances on red blood cells by transfusion, during pregnancy, or in certain vaccination procedures (e.g., immunization with influenza or tetanus vaccine) will normally cause production of "immune" isoantibodies. Typically such antisera show increased agglutinin titers, avidity, and binding constants. Opsonins and hemolysins may appear or increase, neutralization with A or B substance may become difficult, prozone phenomena may occur, incomplete isoantibodies detectable only by antiglobulin testing may develop, optimal reaction temperatures may rise, and the proportion of IgG antibody molecules may increase.

So-called cross-reacting anti-A,B is present in the serum of group O persons. If serum from a group O donor is absorbed with group A red blood cells, an eluate from the group A cells will react with group B as well as group A RBC. Various explanations are offered for this observation: 1) A third antibody ("anti-C") is present in O serum, which reacts with a third ("C") antigen present on both group A and group B red blood cells. 2) Group O serum contains antibody molecules with a double specificity (anti-A and anti-B). 3) Anti-A and anti-B sera each can react with a portion of antigenic determinants common to both. 4) The observation is an example of the Matuhasi-Ogata phenomenon: the nonspecific uptake of a second antibody by RBC specifically sensitized by a different antibody.

Anti-A concentrations are generally higher in sera from group O than from group B donors. It is possible that the similarity of the A and B antigens may restrain immune antibody production when one or the other antigen is present. The fact that the isoantibody in the serum of group A or B people is IgM suggests that the immune response to B or A antigens does not progress very far. The anti-A titer of serum from a group O subject tends to be higher than the anti-B titer. Anti-A and anti-B are often weak in elderly people and may be almost absent from the sera of patients with hypogamma-globulinemia.

Anti-H is present in many animal sera, and a lectin with anti-H activity can be prepared from the seeds of the gorse plant (*Ulex europaeus*). Anti-H reacts with H substance remaining on the red blood cell surface even if some or much of it has been converted to A and/or B substance. Not unexpectedly anti-H is considerably more reactive with group O or A_2 cells and may not react at all with RBC from group A_1 or A_1B donors. Anti-H is found as a saline agglutinin in the sera of group O_h (Bombay) individuals. Anti-H sometimes is encountered as a cold agglutinin in the sera of group A_1 or A_1B persons. There exists a spectrum of antibodies of IH specificity ranging from those that principally recognize H antigen to those that react mainly with I antigen. Antibodies of anti-IH specificity can be separated on the basis of whether they are inhibited by secretor saliva (as a source of H substance). The more common antibody is not inhibited (mostly anti-I) and is found only in secretors; the second (mostly anti-H) is inhibited by H substance and occurs in non-secretors.

Incomplete cold anti-H activity not mediated by antibody in the classic sense of an immunoglobulin is present in essentially all normal sera. If RBC are incubated with large volumes of normal serum at 4 C for two hours or more and then washed with warm saline, they will yield a positive antiglobulin test for bound C4. In the absence of complement incomplete anti-H is not fixed to the red blood cell surface.

RECOMMENDED READING

Dodd, B.E. and Lincoln, P.J.: *Blood Group Topics*. Williams and Wilkins. Baltimore, 1975

Garratty, G.: The ABO blood groups and their relationship to disease. In: *Cellular Antigens and Disease*. Am Assn of Blood Banks. Washington, 1977. p.2

Greenwalt, T.J. and Steane, E.A. (Eds.): *CRC Handbook Series in Clinical Laboratory Science. Section D: Blood banking,* Vol. 1. CRC Press. Cleveland, 1977

Issitt, P.D. and Issitt, C.H.: *Applied Blood Group Serology*, 2nd ed. Spectra. Oxnard, Calif., 1975

Kuhns, W.J.: Naturally occurring agglutinins in health and disease. In: *A Seminar on Polymorphisms in Human Blood*. Am Assn of Blood Banks. Washington, 1975. p.83

Mollison, P.L.: *Blood Transfusion in Clinical Medicine*. Blackwell. Oxford, 1972

Race, R.R. and Sanger, R.: *Blood Groups in Man,* 6th ed. Blackwell. Oxford, 1975

Rosenfield, R.E.: Quantitation of erythrocyte antigens. In: *A Seminar on Performance Evaluation*. Am Assn of Blood Banks. Washington, 1976. p.93

CHAPTER 10

The Lewis System

The unique character of the Lewis blood group system has long been an intriguing puzzle to the immunohematologist. Reference to Figure 10-1 coupled with appreciation of a few basic principles will permit an understanding of the Lewis system as it is currently conceived. It should be noted that the Lewis antigens are soluble plasma and salivary oligosaccharide determinants that are associated with glycoproteins in secretions and only secondarily with glycolipids on RBC surfaces. Thus Lewis antigens are not primarily red blood cell antigens; their attachment to the cell surface is apparently secondary to their secretion into body fluids. Indeed, the Lewis phenotype of a red blood cell can be changed by in vitro or in vivo incubation with plasma containing a Lewis antigen absent from the cells or in plasma lacking a Lewis antigen present on the cells.

The reader will recognize Figure 10-1 as an elaboration of Figure 9-6, Chapter 9, with the addition of the Lewis and secretor genes to the scheme. The Le, le, H, and A/B genes are seen to be structural genes (producing specific glycosyltransferases as will be discussed below). The h and O genes are silent alleles or amorphs, which do not induce changes in their precursor substrate. The Se gene is a regulatory gene that controls the expression of the H gene in secretory cells (but not RBC). Thus, the production of the Lewis antigens is not the consequence of a one-gene, one-antigen relationship but rather the end result of the interaction of three sets of allelic genes acting in concert (Le, Se, and H), one of which (H) has a crucial function in development of the antigens of another blood group system (the ABO system).

The ABO and Lewis antigens are seen in Figure 10-1 to derive from a common precursor substance and as will be discussed, have

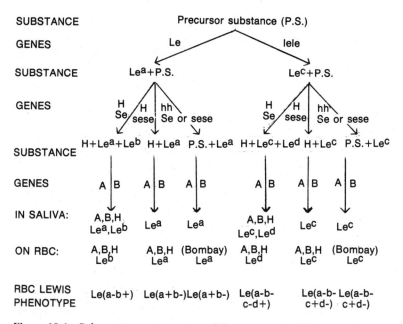

Figure 10-1. *Schematic representation of the interaction of the Le, Hh, Sese and AB genes in the formation of the ABH and Lewis antigens.*

the same basic glycoprotein structure. Modifications of the terminal sugars are responsible for the individuality of the different antigens. Under the influence of the Lewis (Le) gene, precursor substance is partially converted to Le^a substance. Under the regulatory effect of an Se gene, an H gene causes conversion of most of the Le^a substance to Le^b substance and of precursor substance to H substance. The A and/or B genes then function to cause conversion of much of the H substance to A and/or B substance. If an Le gene is present but an Se gene is absent, Le^a substance is produced, but the H gene cannot convert it to Le^b substance. The H gene, however, can cause formation of H substance, permitting subsequent action of A and/or B genes. If an Le gene is present but an H gene is absent, irrespective of whether an Se gene is present, Le^a substance, though made, cannot be converted to Le^b substance nor can H substance be formed, resulting in a Bombay phenotype of Lewis type Le $(a+b-)$. If an Le gene is absent, precursor substance is partially converted to

Le^c substance. Under the regulatory effect of an Se gene, an H gene causes conversion of most of the Le^c substance to Le^d substance and of precursor substance to H substance, with subsequent action of the A and/or B genes. If Le and Se genes are absent, Le^c substance is made, but the H gene cannot convert it to Le^d substance. Again the H gene can cause formation of H substance, permitting subsequent action of A and/or B genes. Finally if Le and H genes are absent, irrespective of Se type, Le^c substance, though made, cannot be converted to Le^d substance nor can H substance be formed, resulting in a second Bombay phenotype, this time of Lewis type Le(a−b−c+d−). It will be noted that the offspring of two Le(a−) parents can be Le(a+) and that the children of two Le(a+) people can be Le(a−).

ABO and Lewis substances as found in secretions are glycoproteins with an average molecular weight of about 300,000, composed of a polypeptide backbone made up of the same 15 amino acids and bearing some 40 to 100 covalently bound oligosaccharide side chains. The side chains are composed of residues of four sugars: N-acetyl-D-galactosamine, N-acetyl-D-glucosamine, D-galactose, and L-fucose. It is the terminal sugar residues that impart ABO and Lewis antigen specificity to the molecules. The action of the Le, le, H, A, and B genes is to determine the synthesis of a series of enzyme proteins known as glycosyltransferases each of which has the capacity to catalyze the addition of a different and specific sugar residue to the terminal portion of the oligosaccharide chains attached to the common polypeptide skeleton. The oligosaccharide chains, or precursor substance, exist in two forms called Type 1 and Type 2 and differ only in the way in which their terminal galactose residue is linked to its neighboring (subterminal) N-acetyl-D-glucosamine. It is thought that blood group I specificity resides in these precursor chains. As illustrated in Figure 10-2, addition of a terminal L-fucose residue by alpha-1,2 linkage to either precursor chain confers H specificity on the molecule. Further addition to the terminal D-galactose of N-acetyl-D-galactosamine by alpha-1,3 linkage masks H and substitutes A specificity, while addition of D-galactose in the same way confers B specificity. In the case of the Lewis substances, if L-fucose is added to the subterminal N-acetyl-D-glucosamine of a Type 1 precursor chain by alpha-1,4 linkage, Le^a specificity results. Further addition of a second L-fucose residue to the terminal D-galactose of an Le^a chain converts it to Le^b. If L-fucose is added to

the subterminal N-acetyl-D-glucosamine of a Type 2 precursor chain by alpha-1,3 linkage, Le^c specificity results. Further addition of a second L-fucose residue to the terminal D-galactose of an Le^c chain converts it to Le^d. It should be noted that these added sugar residues are not responsible for the entire reactivity of the ABH and Lewis antigens and that antibody combining sites appear to include several sugars on the chain. It is also worth remembering that these terminal sugars are not unique to these antigens: for example in addition to A, the Tn and Sd^a antigens also have N-acetyl-D-galactosamine as their immunodominant sugar; the B antigen shares D-galactose as its immunodominant residue with T and P^k.

The A$_1$ gene interferes with the expression of the Le^b antigen in persons with Le and Se genes and also suppresses the Le^a antigen in Le(b+) subjects. Thus A$_1$, Le(a−b+) RBC are often mistyped as Le(a−b−). Group A$_1$, Le(a−b+) RBC will react only with certain anti-Le^b sera (anti-Le^{bL} or anti-A$_1$Le^b), but not with others (anti-Le^{bH} or anti-HLe^b). The latter antiserum reacts only with group O or A$_2$, Le(a−b+) RBC. The amount of Le^a substance on Le(a+b−) RBC is about 30 times as much as the amount on Le(a−b+) cells, and this amount is in turn ten times greater than the quantity on Le(a−b−) cells. The number of Le^a antigen sites on Le(a+b−) red blood cells has been estimated to be in the range of 4,500 to 7,300 per cell.

The distribution of Lewis phenotypes in white and black adult populations is shown in Table 10-1. Note that the phenotype Le(a−b−) is considerably more common in black people than in whites. The expression of the Lewis antigens often weakens during pregnancy, so that RBC may type as Le(a−b−). Anti-Lewis antibodies may even be formed. The RBC of newborn infants generally yield negative reactions with anti-Le^a and anti-Le^b. The Le^a antigen appears rapidly, with 80% of white infants typing as Le(a+) by the age of three months, though in time some of the early reactions disappear and are replaced by age two years with adult Le^b specificity. Thus, Lewis typings in babies may not be reliable indicators of the adult phenotype, with infants destined to become Le(a−b+) passing through stages in which their cells may type as Le(a−b−) and then Le(a+b−) before acquiring their adult reactions. There exists another Lewis antigen called Le^x, which appears to be a direct product of the Le gene, independent of Se status but closely paralleling Le^a in its occurrence and found on Le(a+b−) and Le(a−b+) RBC. Le^x is well developed on RBC at birth and anti-Le^x will detect

TABLE 10-1

Frequency Distribution of Lewis Phenotypes in Adults

Lewis Phenotype	Frequency	
	Whites	Blacks
Le (a+ b−)	22	23
Le (a− b+)	72	55
Le (a− b−)	6	22

Le(a−b−x+) RBC in infants, thereby predicting those who carry the Le gene and are destined to be of Le(a+b−) or Le(a−b+) adult phenotype.

LEWIS ANTIBODIES

The antibodies of the Lewis system are made principally by Le(a−b−) subjects, though occasional Le(a+b−) persons have been shown to produce anti-Le^b. Le(a−b+) persons do not form anti-Le^a, since they possess Le^a substances in their serum and saliva, though not on their RBC. If sufficiently sensitive testing procedures are employed the RBC from some Le(a−b+) persons, especially if group O, can be shown to be Le(a+b+) and may be destroyed by anti-Le^a in vivo. The close similarity of Le^c to Le^a apparently prevents Le(a−b−c+d−) subjects from producing anti-Le^a, so that only Le(a−b−c−d+) persons can make the antibody.

Anti-Le^a and anti-Le^b frequently occur without known foreign red blood cell exposure and are commonly encountered together in the sera of Le(a−b−) subjects. Some sera contain an almost pure anti-Le^a, others anti-Le^b; most commonly there is present an only partially separable mixture of the two in varying proportions. Anti-Le^b antibodies appear to be part of a spectrum of antibody specificity ranging from "pure" anti-H to anti-Le^{bH} to anti-Le^{bL}. Anti-Le^{bH} reacts best with group O or A$_2$ RBC, is made by group A$_1$ or A$_1$B persons, and is inhibited by secretor saliva, even if from Le(a−b−) subjects. Anti-Le^{bL} reacts with all Le(b+) RBC and is neutralized by saliva from Le(b+) secretors but not Le(a−b−) secretors.

Most Lewis antisera are weak saline agglutinins best demonstrated at temperatures below 37 C. Many require the use of enzyme-treated RBC often in combination with antiglobulin testing, for their demonstration. Most Lewis antisera fix complement, and some are detected in antiglobulin tests only by anti-C3 components. Rare examples of immune anti-Le^a are hemolytic in vitro. Anti-Le^x is the most common Lewis antibody after anti-Le^a, and agglutinates both Le(a+b−) and Le(a−b+) RBC. Anti-Le^x reacts with about 90% of RBC from white newborn infants, and can be absorbed from mixtures with other Lewis antibodies by using Le(a−b−x+) cord red blood cells.

Lewis antisera are composed almost completely of IgM molecules, which are not transported across the placenta. For this reason, and because fetal RBC are Le(a−b−), Lewis antibodies do not cause hemolytic disease of the newborn. Potent anti-Le^a antibodies, especially if reactive at 37 C, are clinically significant and are capable of causing hemolytic transfusion reactions. Anti-Le^b antibodies in their usually encountered form as weak cold agglutinins are rarely of clinical importance. The problem of securing blood for transfusion to the patient with anti-Le^a and anti-Le^b is a practical one inasmuch as only one in 16 white donors and one in four or five blacks is Le(a−b−). In emergency situations it has been recommended that Le(a−) blood be given without reference to Le^b type. It has also been suggested that plasma containing Lewis substance(s) first be transfused to neutralize Lewis antibodies before Lewis-incompatible RBC are transfused.

RECOMMENDED READING

Dodd, B.E. and Lincoln, P.J.: *Blood Group Topics.* Williams and Wilkins. Baltimore, 1975

Graham H.A. et al: Genetic and immunochemical relationship between soluble and cell-bound antigens in the Lewis system. In: *Human Blood Groups.* Proc Fifth Intl Convocation on Immunol S. Karger. Basel, 1977. p. 257

Greenwalt, T.J. and Steane, E.A., (Eds.): *CRC Handbook Series in Clinical Laboratory Science. Section D: Blood banking,* Vol. 1. CRC Press. Cleveland, 1977

Issitt, P.D. and Issitt, C.H.: *Applied Blood Group Serology,* 2nd ed. Spectra, Oxnard, Calif., 1975

Mollison, P.L.: *Blood Transfusion in Clinical Medicine,* 5th ed. Blackwell. Oxford, 1972

Race, R.R. and Sanger, R.: *Blood Groups in Man,* 6th ed. Blackwell. Oxford, 1975

CHAPTER 11

The Rh System

Clinically, the most important of the irregular, unexpected or atypical antibodies (antibodies outside of the ABO system) or, as they are also known, alloantibodies, are those of the Rh system. First recognized in 1939 as the result of immunization experiments with the Rhesus monkey (whence the name Rh), this system today counts at least 35 components. The first antigen defined was called Rh_0 or D, and is the single most important antigen of the system. Persons with an Rh_0 (D) gene are said to be Rh_0-positive, or D-positive, or more loosely, Rh-positive. Individuals lacking $Rh_0(D)$ are Rh-negative. The expected allele of $Rh_0(D)$, expected to be named rh or d, does not exist.

Other major components of the Rh system are rh'(C), its allele hr'(c), and rh''(E) and its allele hr''(e). These antigens are assembled in complexes in any of eight different ways: R^1(CDe), R^2(cDE), r(cde), R_0(cDe), r'(Cde), r''(cdE), R^z(CDE), and r^y(CdE). One such complex from each parent is contributed by a genetic locus situated on chromosome number 1. The exact mode in inheritance of the Rh complexes is not settled and has given rise to three sets of nomenclature summarized in part in Table 11-1. The Wiener concept envisions multiple Rh alleles at a single locus, each producing a different complex antigen or agglutinogen bearing several antigenic determinants or factors. In this view one agglutinogen can react with several different antibodies identifying various factors contained within its antigenic makeup. The Fisher-Race theory holds that the genetic control of Rh antigens is effected by three sets of closely linked genes, each with multiple alleles. At one locus is the gene D (or its absence, denoted by d), at a second, C or one of its alleles (c, C^w, C^x, etc.), and at a third E or one of its alleles (e, E^w, E^T, e^s, etc.). Weiner

119

TABLE 11-1

Comparative Nomenclature for Rh Antigens, with Frequencies in
the White Population

Numerical (Rosenfeld et al)	Rh (Weiner)	CDE (Fisher-Race)	Percent of Whites Bearing Antigen
Rh:1	Rh_O	D	85
Rh:2	rh′	C	69
Rh:3	rh″	E	17
Rh:4	hr′	c	81
Rh:5	hr″	e	98
Rh:6	hr	ce or f	64
Rh:7	rh_i	Ce	70
Rh:22	—	CE	< 1
Rh:27	—	cE	30
Rh:8	rh^{w1}	C^W	1
Rh:9	rh^x	C^x	< 1
Rh:10	hr^v	V or ce^s	Very rare (20% of blacks)
Rh:20	—	VS or e^s	Very rare (20% of blacks)
Rh:11	rh^{w2}	E^W	< 1
Rh:12	rh^G	G	85
Rh:13	Rh^A	—	85
Rh:14	Rh^B	—	85
Rh:15	Rh^C	—	85
Rh:16	Rh^D	—	85
Rh:25	—	LW	> 99.9
Rh:29	—	RH	> 99.9
Rh:17	Hr_O	—	> 99.9
Rh:18	Hr	—	> 99.9

postulated for example that the gene R^1 produces the agglutinogen Rh^1 composed of factors rh′, Rh_O, and hr″. In corresponding Fisher-Race terminology, C, D, and e genes produce the antigens C, D, and e. The terminology of Rosenfeld et al is noncommittal about the genetics of the system, making no assumptions about allelic relationships, but merely numbering the antigens, indicating whether they have been tested for, and whether positive or negative reactions were obtained. Thus, a red blood cell suspension giving positive reactions with anti-rh′(C), anti-Rh_O(D), and anti-hr″(e) but negative reactions with anti-hr′(c) and anti-rh″(E) would be designated as Rh:

1,2,−3,−4,5. Each system has advantages, but despite theoretical shortcomings, the CDE terminology of Fisher and Race is more popular, principally because the Rh nomenclature of Weiner is so unwieldy, especially in conversation, and the numerical terminology of Rosenfield is beyond the memories of most of us. Fisher-Race terminology will be used in this volume, except where additional clarification seems desirable.

Terminology and scientific certainty become further confused when an attempt is made to translate what we observe in the form of antiserum reactions into "most probable genotypes". For example, testing of a blood sample might yield positive reactions with anti-C, anti-c, anti-D, and anti-e but not with anti-E. This would be interpreted to mean that the subject's RBC bear the antigens C, c, D, and e and that he carries the corresponding genes. Because his RBC lack E, we presume that he is homozygous for the e gene and thus is genetically CcDee. Because there is no anti-d serum we cannot determine whether the subject is homozygous for the D gene. If we attempt to determine the Rh genotype, we arrive at two possibilities: CDe/cde or CDe/cDe (Table 11-2). Family studies have shown that the gene complex cDe is rare, at least in white people, and therefore we assume the former genotype to be the "most probable." If the subject in the above example were to marry someone of genotype

TABLE 11-2

Common Rh Typing Reactions, Phenotypes, and Genotypes

Anti-C	Anti-c	Anti-D	Anti-E	Anti-e	Phenotype	Most Probable Genotype	Other Possible Genotypes
+	+	+	−	+	CcDee	CDe/cde	CDe/cDe, Cde/cDe
+	−	+	−	+	CCDee	CDe/CDe	CDe/CDe
+	+	+	+	+	CcDEe	CDe/cDE	cDe/CdE, Cde/cDE, CDE/cde, CDe/cdE, CDE/cDe
−	+	+	−	+	ccDee	cDe/cde	cDe/cDe
−	+	+	+	+	ccDEe	cDE/cde	cDe/cdE, cDE/cDe
−	+	+	+	−	ccDEE	cDE/cDE	cDE/cdE
−	+	−	−	+	ccddee	cde/cde	—

cde/cde and have a cde/cde child, he would be proved to carry a cde complex and therefore to be of the genotype CDe/cde.

Another problem with the concept of the "most probable geno-type" lies in the fact that lack of a reaction with an antiserum to one antigen and reaction with one to a second allelic antigen does not prove that the subject is homozygous for the second allele. For example, if an RBC suspension gives a positive reaction with anti-C and a negative reaction with anti-c, it is not proved that the cell donor is homozygous for the C gene: there may be present another allele for which the antigen was not tested, e.g. C^w. Table 11-3 lists the frequency of occurrence of Rh genotypes in the white population, while Table 11-4 gives the frequencies of occurrence of common Rh gene complexes.

Several variant forms of the D antigen have been discovered, the most common of which is called D^u, or variant Rh_0. The D^u antigen is a weak form of D, exhibiting some but not all of the serologic properties expected of D-positive red blood cells. Red blood cells bearing inherited weak forms of D, the so-called "low-grade" D^u type, exhibit weak or absent agglutination by most anti-D sera and require antiglobulin testing to demonstrate anti-D uptake. There also exist "high-grade" D^u types in which the expression of the D gene is only somewhat weakened but still detectable with modern commercial anti-D typing sera. The weakened reactions on such cells are usually a result of suppression of the expression of a normal D gene on one chromosome by the gene complex Cde or CdE on the other. This is an example of a "position effect." If we consider the genotype CDE/cde, we note that the genes C and E are on the same chromosome (cis) while C and e are on different chromosomes (trans). C in trans position, as noted above, weakens the expression of D. D cis to C, E, or e results in the partial suppression of the latter as do D or E trans to C, or D trans to E. An alternative explanation for position effects invokes the location of D sites in such a way that although they are structurally normal and fully expressed chemically, antibody does not have ready access to them (steric hindrance). Weakened expression of D due to position effects is not ordinarily shown by the offspring of affected subjects because of different pairing of haplotypes.

Both blood donors and recipients of D^u type are considered Rh-positive for purposes of transfusion, although D^u testing is not done on recipients. It is doubtful if a D^u-positive transfusion ever induces

TABLE 11-3

Frequencies of Occurrence of Rh Genotypes in the White Population

Genotype		Approximate Frequency in Whites (%)
"Shorthand" Notation	Fisher-Race Notation	
rr	cde/cde	14.4
r'r	Cde/cde	0.5
r'r'	Cde/Cde	0.004
r''r	cdE/cde	0.4
r''r''	cdE/cdE	0.002
r'r''	Cde/cdE	0.006
r^yr	CdE/cde	0.008
r^yr'	CdE/Cde	0.0001
r^yr''	CdE/cdE	0.001
$r^y r^y$	CdE/CdE	0.00001
R^0r	cDe/cde	2.0
$R^0 R^0$	cDe/cDe	0.07
R^1r	CDe/cde	32.7
$R^1 R^0$	CDe/cDe	2.3
R^0r'	cDe/Cde	0.03
$R^1 R^1$	CDe/CDe	18.5
R^1r'	CDe/Cde	0.5
R^2r	cDE/cde	11.4
$R^2 R^0$	cDE/cDe	0.8
R^0r''	cDe/cdE	0.03
$R^2 R^2$	cDE/cDE	2.2
R^2r''	cDE/cdE	0.2
$R^1 R^2$	CDe/cDE	12.9
R^1r''	CDe/cdE	0.4
R^2r'	cDE/Cde	0.2
R_zr	CDE/cde	0.2
$R^Z R^0$	CDE/cDe	0.01
$R^0 r^y$	cDe/CdE	0.0005
$R^Z R^1$	CDE/CDe	0.2
R^Zr'	CDE/Cde	0.02
$R^1 r^y$	CDe/CdE	0.008
$R^Z R^2$	CDE/cDE	0.06
R^Zr''	CDE/cdE	0.002
$R^2 r^y$	cDE/CdE	0.003
$R^Z R^Z$	CDE/CDE	0.0004
$R^Z r^y$	CDE/CdE	0.00004

TABLE 11-4

Approximate Frequencies of Occurrence of Common Rh Gene Complexes in the White Population

Shorthand Notation	Gene Complex	Approximate Frequency in Whites (%)
R^1	CDe	40
r	cde	38
R^2	cDE	16
R^0	cDe	2
r'	Cde	1
r''	cdE	1
R^z	CDE	0.08
r^y	CdE	Very rare

formation of anti-D in an Rh-negative recipient, even if inadvertently given. D^u is a relatively common antigen in black people, though it is quite rare in whites.

It has been observed that rare Rh-positive people, some but not all of whose D antigens react weakly, are capable of making "anti-D" antibody. This observation led to the recognition of the D antigen as a mosaic composed of at least four parts, called Rh^A, Rh^B, Rh^C, and Rh^D, one or more of which may occasionally be congenitally missing. In such subjects, transfusion with or exposure during pregnancy to "complete" D antigen can result in sensitization to the missing part of the mosaic and production of antibody directed against it. Inasmuch as this component will be present on all normal type D red blood cells, the antibody will appear to be "anti-D." Such antibodies may rarely cause hemolytic disease of the newborn or hemolytic transfusion reactions.

Rare Rh antigens known as D^w and Go^a may be "replacement" antigens for parts of the D mosaic. Subjects with these rare types can make antibodies that will react as "anti-D" in response to transfusion with normal Rh-positive RBC.

The discovery of another very rare Rh variation in the form of red blood cells completely lacking conventional Rh antigens (the so-called Rh_{null} type) has led to our further understanding of the complexity of the Rh system. Figure 11-1 shows the scheme by which precursor substance is thought to be modified under the effect of a

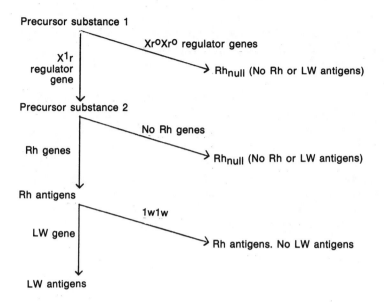

Precursor substance 1

X^1r regulator gene

Xr^oXr^o regulator genes

Rh_null (No Rh or LW antigens)

Precursor substance 2

Rh genes

No Rh genes

Rh_null (No Rh or LW antigens)

Rh antigens

LW gene

1w1w

Rh antigens. No LW antigens

LW antigens

Figure 11-1. *Schematic representation of the synthesis of the Rh and LW antigens.*

regulator gene X^1r to form a second precursor, which is acted upon by Rh structural genes to form the various Rh antigens on the red blood cell membrane. Further action by an LW gene then causes LW substance to be formed as well. The Rh_{null} condition can result either from the absence of an X^1r regulator gene, with production of the so-called regulator type of Rh_{null} or more rarely, from absence of Rh genes, with a resulting Rh amorph. Absence of an LW gene does not affect development of normal Rh antigens but prevents formation of LW antigens. Rh_{null} types due to abnormality of regulator genes cannot be distinguished clinically or serologically from those due to absent (or silent) Rh genes. Regulator-type Rh_{null} patients, however, have parents or children with normal Rh antigens (e.g., both C and c, or both E and e).

The red blood cells of Rh_{null} patients exhibit a membrane defect characterized by abnormal exchange of Na^+ and K^+ ions. Patients with the so-called Rh_{null} syndrome exhibit a chronic hemolytic anemia, usually compensated, with decreased RBC life span, intermittently increased serum bilirubin levels, increased reticulocyte counts, decreased serum haptoglobin concentrations, increased RBC osmotic fragility, peripheral blood stomatocytes, increased RBC F hemoglobin content, and splenomegaly. The syndrome is found in both the regulator gene and amorph varieties of the condition, and is very rare, with an estimated incidence of one in 6,000,000 persons. An allied condition in which all Rh genes exhibit decreased expression (Rh_{mod}) has a similar clinical presentation and may represent the heterozygous condition of the $X^{o}r$ gene. It has been found that Rh_{null} red blood cells often exhibit suppression of their reactions for S, s, and U antigens in antiglobulin tests. Rh_{null} subjects sensitized by blood transfusion make an antibody known as anti-total Rh, or anti-RH (anti-Rh 29). The Rh antigens are known to be lipoproteins and would appear from the evidence noted above to be intrinsic portions of the red blood cell membrane, essential to its integrity. This observation is in contrast to the situation in the Bombay (O_h) blood group, in which absence of ABH antigens appears to be of no physiologic consequence, and the antigens of no structural importance to the function or integrity of the cell membrane.

The observation that rare D-positive people make "anti-D" that can be absorbed by Rh-negative red blood cells led to the concept of the LW antigen. A very common gene, LW (and its allele lw) segregate separately from the Rh genes (see Figure 11-1) and control the production of LW antigen from Rh substance. The LW antigen is weaker on Rh-negative than on Rh-positive RBC, the stronger form being called LW_1 and the weaker LW_2. The gene lw, although not silent, when homozygous determines formation of still weaker forms of LW called LW_3 and LW_4. Subjects with weak forms of LW can produce antibodies that react with stronger forms of the antigen and that initially may be misinterpreted as "anti-D." Pregnant women have weakened expression of the LW antigen on their RBC and may make anti-LW (possibly as a first reaction to Rh sensitization, preceding formation of anti-D by Rh-negative women.)

The number of D antigen sites on red blood cells of various phenotypes varies considerably, a fact of importance when comparing serologic studies, including titers (Table 11-5). Enhanced reactions with anti-D sera are found on the RBC of two rare types of subjects: 1) Persons with weak or absent expression of C and/or E alleles, e.g., –D–, CD–, C^wD–, (C)D(e) and subjects whose RBC are Go^a-positive. 2) Persons with Rh-positive RBC who are also of types

TABLE 11-5

Numbers of Various Rh Antigen Sites on RBC of Different Phenotypes
(The number of c sites on heterozygous (Cc) RBC has been estimated between 37,000 and 53,000 per cell, and the number on homozygous (cc) cells, from 70,000 to 85,000 per cell.)

Phenotype	Probable Genotype	No. of D Antigen Sites per RBC	No. of E Antigen Sites per RBC	No. of e Antigen Sites per RBC
CcDee	R^1r	9,900–14,600	—	24,400
ccDee	R^0r	12,000–20,000	—	—
ccDEe	R^2r	14,000–16,600	11,800	—
CCDee	R^1R^1	15,500–19,300	—	—
CcDEe	R^1R^2	23,000–31,000	1,680–8,000	14,500
ccDEE	R^2R^2	15,800–33,300	5,560–25,600	—
-D-	—	110,000–202,000	—	—
ccddEE	$r''r''$	—	5,100–22,400	—
ccddee	rr	—	—	18,200

Ena-negative, Mg, or Mk. In the first situation there appears to be either extra precursor substance available to be converted to D antigenic material or a lack of steric hindrance by other Rh antigens. Persons with heterozygous Rh deletions may show enhanced D reactivity. In the second case the cell membranes of the RBC have reduced sialic acid levels, rendering them unusually easily agglutinable.

The serologic reactions of anti-D are representative of those of many of the antibodies of the Rh system. Although it is traditionally taught that anti-D produced after primary immunization is an IgM saline agglutinin, anti-D is more usually encountered in an incomplete IgG form mixed with a varying amount of IgM antibody. The reaction characteristics of mixed IgG-IgM anti-D depend on the proportions of the two forms. The presence of even small amounts of incomplete anti-D decreases the ability of IgM anti-D to agglutinate weakly reactive D-positive RBC. It is possible that the prozones exhibited by certain anti-D sera may be as much a result of an excess of incomplete antibody as of excess of saline agglutinins.

Anti-D sera are optimally reactive at 37 C. Their reactions are enhanced in albumin but best demonstrated using enzyme or antiglobulin techniques. Anti-D does not fix complement, is not hemolytic in vitro, and is a poor opsonin. The failure of anti-D to bind complement appears to be a result of the fact that D antigenic determinants on the red blood cell surface are too far apart to collaborate. If there are 10,000 D sites on a cell and they are evenly distributed, the distance between sites will be about 130 nm. Since the greatest dimensions of an IgG molecule are about 10 x 25 nm, collaboration is not possible, and the formation of the "doublet" necessary to complement fixation by IgG molecules cannot occur.

In some cases anti-D can only be detected by enzyme-treated RBC, especially when first produced. IgG anti-D occurs principally in the subclasses IgG1 and IgG3, although a few examples are IgG4 and some partly IgG2. In a typical anti-D serum with a typical binding constant, an antiglobulin titer of one corresponds to an antibody concentration of about 0.02 μg/ml. The lowest detectable concentration of IgM anti-D in saline using manual methods is about 0.03 μg/ml. The binding constant of IgM anti-D is generally substantially higher than that of IgG anti-D.

The relative frequency of occurrence of various alloantibodies detectable at room temperature and above in one large study is shown in Table 11-6. It will be seen that anti-D and anti-CD (G) together comprised almost half of the antibodies encountered, though it should be noted that the prevalence of anti-Lewis antibodies is dependent on the sensitivity of the detection techniques used and the proportion of blacks in the population studied. With the decrease in recent years in D sensitization after Rh-incompatible pregnancy owing to the use of Rh-immune globulin (see Chapter 21), Lewis antibodies are now the most commonly encountered specificities in the author's practice. Nevertheless, as a practical problem, anti-D deserves a large share of our attention in the blood bank. The contribution of anti-D as a cause of hemolytic transfusion reactions and hemolytic disease of the newborn will be returned to in Chapters 19 and 21, but, at this time, consideration should be given to why this antibody is so significant. Part of the answer lies in the fact that D is a potent antigen, which in rather small amounts and with reasonable regularity is capable of inducing anti-D formation in Rh-negative subjects. A single transfusion of 1 ml of Rh-positive blood to Rh-negative recipients will cause detectable anti-D production within six months in 15% of subjects. If 25 ml are administered the figure rises to 50% and with 500 ml transfu-

TABLE 11-6

Occurrence of Alloantibodies in Approximately 200,000 Persons
(Kissmeyer-Nielsen, *Scand J Hematol* 2:331, 1965.) A variety of detection techniques
was used, including enzyme and antiglobulin testing. Antibodies not detectable at
room temperature or 37 C are not included.

Antibody Specificity	Number of Times Found
Anti-D	1,425
Anti-P$_1$	817
Anti-CD	552
Anti-Le^a	522
Anti-E	260
Anti-K	116
Anti-H	107
Anti-Le^a + Le^b	57
Anti-c	49
Anti-Le^b	34
Anti-DE	34
Anti-CDE	27
Anti-M	27
Anti-cE	25
Anti-Fy^a	19
Anti-Lu^a	17
Anti-Ce	16
Anti-C^w	15
Anti-Jk^a	10
Other	38
Total	4,168

sions, production exceeds 50%. With multiple exposures to the D antigen up to 70% of Rh-negative people will produce anti-D. The time of initial antibody appearance with repeated restimulation ranges from a few weeks (or even less if techniques are sensitive) to more than two years. The minimum dose of Rh-positive RBC required for primary immunization of a susceptible subject is no greater than 0.03 ml, and possibly less than 0.01 ml. Transfusion of ABO-incompatible RBC reduces the likelihood of sensitization to the D antigen and results in formation of antibodies of low titer in those persons who do respond. The reason for this fact is not clear but may relate to sequestration of ABO-incompatible RBC in the liver, an apparently inefficient site for induction of the immune response. A secondary immune reaction to D antigen in a subject already sensitized will occur in response to a single injection of 0.2 to 2 ml of RBC, with maximal antibody production within three weeks. IgM anti-D tends to disappear rapidly, but IgG anti-D has persisted for 30 years. The subject who forms anti-D often later produces blood group antibodies to antigens outside of the Rh system. It has been suggested that various Ir (immune response) genes may be linked. It is also possible that blood group antigens are concentrated during immunization, facilitating response to antigens that might not be able to initiate an immune reaction in unconcentrated form.

Rh-negative mothers with Rh-positive infants incur a special risk of immunization to the D antigen as a consequence of fetal-maternal hemorrhage at the time of delivery. About 1% of mothers have 3 ml of fetal RBC in their circulation immediately after delivery, and 0.3% have 10 ml or more. The risk of fetal-maternal hemorrhage is increased by such procedures as amniocentesis, cesarean section or manual extraction of the placenta. As discussed in Chapter 21, immunization beginning at the time of delivery (or, on occasion, beforehand) may result in damage to a subsequent Rh-positive fetus by maternal anti-D. About 10% of pregnancies resulting from matings of white parents yield an Rh-negative mother with an Rh-positive baby. Six percent of untreated Rh-negative women (1% of all women) with a second Rh-positive pregnancy will have an affected infant.

The likelihood of immunization to the D antigen may be in part related to the numbers of antigen sites on the red blood cell surface: D sites are four times as numerous as K sites and ten times more numerous than Fy^a sites, but only a fiftieth or a hundredth as numerous as A_1 sites. This is not the only factor involved, however, as shown in Table 11-5, E and e sites are often as numerous as D sites and c sites, two or three times as numerous, although these antigens are far less effective in eliciting antibody formation.

The frequency of sensitization to a blood group antigen is influenced by the relative proportions of persons who possess and who lack the antigen. Without resorting to mathematical argument, we can appreciate at once that if the red blood cells of almost everyone carry a given antigen, transfusion of random units of blood (almost all of which will possess that antigen) will not cause immunization very often. Conversely, if an antigen is very rare, no matter how potent, the likelihood of a random transfusion causing sensitization is remote. In the case of the D antigen, 85% of the white population is D-positive and 15% is D-negative. Hence, there is a considerable chance of a random transfusion supplying the antigen and a sufficiently large population at risk to create the statistical conditions for frequent sensitization. Indeed, the incidence of sensitization of D-negative recipients transfused with D-positive blood is sufficiently great that in selecting blood for transfusion, D-compatible as well as ABO-compatible units are required.

OTHER ANTIGENS AND ANTIBODIES IN THE Rh SYSTEM

The remainder of the antigens in the Rh system are considerably less antigenic than D, and, as seen in Table 11-6, their corresponding antibodies are less common. "Anti-CD" is the next most common Rh antibody and is found three to seven times less frequently than anti-D, followed among Rh antibodies by anti-E and anti-c. The serologic reactions of most antibodies in the Rh system are similar to those already described for anti-D. An exception is occasionally encountered in the case of anti-E, some examples of which are non-red blood cell immune IgM antibodies reactive at room temperature, often as saline agglutinins. Some anti-E antibodies are not detected by antiglobulin testing but are reactive with enzyme-treated RBC.

The antigen C^w is the product of an important though moderately rare gene occurring as an allele at the C locus. C^w is found on the RBC of about 1% of white subjects. Like anti-E, anti-C^w may also be naturally occurring, and is often found in sera containing antibodies to other low-incidence antigens. For unknown reasons R^1R^1 people who produce anti-c often also form anti-C^w. Similarly, most anti-C sera are anti-C+C^w, despite the absence of identifiable exposure to the C^w antigen. It has been suggested that the C^w gene produces the antigens C plus C^w in a fashion analogous to the determination of A plus A_1 antigens by the A_1 gene. Of practical importance is the fact that many IgM saline agglutinating anti-C sera contain incomplete IgG anti-D as well. As typing reagents such sera may be quite satisfactory if used according to the manufacturer's directions, but they will yield misleading and inaccurate results if not used correctly.

C^x is another even rarer allele at the C locus, with properties similar to those of C^w. Anti-C^x may also be naturally occurring and is often found, as are anti-Wr^a, anti-Sw^a, and other antibodies to low-incidence antigens in the sera of patients with autoimmune acquired hemolytic disease. The genes C^W or C^X paired with C will not be detected by usual RBC typing procedures employing anti-C and anti-c; such RBC are generally misclassified as homozygous C cells. If paired with c, C^W or C^X may be suspected because of the weak agglutination produced by those anti-c sera exhibiting a dosage effect. Dosage effects are normally encountered in antisera of the specificities anti$-M$, $-N$, $-c$, $-C^W$, $-E$, $-e$, and $-f$ but not $-C$.

The c antigen bears a component known as Rh26, which is occasionally missing on c-positive RBC. Rh:-26 subjects can produce anti-Rh26, and anti-Rh26 activity is present in most anti-c sera. E^W is a rare allele at the E locus analogous to C^W, but anti-E sera do not usually contain anti-E^W. The antigen E^T is a component of E and E^W antigens. Anti-E^T activity is present in most anti-E sera. The e antigen has been shown to be a complex mosaic with parts named hr^S and hr^B, the absence of which permits the formation of the corresponding antibodies. Anti-Hr^S and anti-hr^B are present in most anti-e sera. The antigens e^S (VS) and ce^S (V) are low-frequency antigens almost unique to people of the black race. They have been thought to be a part of the e antigen, but recent evidence suggests that they are more likely part of the D mosaic.

Of considerable interest is the occurrence of so-called compound Rh antigens involving the C and E loci. All four combinations, Ce, cE, CE, and ce (or f) can elicit the formation of antibodies reacting with a joint gene product formed when both genes occur on the same chromosome. Antibodies to compound antigens will not react with either component alone. Thus anti-ce sera will not react with CDe/cDE red blood cells. Such sera are useful in distinguishing among CcDEe phenotypes, anti-ce making a distinction between CDe/cDE and CDE/cde cells. Whenever anti-c or anti-E is detected in the serum of R^1R^1 subjects, anti-cE should be sought. Similarly the other antibodies to compound antigens should be suspected in the sera of patients with appropriate phenotypes of C/c and E/e. Anti-ce (f) is present in most anti-c and anti-e sera and confuses the interpretation of dosage effects obtained when using them. Anti-C sera often contain anti-Ce or anti-CE, and anti-E sera frequently contain anti-CE also. For reasons unknown, anti-ce reacts with CD–/CD– RBC.

The Rh antigen called G is of particular interest, occurring on essentially all RBC that bear C and/or D antigens. Many antisera reacting with C or D antigens contain anti-G as well, thus explaining such phenomena as the ability of some anti-D sera to react with Cde cells, the ability of cDe red blood cells to absorb both antibodies from an "anti-CD" serum, or the formation of "anti-CD" by a mother whose fetus is D-positive but C-negative. Thus most "anti-CD" sera are anti-D plus G, anti-C plus G, or anti-C plus D plus G. Rare cDE and cDe persons lack the G antigen and can make anti-G. People who are of genotype cde/cde lack G, but the very rare r^G subject produces G in the absence of C and D.

People with deleted Rh genes can produce, in response to transfusion with normal Rh blood, an antibody with very broad Rh reactivity called anti-Hr_0. In its usual form this antibody reacts with an antigen present on the RBC of all nondeleted Rh phenotypes, irrespective of CcDEe type. A second separable antibody called anti-Hr also occurs in such sera and similarly reacts with a high-incidence Rh antigen.

RECOMMENDED READING

Fletcher, J.L.: Rh-Hr blood group system. In: *Blood Group Immunology: Theoretical and Practical Concepts*. Dade. Miami, 1976. p.47

Huestis, D.W. et al: *Practical Blood Transfusion*, 2nd ed. Little, Brown and Co. Boston, 1976

Issitt, P.D. and Issitt, C.H.: *Applied Blood Group Serology*, 2nd ed. Spectra. Oxnard, Calif., 1975

Kissmeyer-Nielsen, F.: Irregular blood group antibodies in 200,000 individuals. *Scand J Hematol* 2:331, 1965

Mollison, P.L.: *Blood Transfusion in Clinical Medicine*, 5th ed. Blackwell. Oxford, 1972

Nichols, M.E.: Red cell antigens in health and disease. In: *A Seminar on Polymorphisms in Human Blood*. Am Assn of Blood Banks. Washington, 1975. p.59

Race, R.R. and Sanger, R.: *Blood Groups in Man*, 6th ed. Blackwell. Oxford, 1975

Schmidt, P.J.: The hemolytic anemia of the Rh_{null} blood group. In: *Cellular Antigens and Disease*. Am Assn of Blood Banks. Washington, 1977. p.31

CHAPTER 12

The Kell, Duffy, and Kidd Systems

The Kell, Duffy, and Kidd blood group systems are considered together because of similarities in serologic characteristics and clinical significance. All were named after the patient in whom the first antibody in the system was identified (the propositus). The antibodies of the Kell, Duffy, and Kidd systems are potentially dangerous as causes of hemolytic disease of the newborn and hemolytic transfusion reactions. In general, the antibodies of these three systems are formed as a result of exposure to foreign red blood cell antigens in consequence of transfusion or pregnancy. They are generally IgG (rarely IgM), react best at 37 C, and are nonagglutinating in saline, requiring antiglobulin testing for detection. Some examples, particularly Kidd antibodies are complement fixing. The relative frequency of occurrence of the more common antibodies in these systems is illustrated in Table 11-6.

THE KELL SYSTEM

Clinically, the most significant antigens in the Kell blood group system are those determined by the allelic genes K (Kell, or Kl) and k (Cellano, or K2). The distribution frequency of the common Kell genotypes is given in Table 12-1. Both K and k are potent antigens, ranking behind D, though K is six to ten times less effective that D in eliciting antibody production. Anti-Kell is the most common red blood cell immune alloantibody outside of the Rh system, occurring in up to one in 700 patients. Transfusion of a unit of K-positive blood will elicit formation of anti-K in about 5% of K-negative recipients. The calculated incidence of hemolytic disease of the newborn due to a second K-positive pregnancy in a K-negative woman is one in

TABLE 12-1

Frequency Distribution of Kell Phenotypes

Genotype	Frequency (%)	
	Whites	Blacks
KK	0.2	< 0.1
Kk	8.6	2.0
kk	91.2	98.0
K_O	Very rare	—
Kp (a+ b−)	< 0.1	< 0.1
Kp (a− b+)	98.0	> 99.9
Kp (a+ b+)	2.0	< 0.1
Js (a+ b−)	< 0.1	1.1
Js (a− b+)	> 99.9	80.5
Js (a+ b+)	< 0.1	18.4

4,000. Homozygous (KK) Kell-positive RBC possess about 6,100 K sites per cell; heterozygous (Kk) cells, about 3,500 per cell.

Because less than 9% of white subjects are K-positive, opportunities for immunization by blood transfusion or pregnancy are not as common as in the case of the D antigen. Anti-k is very rare, with only one white person in 500 homozygous for K and therefore capable of producing the antibody. On the other hand, in the case of that rare person who is a genotype KK, the chance of a random transfusion being k-positive is 998 in 1,000, and the opportunity for sensitization by k is thus considerable. From a practical viewpoint, routine Kell typing and blood donor-recipient matching are not carried out when selecting blood for transfusion to the patient who has not made Kell-system antibodies.

A total of 18 antigens belonging to the Kell system have been discovered, together with their corresponding antibodies. Table 12-2 lists the allelic relationships that have been established. The amorph K_O lacks all of the identifiable Kell antigens. The genes for various Kell system alleles such as Kp^a and Kp^b, Js^a and Js^b, or K11 and K17 are postulated to bear the same relationship to K and k that C and c or E and e alleles of the Rh system have to D. A numerical system of notation for the Kell antigens is shown in Table 12-3.

TABLE 12-2

Known Alleles in the Kell System

Common:	k	Kp^b	Js^b	K11	?		K12	K13	K14	K18
Rare:	K	Kp^a	Js^a	K17	Ul^a	?	?	?	?

The gene Kp^a is almost exclusively found in the white race, whereas Js^a occurs only in blacks. Anti-Kp^a and anti-Js^a are relatively uncommon antibodies in white people because most donor blood from whites is Kp^a-negative and Js^a-negative. Hence, transfusion problems involving these antibodies are unusual. Anti-Kp^b and anti-Js^b, like anti-k are rare antibodies, but when they are encountered can pose major problems in securing compatible blood for transfusion. As is evident from Table 12-1, black donors should be screened to find Js^b-negative blood, whites to find Kp^b-negative types. To find donors for patients of K_O phenotypes who have made

TABLE 12-3

Kell System Nomenclature and Antigen Frequency

Antigen	Symbol	Numerical Designation	Antigen Frequency (Whites)
Kell	K	K1	9.0
Cellano	k	K2	99.8
Penny	Kp^a	K3	2.0
Rautenberg	Kp^b	K4	99.9
Peltz	K_u	K5	> 99.9
Sutter	Js^a	K6	20.0 (blacks)
Matthews	Js^b	K7	99.0 (blacks)
—	K^w	K8	5.0
—	KL	K9	> 99.9
—	Ul^a	K10	2.6 (Finns)
Cote	—	K11	> 99.9
Boc	—	K12	> 99.9
Sgro	—	K13	> 99.9
San	—	K14	> 99.9
—	Kx	K15	> 99.9
k-like	—	K16	> 99.9
—	Wk^a	K17	0.3
—	—	K18	> 99.9

anti-Ku (an antibody reacting with all of the known Kell system anti-gens), siblings should be screened or the assistance of a rare donor file or frozen blood depot enlisted. The same holds true for patients of McLeod type with anti-KL (discussed below).

Some of the theoretically possible gene complexes involv-ing combinations of the three common pairs of Kell alleles have not been detected. Those that have been found are KKp^bJs^b, kKp^bJs^b, kKp^aJs^b, and kKp^bJs^a. It has been suggested that the gene complex kKp^bJs^bKll is the primordial Kell form and that com-plexes bearing K, Kp^a, Js^a, or K17 represent mutations. It has been noted that the presence of Kp^a seems to suppress the expression of k. In the scheme presented by Marsh (see Figure 12-1), a single Kell gene complex produces one of each pair of alleles but only one rare allele. Thus a gene that produces K also produces Kp^b, Js^b, and Kll but never Kp^a, Js^a, or K17. The biosynthetic pathway illustrated in Figure 12-1 postulates a series of allelic X-linked genes (Xk genes) that control the transformation of precursor substance into an inter-mediate called Kx, produced on both RBC and phagocytic leuko-cytes. Kx remains unaltered on WBC but is transformed by the ac-tion of alleles at the autosomal Kell gene locus into the various Kell antigens on RBC. In the absence of functional autosomal Kell genes (K_O type) Kx remains on red blood cells. If the K_O patient is trans-fused, he may produce anti-Ku, which reacts with RBC of all Kell phenotypes but K_O. K_O phenotypes are very rare, occurring with a frequency of 0.0006. Race and Sanger feel that K_O red blood cells result from the presence of a rare allele at an operator site that switches off all activity at the Kell structural loci.

Fascinating recent work has elucidated the role of aberrant Xk genes in the production of chronic granulomatous disease. This con-dition is X-linked and genetically determined, affects male children, and is inherited from the mother who is a carrier of a variant Xk gene. The neutrophils and monocytes of affected boys exhibit defec-tive bactericidal activity, which results in repeated infections by low-grade pathogenic bacteria despite the presence of a normal immune system. Kx substance is a cell membrane glycoprotein required for normal function of phagocytic WBC and is specifically required for transmembrane transport of cell metabolites into the phagosome surrounding ingested bacteria. Figure 12-1 shows that replacement of the normal X^1k gene by X^2k results in failure to convert Kell pre-cursor substance to Kx. On RBC this results in failure of normal production of usual Kell antigens, while on phagocytic WBC the absence of Kx is associated with defective phagocytosis. The RBC produced in this situation are of the so-called McLeod type, exhibiting very weak k, Kp^b, Js^b, and Kll antigens. Kx substance on the red blood cell is used by Kell genes for the production of membrane structures with Kell blood group specificities. Clinically, patients with McLeod red blood cells exhibit a usually compensated chronic hemolytic anemia, with decreased RBC life span, acanthocytes in the peripheral blood smear, increased reticulocyte counts, decreased serum haptoglobin levels, and splenomegaly.

Substitution of X^3k at the Xk locus causes the production of phagocytes with absent Kx and resultant chronic granulomatous disease, but of RBC with normal Kell system antigens and no decrease in survival. The opposite situation is brought about by an X^4k gene: Kx is normal on phagocytes and there is no chronic granulomatous disease, but the RBC are of the McLeod type with weak Kell system antigens and shortened survival. It is evident that the cell membrane structure that carries Kx is of vital importance to RBC integrity. This is in contrast to the situation in K_O red blood cells, which carry an abundance of Kx substance though lacking other Kell antigens and exhibit no evidence of defective function or decreased life span. Patients whose RBC are of the McLeod type can make an antibody called anti-KL in response to transfusion of normal RBC. Anti-KL is directed against Kell system precursor substance and reacts with all but McLeod RBC, including reaction with K_O cells. The female carriers of the abnormal Xk genes determining the above conditions have been shown to have dual populations of Kx-positive and Kx-negative phagocytes and/or McLeod and normal RBC as the result of the phenomenon of Lyonization. The term Lyonization refers to the normal inactivation of one X chromosome in each somatic cell of a woman. If the process occurs randomly in bone marrow cells, the X chromosome carrying an X^1k gene and determining normal RBC and phagocytes will be active in half of her cells, and the X chromosome carrying an abnormal Xk gene and determining defective phagocytes and/or RBC will be active in the other half, thereby producing a mosaic cell population.

Most of the antibodies of the Kell blood group system are immune, IgG, incomplete, warm-acting and best demonstrated by antiglobulin testing. Occasional Kell system antisera, particularly anti-K, are partially IgM, and a few fix complement. Very rare examples gens are readily inactivated by enzymes of plant origin, such as papain or ficin, but in contrast to the M and N antigens are resistant to degradation by neuraminidase. A mutant weak allele at the Duffy locus called Fy^x determines the production of a weak form of the Fy^b antigen and is responsible for most instances of apparent Fy(a−b−) phenotypes in white subjects.

An antibody occasionally formed in Fy(a−b−) persons called anti-Fy3 is capable of reacting with Fy^a-positive and/or Fy^b-positive RBC and would appear to be inseparable anti-Fy^aFy^b but for the fact that its antigenic determinant is not inactivated by enzyme treatment. All Fy(a−b−) RBC also lack Fy3. Thus all Fy^a-positive or Fy^b-positive RBC are Fy:3.

A rare Duffy antibody named anti-Fy4 apparently recognizes an allele to the Fy3 gene variously called Fy or Fy4. The Fy gene is found almost exclusively in black persons and if homozygous results in the phenotype Fy(a−b−). Red blood cells from black subjects of phenotype Fy(a−b−) are always Fy:4, as are many RBC from blacks with the phenotypes Fy(a+b−) (= Fy^aFy) and Fy(a−b+) (= Fy^bFy). Anti-Fy4 will not react with Fy(a+b+) cells. The Fy4 antigen is resistant to enzyme treatment.

Anti-Fy5 somewhat resembles anti-Fy3 in its activity, reacting with Fy^a-positive and/or Fy^b-positive RBC but only in the presence of normal, fully expressed Rh genes. Rh_{null} RBC are Fy:-5. The relationship between Rh and Duffy antigens is a matter for speculation, but it is intriguing to recall that the genes determining both systems are located on chromosome number 1.

A biosynthetic pathway postulated to explain the various relations observed in the Duffy system is shown in Figure 12-2. Two mechanisms of production of Fy(a−b−) cells are shown, one type resulting from the presence of the silent allele Fy (Fy4) and analogous to group O, the other the consequence of a lack of conversion of precursor substance to Duffy precursor substance, and analogous to group O_h. Both paths are required to explain the ability of some Fy(a−b−) persons to make Duffy blood group antibodies and others not. There could be enough similarity between Fy substance and Fy^a and/or Fy^b to prevent Fy(a−b−) persons who are genetically FyFy from making the antibodies, while other, rarer Fy(a−b−) subjects who do not convert precursor substance to Fy substance would be able to do so.

Most anti-Fy^a and anti-Fy^b sera are IgG, incomplete antibodies reactive at 37 C and best detected by antiglobulin testing. Trypsin, papain, ficin, and bromelin may inactivate Fy^a and Fy^b antigenic determinants. Occasional anti-Fy^a sera fix complement and rare examples are saline agglutinins. Some examples show dosage effects. Anti-Fy^a and anti-Fy^b are capable of causing hemolytic transfusion reactions and mild cases of hemolytic disease of the newborn. Recent work has demonstrated an RBC surface receptor in the Duffy system for *Plasmodium vivax* suggesting an explanation for the relative resistance of Fy(a−b−) black people to Vivax malaria.

THE KIDD SYSTEM

In comparison with the Kell and Duffy systems, the Kidd blood group system still seems relatively simple. Two allelic genes, Jk^a and Jk^b, plus a silent allele, Jk, comprise the Kidd system, determining the phenotypes listed in Table 12-5. Homozygous JkJk subjects may make an inseparable anti-Jk^aJk^b antibody, which reacts with a high frequency antigen (Jk3) present on both RBC and phagocytic leukocytes of Jk^a-positive and Jk^b-positive persons. In contrast to the situation with Kell, however, absence of this shared, possibly precursor antigen causes no cell dysfunction.

Antibodies in the Kidd system are incomplete, IgG (often plus IgM), generally complement-fixing, react only at 37 C, and are best demonstrated by antiglobulin techniques, often requiring enzyme

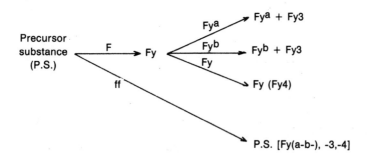

Figure 12-2. *Schematic representation of a possible biosynthetic pathway for development of the Duffy antigens.*

TABLE 12-5

Frequency Distribution of Kidd Phenotypes

	Frequency (%)	
Phenotype	Whites	Blacks
Jk (a+b−)	26	57
Jk (a+b+)	50	34
Jk (a−b+)	24	9
Jk (a−b−)	0*	0*

*Reported primarily in Polynesian and Chinese persons.

pretreatment of the test RBC for detection. Use of an antiglobulin serum containing potent anti-C3b activity sometimes enhances reactions involving Kidd antibodies. Kidd antisera are often weakly reactive and store poorly, with loss of potency. Similarly, Kidd antibodies usually persist for but short periods in vivo and disappear in the space of weeks to months from the patient's serum, so that they are no longer detectable using routine techniques. Transfusion of Kidd-incompatible blood results in their rapid reappearance, with subsequent destruction of the transfused RBC a few days after their administration, a phenomenon known as a delayed transfusion reaction. Delayed transfusion reactions occur in similar situations involving other blood group systems, but are most common with Kidd antibodies. As a general principle it is important to remember that blood group antibodies may not persist indefinitely in detectable form, but that once sensitized, a patient may respond in exaggerated fashion upon re-exposure to the antigen, with possibly disastrous consequences including renal failure and even death from a delayed hemolytic reaction. Several practical points arise from this observation:

1) The patient's clinical records and the blood bank records should include information about known sensitization to blood group antigens. The patient and his physician should be appraised of the existence and significance of such sensitization. Many blood banks provide sensitized patients with wallet-sized cautionary cards bearing the appropriate information.

2) Before blood is selected for compatibility testing the records

of all patients to be transfused should be searched for information indicating prior blood group sensitization or transfusion problems.

3) A nonreactive compatibility test does not provide assurance that a delayed transfusion reaction will not occur.

Anti-Kidd antibodies can also cause immediate hemolytic transfusion reactions and generally mild hemolytic disease of the newborn.

RECOMMENDED READING

Issitt, P.D. and Issitt, C.H.: *Applied Blood Group Serology*, 2nd ed. Spectra. Oxnard, Calif., 1975

Marsh, W.L.: The Kell Blood Group. In: *Advances in Immunohematology*. Vol. 4, No. 2 & 3 Spectra. Oxnard, Calif., N.D.

Marsh, W.L.: The Duffy blood group system. In: *Advances in Immunohematology*. Vol. 3, No. 3. Spectra. Oxnard, Calif., 1975

Marsh, W.L.: The Kell blood groups and their relationship to chronic granulomatous disease. In: *Cellular Antigens and Disease*. Am Assn of Blood Banks. Washington, 1977. p. 52

McGinniss, M.H. and Miller, L.H.: Malaria, erythrocyte receptors and the Duffy blood group system. In: *Cellular Antigens and Disease*. Am Assn of Blood Banks. Washington, 1977. p. 67

Mollison, P.L.: *Blood Transfusion in Clinical Medicine,* 5th ed. Blackwell. Oxford, 1972

Nichols, M.E.: Red cell antigens in health and disease. In: *A Seminar of Polymorphisms in Human Blood*. Am Assn of Blood Banks. Washington, 1975. p. 59

Race, R.R. and Sanger, R.: *Blood Groups in Man*. 6th ed. Blackwell. Oxford, 1975

CHAPTER 13

The MNSs, P, and Lutheran Systems

The blood groups described in this chapter are of relatively minor clinical significance as compared to those detailed in previous chapters, and although of considerable theoretical interest, are of less concern in the blood bank as causes of hemolytic transfusion reactions and hardly ever cause hemolytic disease of the newborn. This is not to dismiss these groups, for serious problems involving them may occur, but rather to indicate the relatively low frequency with which they cause difficulty in the patient. Most of the antibodies recognizing antigens in these groups are non-red blood cell immune, although immune forms secondary to blood transfusion or pregnancy are occasionally encountered.

THE MNSs SYSTEM

The MNSs genes plus their variants and rare alleles determine a blood group system that has been compared to the Rh system in its complexity. The MNSs genes reside on chromosome number 2. At the simplest level of conceptualization, human red blood cells carry either M or N antigens, or both, or one of their rare alleles, so that the RBC of most people type as M, MN, or N. Closely associated with the M and N antigens in much the same way as C and c relate to D are the antigens S and s, resulting in the formation of four complexes: MS, Ms, NS, and Ns. Table 13-1 shows the frequency distribution of the common phenotypes.

The U antigen is produced by all gene complexes making S or s, and occasionally by those that make neither. All U-negative RBC are from black subjects and are also S-negative and s-negative. Of RBC from black donors that are (S–s–), 86% are U-negative, 14%

TABLE 13-1

Frequency Distribution of Common MNSs Phenotypes in White Subjects

Phenotype	Frequency (%) in Whites
MS	6
Ms	10
MSs	14
NS	0.3
Ns	16
NSs	5
MNS	4
MNs	23
MNSs	22

are U-positive. One percent of black persons in the United States are U-negative.

N is not an allele of M, but rather N substance is thought to be the precursor of M. The M and N antigens are glycoproteins, and their specificities are determined by a combination of short repeating chains of specific amino acid sequences and N-acetylneuraminic acid (NANA, a sialic acid) residues. These are attached to a polypeptide backbone that is an integral part of the RBC membrane. Neuraminidase and plant enzymes (e.g., papain) remove NANA and denature the M, N, and S, but not the s or U, antigens. "Defective" forms of the glycoprotein comprise the T and Tn antigens (see Chapter 14 and the discussion of polyagglutination). N substance as a precursor is partly (in heterozygotes) or mostly (in homozygotes) converted to M by the action of the M gene. Almost all group M red blood cells bear some N antigen and even MM cells will absorb anti-N, especially at 4 C, the exception being cells of type (M+S–s–U+) or (M+S–s–U–). The M, N, S, s, and U antigens are well developed on the red blood cells of newborn infants.

A wide variety of aberrant antigens occurs within the MNSs system, some representing the products of rare alleles at the MN or Ss loci that yield weak or negative reactions with standard typing sera. Others are apparently satellite antigens linked to a normal MNSs locus and are detectable only by specific antisera. Among these variant forms may be mentioned the following:

1) M_1. This is an extra potent M antigen related to the standard M as A_1 is to A, though with some difference. M_1 is a gene predominantly found in black subjects, with about 17% of RBC samples from M-positive black people reacting with anti-M_1 as opposed to less than 1% of RBC from white donors.

2) M^g. M^g is a rare allele of M said to be unique to Swiss and Sicilian white persons. The antigen M^g does not react with anti-M or anti-N. M^g-positive RBC have reduced levels of sialic acid. Anti-M^g is a common non-red blood cell immune antibody. In the absence of an anti-M^g typing serum, M^g may be suspected on apparently MM cells that yield single-dose agglutination reactions with anti-M.

3) M^k. The M^k gene is viewed as an operator gene for the production of the M, N, S, and s antigens, none of which are produced on M^k-positive RBC. M^k substance is probably a precursor to N (and thus M) antigens. In this view M^k cells are amorphs analogous to Rh_{null} or K_0 RBC. Decreased sialic acid concentrations are present on M^k-positive RBC, and as is the case with other such cells, both M^g- and M^k-positive red blood cells are agglutinated in saline by appropriate incomplete Rh antibodies. No anti-M^k serum is presently available.

4) M^v. The M^v antigen appears to be a determinant shared between M and N. M^v is produced whenever N is present and reacts with all anti-M sera. Anti-M^v reacts as if it were anti-N.

5) M^c. The M^c antigen is an intermediate between M and N, reacting with most anti-M and some anti-N sera.

6) M_2, N_2. These antigens are weakened forms of M and N and not necessarily the products of alleles to the M and N genes. M_2 and N_2 RBC have decreased sialic acid levels and may exhibit positive direct antiglobulin tests.

Anti-M and anti-N sera for typing purposes are usually produced commercially in animals, though occasionally anti-M of human origin is offered. Lectins can be produced with anti-M activity from the seeds of *Iberis amara* (candytuft) and anti-N activity from the seeds of *Vicea graminea* or *Bauhinea purpurea*. Anti-M, anti-S, and the very rare anti-N of human origin are usually non-red blood cell immune, though all may be produced as immune antibodies after blood transfusion or, very rarely, pregnancy. Anti-s and anti-U are immune antibodies. Naturally occurring anti-M, -N, and -S are usually IgM saline agglutinins reactive at room temperature, while immune anti-M, -S, -s, and -U are IgG (with or without IgM) usually incomplete antibodies optimally reacting at 37 C and often requiring antiglobulin testing for demonstration. Complement fixation by immune antibodies in the MNSs group may occur. Both anti-M and anti-N sera almost always show dosage effects, as may some anti-S sera. About one third of anti-M sera contain anti-M_1 activity. About 3% of random donor sera contain naturally occurring anti-M^g. Anti-M antibodies often exhibit enhanced reactivity at acid pH values. Although anti-N is very rare because of the residual N substance present on almost all RBC, anti-N may rarely be found as an autoantibody in the sera of patients receiving hemodialysis. This occurrence may be caused by alteration of the residual RBC in the machine when its tubing is formalin-sterilized between patient treatments. In other cases "anti-N" may be formed by patients whose RBC lack part of the N mosaic. Anti-N activity may occasionally be found in the autoantibodies produced by patients with autoimmune acquired hemolytic disease.

All of the antibodies of the MNSs system have been implicated as rare causes of hemolytic transfusion reactions and very rare weak forms of hemolytic disease of the newborn.

THE P SYSTEM

The P blood group system is represented by two common phenotypes, P_1 and P_2, and two very rare ones, P^k and p. The proposed biosynthetic pathway for the development of the P antigens is shown in Figure 13-1. A precursor substance p^k is converted under the influence of a Y gene to p substance. The P_1 and P_2 genes convert p substance to P, and in the presence of the P_1 gene P_1 substance is also formed. The amorph p results from the absence of a functional P_1 or P_2 gene. If a Y gene is not present, precursor substance is not converted to p substance. The P_1 and P_2 genes then cause production of P^k plus, in the presence of a P_1 gene, P_1^k substance. Note that P^k phenotypes lack P antigen, and can be separated into P_1^k and P_2^k by anti-P_1. The frequency distribution of P phenotypes is shown in Table 13-2.

There is considerable similarity between the relationships of the A_1, A_2, and O blood group antigens on the one hand and P_1, P_2, and

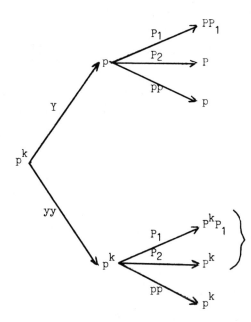

Figure 13-1. *Schematic representation of the production of the P blood group antigens.*

p on the other, summarized in Table 13-3. Anti-P₁ recognizes wide variations in the agglutinability of P₁ RBC, but it is not possible to subdivide these cells further into distinct categories. Homozygous P₁ subjects' red blood cells react more strongly than do those of hetero-

TABLE 13-2

Frequency Distribution of P Phenotypes

Phenotype	Frequency (%)	
	Whites	Blacks
P_1	79	94
P_2	21	6
p	Rare	Rare
p^k	Rare	Rare

zygotes. The P_1 antigen is not fully developed at birth, and its reactions are often weak on the cells of young children. The In(Lu) gene (see Lutheran blood groups), a dominant inhibitor of expression of the Lu^a and Lu^b genes also suppresses formation of the P_1 antigen. The variability of expression of the P_1 antigen on RBC occasionally causes problems in antibody identification if all P_1 red blood cell samples in a panel do not react well. It should also be noted that the P antigens deteriorate on storage. The P antigens are glycoproteins, with alpha-D-galactose the immunodominant sugar. Close interaction exists among the P and I blood group systems as evidenced by the formation of compound antigens such as IP and iP.

Anti-P_1 is present in the serum of all persons of phenotype P_2; anti-P is found in the serum of all P^k subjects, and anti-$P+P_1+P^k$ (anti-Tj^a) occurs in the serum of individuals of genotype pp. Anti-P_1 is usually a weak, IgM saline agglutinin often not reactive above 4 C. Patients with potent immune anti-P_1 antibodies active at room temperature or above should receive P_1-negative blood because of the possibility of a transfusion reaction, but most experts ignore weak, cold-reactive anti-P_1 as not clinically significant. Anti-Tj^a is a hemolysin active at 37 C and is almost certain to cause transfusion reactions if the rare homozygous group pp RBC are not administered. Patients with an unusual hemolytic disease known as paroxysmal cold hemoglobinuria exhibit the Donath-Landsteiner antibody in their serum. This is an IgG autoantibody usually of anti-

---

TABLE 13-3

Similarities Between the P System and the A Portion of the ABO System

ABO SYSTEM			P SYSTEM		
RBC Phenotype	RBC Antigens of Group A	Serum Antibodies Present	RBC Phenotype	RBC Antigens of Group B	Serum Antibodies Present
A_1	$A + A_1$	None	P_1	$P + P_1$	None
A_2	A	Sometimes anti-A_1	P_2	P	Sometimes anti-P_1
O	None	Anti-A + A_1	p	None	Anti-P + P_1 + P^k

P (occasionally of anti-IH) specificity that binds to red blood cells in the cold and upon rewarming to 37 C fixes complement with resultant cell hemolysis.

THE LUTHERAN SYSTEM

The Lutheran system is extensive, with 17 antigens recognized at the time of this writing. The most important Lutheran antigens are determined by two alleles called Lu^a and Lu^b, located on the same chromosome as the secretor genes. The zygosity of a Lutheran gene may sometimes be determined because of dosage effects demonstrable with anti-Lu^a or anti-Lu^b. There is, however, considerable variability in the strength of expression of the Lu^a gene among Lu^a-positive subjects. The Lu^a and Lu^b antigens are present but weak on the red blood cells of newborn infants. The distribution frequency of the common Lutheran phenotypes is shown in Table 13-4. Two relatively uncommon Lutheran genes other than Lu^a have been identified (Lu9 and Lu14) along with very common alleles (Lu6 and Lu8, respectively) plus a number of other common Lutheran genes without identified alleles. The known situation is summarized in Table 13-5.

Two rare but informative types of Lutheran amorphs [Lu(a–b–)] have been found, one the result of the presence of homozygous silent Lu genes (the "recessive" type) and the other caused by the presence of a dominant, nonlinked inhibitor gene called In(Lu). The In(Lu) gene also suppresses expression of the antigens Au^a, P$_1$, and i. These antigens are normally expressed on the recessive type of Lu(a–b–) RBC. RBC from persons of the dominant form of Lu(a–b–) will ab-

TABLE 13-4

Distribution Frequency of Lutheran Phenotypes in the White Population

Phenotype	Frequency in Whites (%)
Lu (a+ b−)	0.15
Lu (a+ b+)	7.5
Lu (a− b+)	92.5
Lu (a− b−)	Very rare

TABLE 13-5

Known Alleles in the Lutheran System

(Approximately 8% of RBC from white persons are Lu(a+), 2% Lu:9, and 2.4% Lu:14.)

	Alleles	Allele Unknown
Common (frequency > 99%)	Lu^b Lu6 Lu8	
		Lu3 Lu4 Lu5 Lu7 Lu8 Lu10
		Lu11 Lu12 Lu13 Lu15
Rare	Lu^a Lu9 Lu14	

sorb small amounts of anti-Lu^b and anti-Lu^{a}Lu^b. The proposed biosynthetic pathway for the development of the Lutheran system is shown in Figure 13-2.

Anti-Lu^a antibodies are generally non-red blood cell immune saline agglutinins of classes IgM and/or IgA, most reactive at 12 C to 18 C and rarely at 37 C. They may show dosage effects, are usually not reactive by antiglobulin testing with commercial broadspectrum reagents, rarely bind complement, and are not enhanced by enzyme testing. Anti-Lu^a, though reasonably common, is usually not detected in practice because most commercially obtainable screening cells are Lu^a-negative. Its usual in vitro reaction conditions are such that it is not detected on compatibility testing. Anti-Lu^a typically produces mixed-field agglutination in laboratory tests and may be suspected on this basis. (Anti-Sd^a also produces mixed-field agglutination, as does anti-A with A$_3$ and A$_{end}$ RBC.) It is thought that the reason for this occurrence is the variation in Lu^a antigen strength from cell to cell in a given subject. Anti-Lu^b is a rare, usually immune antibody, typically of class IgA (sometimes mixed with IgG and/or IgM) and is most reactive at 37 C by antiglobulin or enzyme testing. Anti-Lu^b may fix complement and exhibit dosage effects. Anti-Lu3 is an immune antibody with inseparable anti-Lu^{a}Lu^b activity formed in the recessive type of Lu (a–b–) subject. Antisera to the other Lutheran antigens have generally comprised warm-reacting, IgG antibodies demonstrated by antiglobulin testing.

The Lu^a and Lu^b antigens are rather weakly immunogenic. Naturally occurring anti-Lu^a may cause no significant effects in vivo or at most a slight decrease in survival of transfused incompatible

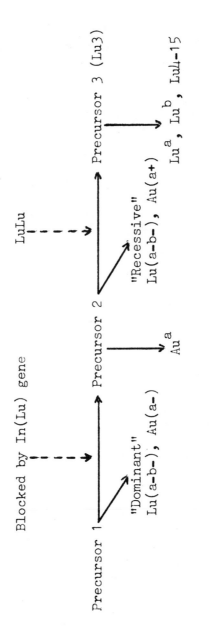

Figure 13-2. *Schematic representation of a theoretical pathway for development of the Lutheran system.*

RBC. Immune anti-Lu^a or anti-Lu^b may potentially cause mild transfusion reactions and hemolytic disease of the newborn. The antibodies of the Lutheran system do not ordinarily persist in vivo and are often formed only by "good responders" who have produced other alloantibodies as well.

RECOMMENDED READING:

Greenwalt, T.J. and Steane, E.A., Eds.: *CRC Handbook Series in Clinical Laboratory Science. Section D: Blood banking,* Vol. 1. CRC Press. Cleveland, 1977

Issitt, P.D. and Issitt, C.H.: *Applied Blood Group Serology,* 2nd ed. Spectra. Oxnard, Calif., 1975

Kaczmarski, G. and Wilson, J.: Other blood groups. In: *Blood Group Immunology. Theoretical and Practical Concepts.* Dade, Miami, 1976. p.69

Mollison, P.L.: *Blood Transfusion in Clinical Medicine,* 5th ed. Blackwell. Oxford, 1972

Race, R.R. and Sanger, R.: *Blood Groups in Man,* 6th ed. Blackwell. Oxford, 1975

Reid, M.E.: The Lutheran blood group system. In: *Advances in Immunohematology.* Vol. 2, No.1 & 2. Spectra. Oxnard, Calif., 1973

CHAPTER 14

The I and Other Blood Group Systems

The existence of "nonspecific" cold agglutinins has always posed a problem to immunologists: there is a contradiction implicit in calling an antibody nonspecific when by definition antibodies are produced in response to a definable antigenic stimulus and possess limited and specific reactivity. The question was at least partially resolved by the discovery of the I blood group system.

The I antigen is only weakly detectable on the red blood cells of infants at birth. Cord RBC are uniformly of group i and only during the first 18 months of life does the I antigen reach adult strength. Marked differences in the I reactivity of red blood cells are present even then and persist as such throughout adult life. Weakly reactive, or I_{int}, RBC are thought to result from the heterozygous genotype Ii or to occur as the result of partial suppression of the expression of I genes, while strongly reactive cells are normally found in homozygous I subjects. The reason for the tardy recognition of the I blood group system is found in the almost universal occurrence of the I antigen on adult red blood cells. In the original studies the RBC of only five persons of 22,000 tested failed to react when tested with a potent anti-I serum. Such I-negative cells from adults are classified as group i_{adult} and have been shown to be of two types: i_1, which possess the most i and least I substance of any RBC type and are found as a rare variant in white people; and i_2, which possess slightly less i and slightly more I and occur rarely in black subjects and very rarely in white persons. RBC of i_{adult} type are found in less than one in 10,000 persons. The i_{adult} phenotype is thought to be the result of the lack of a Z gene necessary for conversion of i substance of I on RBC. Thus the zz genotype results in formation of i_{adult} RBC but does not affect formation of I substance in body fluids. The sera of

155

both i_{adult} types contain anti-I, which reacts with cord RBC; the anti-I from i_1 subjects will react with i_2 cells. Cord red blood cells contain slightly less i substance and somewhat more I than do the cells of either of the i_{adult} types, although the amounts of i and I substances on cord RBC are variable. Anti-I is not present in cord sera. I_{int} cells contain still less i and more I than do cord RBC. The differences in the various types of i red blood cells are apparently quantitative, with development of I substance occurring at the expense of loss of i.

The I antigen is thought to be a mosaic composed of I^F (fetal) and I^D (developed). The I^D component is absent at birth and normally develops during the first 18 months of life. I^D is absent on i_{adult} RBC. I^F occurs on all red blood cells, including cord cells. A third component called I^T, plus some residual i is found on all adult RBC. It has been speculated that I^T might be a transitional form between i and I^D substances.

An inverse relationship has been demonstrated between bone marrow transit time for developing RBC and the amount of i substance on peripheral red blood cells. Patients with diseases causing bone marrow stress such as acute leukemia, chronic hemolytic anemias (e.g., thalassemia major), and some hypoplastic anemias bear increased amounts of i antigen on their RBC. In acute leukemia, the amount of I^D antigen on the patient's red blood cells may decrease. The I and i determinants are situated at an unknown location on the internal structure of the ABH and Lewis substances. The ABO group of a test cell may influence the strength of anti-I reactions: i.e., many anti-I sera react best with group O or A_2 red blood cells, and are at least in part anti-IH, while others (anti-IA or -IB) react preferentially with the I antigens on group A or group B cells. The weak agglutination of cord or i_{adult} red blood cells by anti-I has been shown to be a result of differences in membrane structure (molecular configuration) and not to lack of I antigenic sites. There are about 500,000 I sites on each of the RBC of an adult. I and i substances are found in soluble form in milk, saliva, amniotic fluid, and serum. I substance has also been demonstrated in urine. Saliva is quite rich in I substance. There is no correlation between secretor status or amounts of Lewis or Sd^a substance and the amount of I substance present in body fluids.

Anti-I may be found in human sera in several different situations. Anti-I occurs as a weak complete or incomplete complement-fixing autoantibody reactive at 4 C in the sera of most normal people. It may be found in markedly increased quantities in the serum of patients with mycoplasmal pneumonitis. The anti-I is IgM and upon acidification of the serum may be hemolytic. Usually the form of the anti-I is anti-I^D. Anti-I also occurs regularly in the serum of i_1 and i_2 adults. It should be noted that some anti-I sera react quite strongly with cord RBC, so that dilution may be required to demonstrate the difference in their reactions with cord and adult RBC. Anti-I (or anti-IH) is also found, usually as a mixture of anti-I^D and anti-I^F, or rarely as anti-I^F only, in the sera of patients with cold agglutinin disease or cold antibody-mediated autoimmune acquired hemolytic disease. Anti-I^D can be inhibited by the I substance in saliva or other body fluids.

Weak, cold agglutinating autoanti-I is of no clinical importance, although its presence may complicate compatibility testing requiring that the anti-I be autoabsorbed by the recipient's (preferably enzyme-treated) RBC before satisfactory crossmatching can be accomplished. In contrast, anti-I occurring in true i_{adult} recipients can cause significant clinical reactions if group I RBC are administered. I-negative blood must be secured for transfusion to such patients. The typing of a patient as i_{adult} (I-negative) must be confirmed by using RBC drawn into EDTA and maintained at 37 C until testing is finished to prevent incomplete anti-I from masking I sites on the cells.

Anti-i is a cold agglutinin commonly found in sera of patients with infectious mononucleosis. Occasionally, incomplete IgG anti-i occurs in association with IqM anti-IgG or as a mixture of anti-i plus anti-I. As indicated previously, a relationship between the ABO, I and P systems is apparent in the form of antibodies requiring the presence of determinants from two of these blood groups to react. Anti-IH sera will, for example, not react with O_h, I-positive RBC, agglutinating only cells bearing both I and H determinants. Antisera of specificities IA, IB, IP_1, iP_1, and iH have been identified. It is emphasized that antibodies in the I system may mask the presence of clinically significant antibodies if care is not taken. Similarly they must be differentiated from antibodies to high-incidence antigens, some of which may be poorly developed at birth and therefore not distinguishable from I by using cord RBC. It is useful to recall that autocontrols are usually positive with sera that contain strong anti-I activity.

OTHER BLOOD GROUP SYSTEMS

Several additional blood group systems and a large number of related and unrelated, common and rare red blood cell antigens have been described. Only a few of those of practical or theoretical interest will be mentioned here, and the interested reader is referred to the works listed at the end of this chapter for more complete information. The publications of Race and Sanger and of Issitt and Issitt are particularly recommended. The characteristics and frequency of some of the more common antibodies of possible clinical significance are listed in Table 14-1.

The Diego blood group is of interest principally because the antigen Di^a is almost exclusively found in Mongoloid peoples (up to 12% of whom are Di^a-positive), and is not encountered in the black or white races. Antibodies in the Diego system are usually IgG and react best in antiglobulin tests.

The Xg^a antigen is mentioned only because of its genetic interest and has no clinical significance. The Xg^a gene occurs on the X chromosome, and thus its inheritance is sex-linked. In simplest terms, it will be recalled that the male sex chromosomes are X and Y, the female both X, and hence male sex cells are X or Y and female sex cells all X. When an X sperm fertilizes an egg (X), the offspring will be female (XX) and if a Y sperm fertilizes it, the baby will

TABLE 14-1

Miscellaneous Blood Group Antibodies of Possible Clinical Significance

Antibody	Usual Reaction Conditions	Clinical Significance	Frequency in Whites (%)
Anti-Xg^a	AGT	None (see text)	87 (female); 64 (male)
Anti-Do^a	AGT, Enz.	HDN	67
Anti-Yt^a	AGT	? HTR	> 99
Anti-Di^a	AGT	HDN	< 0.1
Anti-Di^b	AGT, Enz.	HDN	100
Anti-Wr^a	AGT	HDN, HTR	0.1
Anti-Co^a	AGT, Enz.	HDN, ?HTR	> 99
Anti-Vel	AGT	HTR	> 99.9

AGT = antiglobulin test; Enz = enzyme testing; HDN = hemolytic disease of the newborn; HTR = hemolytic transfusion reaction.

be male (XY). If an Xg^a-positive man (Xg^{a}Y) is married to an Xg^a-negative woman (XgXg), all of their male children will be Xg^a-negative (XgY) and their female children all Xg^a-positive (XgXg^a). The Xg^a antigen is useful in studying patients with abnormal sex chromosome karyotypes such as XXY (Klinefelter's syndrome), XO (Down's syndrome), and the like. Anti-Xg^a is usually IgG and reacts best by antiglobulin testing.

The Cartwright system is of little clinical importance, but is mentioned because Yt^a is a relatively potent antigen and anti-Yt^a is reasonably common, causing occasional problems in compatibility testing. Yt^a-negative RBC occur in only 0.2% of white adults and may be difficult to secure for use in identifying a problem antibody. The Yt^a antigen is poorly developed on the red blood cells of newborn infants, and cord cells may be useful here. Anti-Yt^a is always IgG and reacts in the antiglobulin test.

The Wright blood group system is of considerable theoretical interest and practical concern. The Wr^a antigen is rare (about one in 1,500 random white subjects is Wr^a-positive) but naturally occurring anti-Wr^a is very common, being detectable in the serum of about one in 50 random blood donors and more frequently in the sera of pregnant women and multitransfused patients. Anti-Wr^a occurs in up to 12% of sera containing other alloantibodies and in 25% of sera from patients with positive direct antiglobulin tests on their RBC. Inasmuch as screening and panel cells almost never are Wr^a-positive, anti-Wr^a usually goes undetected and only rarely causes crossmatch incompatiblity because of the rarity of Wr^a-positive donor blood. Anti-Wr^a is usually best detected at 37 C by the antiglobulin test. The antibody has caused both hemolytic disease of the newborn and hemolytic transfusion reactions.

Although of no apparent clinical significance in its common form, the Sid (Sd^a) antigen is found on RBC in a spectrum of strengths, with about 1% of white subjects exhibiting Sd^a on their RBC in a very strong form [Sd(a++) or "super-Sid"], 90% exhibiting moderately strong to barely detectable Sd^a, 5% apparently Sd^a-negative but secreting Sd^a substance into body fluids, and perhaps 4% truly Sd^a-negative. Depending on the sensitivity of the testing techniques used, anti-Sd^a can be found in 1% to 10% of normal sera if normal Sd^a-positive test RBC are used, but if super-Sd^a (Cad-positive) RBC are used, reaction can be demonstrated with essentially all human sera – an example of polyagglutinability. Anti-Sd^a is usually IgM, reacts at room temperature or 37 C, and is best detected in antiglobulin tests. Many transfusions of Sd^a-positive blood have been administered to patients with anti-Sd^a without incident, but Sd(a++) RBC may be destroyed prematurely. The blood bank staff should be alert to the frequent occurrence of anti-Sd^a as a cause of weak reactions in screening and compatibility tests. A hint of the cause of the problem may be given by the mixed-field character of the agglutination microscopically and the "red-refractile" character of the agglutinates. Neutralization of the antibody by urine from a strongly Sd^a-positive subject aids in confirming its specificity.

The Sd^a antigen has a terminal N-acetyl-D-galactosamine residue as its immunodominant group, just as do the antigens A and Tn, and may react with anti-A$_1$ lectin (*Dolichos biflorus* seed extract) yielding the apparent contradiction of an anti-A$_1$ reagent agglutinating group O or B (though Sd^a-positive) RBC. The Sd^a antigen is absent from cord RBC and is weakened on maternal RBC during pregnancy, reappearing in normal strength after delivery. Sd^a substance is secreted into body fluids including serum, saliva, tears, and urine.

There are a large number of so-called public and private antigens, occurring so commonly as to be almost universal or so rarely as to be confined to a single family or kindred. A totally unexplained phenomenon is the occurrence in many sera, both from normal donors but especially from patients with autoimmune acquired hemolytic disease, of antibodies to rare antigens to which the subject has never been exposed by pregnancy, transfusion, or other known means. Antibodies occurring in this group include anti-By (Batty), anti-Sw^a (Swann), anti-To^a (Torkildsen), anti-Wr^a, anti-C^x, anti-C^w, anti-Mi^a, and anti-M^g as well as others.

ANTI-LEUKOCYTE ANTIBODIES REACTIVE WITH RBC

Several primarily leukocyte antigens occur in small amounts on red blood cells, enabling the RBC to react, albeit usually in nebulous fashion, with antibodies formed against the shared determinants. Many of these antibodies have no clinical significance but may present problems during compatibility tests. Characteristically the reactions are easily dispersed, but the antibodies are still reactive after considerable dilution, whence the term "high-titer, low-avidity" (HTLA) antibodies. As will be seen below, some of these antigens are also present in soluble form in plasma, and some of the HTLA antibodies are inhibited by incompatible serum. Lymphocyte cytotoxicity tests with HTLA-containing sera are not always positive. On red blood cells the shared antigens are found in greatest strength on reticulocytes, and disappear in unpredictable and variable fashion as the RBC mature.

One such group of shared determinants are the Bg (Bennett-Goodspeed) antigens, which are related to but not identical to certain HLA antigens. Bg^a is closely related to HLA-B7, Bg^b to HLA-BW17, and Bg^c to HLA-A28. Antibodies to one or more of the Bg antigens can be found in the sera of up to 1.5% of hospitalized patients and in up to a third of sera with potent RBC alloantibodies. Anti-Bg antibodies are of doubtful clinical significance, but if present in typing sera can cause false-positive test results. Bg antigens can be detected on the RBC of up to 30% of blood donors using Autoanalyzer technique, but with manual methods only very occasional cell samples are reactive.

Some of the features of a number of antibodies to weak, high-frequency antigens shared by RBC and WBC are shown in Table 14-2. The antigens Chido and Rogers (Ch^a and Rg^a) are found in plasma even at birth though not on cord RBC. Ch^a and Rg^a are not present in secretions. One of these two antibodies should be suspected if a serum agglutinates all RBC tested but the agglutination is fragile, is weak with cord or enzyme-treated cells, and is inhibited by sera from group AB donors but not by saliva samples from the same donors. Table 14-3 summarizes the occurrence of the soluble blood group antigens. In the case of each antigen shown, plasma transfusion may sensitize the recipient to produce antibodies reactive with it. It has been demonstrated that lymphocytes adsorb many plasma blood group antigens, including A, Le^a, Le^b, I, and i. Anti-Lewis and anti-I antibodies may be lymphocytotoxic. It should be noted in passing that while many of the antigens derived from common precursors and shared between WBC and RBC appear to be primarily WBC or plasma antigens incidentally present on RBC, the opposite is also true: the ABH, MN, P, I, and other RBC antigens (though not the Rh antigens) have also been demonstrated on leukocytes.

TABLE 14-2

Some Characteristics of HTLA Antigen-Antibody Systems

Antigen	Symbol	Frequency in Whites (%)	Antibody Inhibited by Plasma Antigen	Antigen Present on Cord RBC	RBC Reactions Decreased by Enzyme Treatment	Clinical Significance
Chido	Ch^a	98.3	Yes	Weak	Yes	No
Rogers	Rg^a	97	Yes	Weak	Yes	No
Cost-Sterling	Cs^a	97	No	Normal	No	No
York	Yk^a	88	No	Normal	Yes (ficin)	No
Knops-Hegelson	Kn^a	99.8	No	Normal	No	No
McCoy	McC^a	99.3	No	Normal	No	Yes
Holley	Ho	99.7	No	Normal	No	Yes

TABLE 14-3

Occurrence of Soluble Blood Group Antigens

	A/B	H	Le	I	i	Ch^a	Rg^a	Sd^a
Antigens on adult RBC and in plasma	Yes	No	Yes	No	Yes	Yes	Yes	No
Antigens in secretions	Yes*	Yes	Yes	Yes	Yes	No	No	Yes
Antigens on cord RBC	Yes**	Yes	No	No**	Yes	No	No	No
Reactions of enzyme-treated RBC	N.C.	N.C.	Inc.	Inc.	Inc.	Dec.	Dec.	N.C.

Le includes Le^a, Le^b, Le^c, and Le^d. * = secretor only; ** = weak reactions; Inc. = increased; Dec. = decreased; N.C. = no change.

RBC ANTIGENS RELATED TO ABNORMALITIES OF THE MEMBRANE SURFACE

Red blood cells of the types designated Tn, En^a-negative, Mg, M^k, and Mi-V are characterized by genetically determined, or in the case of Tn, acquired, abnormalities of the cell surface associated with decreased numbers of sialic acid residues. These cells share decreased expression of their M and N antigens and show increased agglutinability by most antisera, including agglutination in saline by appropriate incomplete Rh antisera, thus resembling RBC after enzyme treatment. Survival in vivo of En^a-negative, Mg, and M^k RBC is normal, but Tn cells show a decreased lifespan. En^a is a high incidence antigen, and En^a-negative RBC, like the others mentioned above, are very rare.

The term polyagglutination is used to describe the agglutination of altered or defective red blood cells by normal sera. Polyagglutination must be distinguished from panagglutination, which is the agglutination of normal RBC by serum substances that may or may not be antibodies, e.g., autoagglutinins, agglutinins reacting with high-incidence antigens, sera containing multiple alloantibodies, albumin autoagglutinins and sera that are contaminated by bacteria or chemicals such as detergents, silica, or metallic cations. Four major categories of polyagglutination are recognized:

1) T-activation. Bacterial or viral neuraminidase either in vivo or in vitro may remove N-acetylneuraminidase (sialic acid) residues

from the red blood cell surface, exposing normally hidden T-receptors to the action of the anti-T present in all normal adult sera. The numbers of receptors exposed is variable, so that the degree of T-activation ranges from partial to complete. If T-activation is partial, only potent anti-T sera will react; if complete, nearly all adult sera react. In vivo T-activation may result in a pseudoautoimmune hemolytic anemia early in the patient's clinical course. Cord sera and the patient's own serum will not react with T-activated RBC. Typing should be carried out with suitably absorbed or aged typing sera (anti-T deteriorates on prolonged storage), with cord sera, or with typing sera treated with 2-mercaptoethanol to destroy IgM antibodies. (Anti-T is IgM.) In cases of in vivo T-activation, blood transfusion should be carried out only with washed RBC to avoid infusion of anti-T, which could cause a transfusion reaction. In vivo T-activation is a transient and reversible phenomenon, disappearing with the sepsis that initiated it. Tk-polyagglutinability resembles T-activation but can be differentiated by the use of appropriate plant seed extracts.

2) Tn-activation. The mechanism of Tn-activation is not known. The alteration occurs only in vivo and is usually permanent. Decreased sialic acid levels are found on Tn-activated RBC and there is shortening of the red blood cell life span in vivo, with chronic hemolytic anemia. Associated leukopenia and thrombocytopenia are common. Tn-activated red blood cells show mixed-field agglutination in vitro and react with the anti-Tn found in essentially all sera from adults. The M and N reactions of Tn-RBC are weak. Typing of Tn-cells for other antigens can be accomplished by enzyme pretreatment, which destroys the Tn receptors, or by use of the same maneuvers as noted above to obtain typing sera free from anti-T. The reaction of Tn-cells with *Dolichos biflorus* seed extract has been noted previously.

3) Cad polyagglutinability. As discussed in connection with the Sd^a antigen, the Cad antigen is a genetically determined very strong form of Sid. All Cad-positive RBC are Sd^a-positive, some will react with *Dolichos biflorus* seed extract (because of the terminal N-acetyl-D-galactosamine residue on the Sd^a antigen), and a few are polyagglutinable. Cord or typing sera treated with 2-mercapto-ethanol can be used for typing Cad-polyagglutinable RBC.

4) Polyagglutinability associated with acquired B antigen. Group A red blood cells with acquired B antigens may be polyagglutinable,

and may or may not also be T-activated. The acquired B phenomenon is of low incidence because the serum of most group A₁ and A₂ subjects can destroy RBC with acquired B antigens in vivo. The RBC of patients with the rare condition known as hereditary erythrocytic multinuclearity with positive acidified serum test (HEMPAS) are also polyagglutinable owing to RBC membrane defects.

Although an A-like antigen is present on both Tn and Cad-poly-agglutinable RBC, as determined by reactions with the lectin from *Dolichos biflorus* seeds, the reactions obtained with other lectins and extracts vary, probably reflecting the influence of subterminal sugar residues on the configuration of the terminal N-acetyl-D-galacto-samine or possibly a reaction with more than one residue.

Polyagglutinins may be present in typing sera but are not always present in sufficient strength to be detectable because of dilution during manufacture. They are frequently discovered as the result of a discrepancy between ABO cell and serum grouping results. Poly-agglutinins are IgM antibodies and react best in saline at room temperature or below. Tests with sera from group AB adults and ABO-compatible cord sera serve as useful screening procedures. A negative autocontrol differentiates polyagglutinins from cold ag-glutinins. The definition of the type of polyagglutinability can be ac-complished with reference to a scheme like the one shown in Table 14-4. Polyagglutinable RBC with sialic acid deficiency include T, Tn, and some acquired B types. Nonpolyagglutinable cells with sialic acid deficiency, as previously noted, include Enᵃ-negative, Mg, Mᵏ, and Mi-V types.

TABLE 14-4

Reactions of Polyagglutinable RBC

	T	Tn	Cad	Acquired B
Papain effect	None	Destroyed	Enhanced	—
Polybrene aggregation	No	No	Yes	Yes or no
Agglutination by lectins:				
Arachis hypogaea	Yes	No	No	Yes or no
Salvia sclarea	No	Yes	No	No
Salvia horminum	No or weak	Yes	Yes	No
Dolichos biflorus	No	Yes	Yes	Yes

RECOMMENDED READING:

Beck, M.L.: The polyagglutinable red cell. In: *The Investigation of Typing and Compatibility Problems Caused by Red Blood Cells.* Am Assn of Blood Banks. Washington, 1975, p.1

Crookston, M.C.: Soluble antigens and leukocyte-related antibodies. In: *Transfusion with Crossmatch-Incompatible Blood. A. Blood Group Antigens in Plasma.* Am Assn of Blood Banks. Washington, 1975. p.17

Dorner, I.M. and Sherman, L.A.: The cold-reacting antibodies, poly-agglutinability and panagglutinability. In: *Transfusion with Crossmatch-Incompatible Blood.* Am Assn of Blood Banks. Washington, 1975. p.59

Greenwalt, T.J. and Steane, E.A. (Eds): *CRC Handbook Series in Clinical Laboratory Science. Section D: Blood banking,* Vol. 1. CRC Press. Cleveland, 1977

Issitt, P.D. and Issitt, C.H.: *Applied Blood Group Serology,* 2nd ed. Spectra. Oxnard, Calif., 1975

Mollison, P.L.: *Blood Transfusion in Clinical Medicine,* 5th ed. Blackwell. Oxford, 1972

Race, R.R. and Sanger, R.: *Blood Groups in Man*, 6th ed. Blackwell. Oxford, 1975

Reid, M.E.: The Sd blood group system. In: *Advances in Immuno-hematology*, Vol. 3, No.4. Spectra. Oxnard, Calif., 1975

CHAPTER 15

Autoimmune Acquired Hemolytic Disease

On occasion the general principle that an organism does not form antibodies against its own tissue antigens is broken and autoantibodies are produced. Autoantibodies may or may not initiate or aggravate disease, and indeed in many cases it appears that they are formed as a consequence of a disease rather than being causative. It has been postulated that in such situations tissue antigens that do not normally come in contact with the immunologic system are released. Not being recognized as "self" these substances may induce antibody formation, which may or may not contribute to further damage. We now recognize that a series of suppressor systems regulate immunologic processes, and that disorders of these systems occur in association with certain disease states. Compelling recent evidence indicates that a reduction in functional activity of suppressor T-cells is involved in the pathogenesis of autoimmune diseases. Autoantibodies have been identified in numerous pathologic conditions, including pernicious anemia, rheumatoid arthritis, disseminated lupus erythematosus, chronic active hepatitis, ulcerative colitis, acute glomerulonephritis, and lymphocytic thyroiditis, as well as in autoimmune acquired hemolytic disease (AHD).

AHD may occur as an idiopathic condition, unrelated to another currently identifiable abnormality in the patient or may develop as a part or complication of a more general disease, especially a collagen-vascular disease or a malignancy of the lymphoid system. The diagnosis of AHD depends on the demonstration of a positive direct antiglobulin test in the presence of a hemolytic process in the patient. The hemolysis may occasionally be brisk, with abrupt appearance of jaundice, fever, splenomegaly, and peripheral blood spherocytosis, but more usually the onset of AHD is insidious, with complaints of fatigue and pallor but no evidence of acute red blood cell destruction. The degree of anemia may range from none to severe, depending on the severity and chronicity of the process (i.e., the amount of shortening of the peripheral RBC life span and the duration of the disease) and the effectiveness of the compensatory efforts of the bone marrow to make additional RBC. Occasionally the marrow can make enough extra RBC to prevent any fall in hematocrit (whence the term acquired hemolytic *disease*, not "anemia").

The autoantibodies produced in AHD may be either warm or cold-reacting types and may or may not fix complement. In some cases only complement is detectable on the cell surface, and in a few instances routine methods detect neither bound IgG nor complement, though more sophisticated techniques may do so. The pattern of cell sensitization by immunoglobulin versus complement has no prognostic significance, and there is also poor correlation between the strength of a positive direct antiglobulin test and the severity of the hemolytic process in the patient. Patients whose RBC yield strongly positive direct antiglobulin tests may suffer no hemolysis, while the red blood cells of 2% to 4% of patients with AHD show negative direct antiglobulin tests, at least by conventional methods. Sensitive research techniques have shown fewer than 35 immunoglobulin molecules on the surface of a normal red blood cell and between 60 and 470 on cells of patients with AHD and negative conventional direct antiglobulin tests. (The usual direct antiglobulin test requires over 500 bound immunoglobulin molecules to be detectably positive.) In individual patients the amount of bound immunoglobulin tends to parallel the severity of hemolysis, the two changing in tandem.

Both warm- and cold-reacting red blood cell autoantibodies may or may not exert harmful effects in vivo. Most normal sera, both adult and newborn, contain weak, complement-fixing, cold-reactive, incomplete autoanti-H activity that is not due to an immunoglobulin. Sera from adults also usually contain low-titered, IgM, cold-reactive, saline-agglutinating autoanti-I. Neither is of physiologic significance. Normal adult RBC incubated at 4 C with a large excess of complement-containing fresh normal serum and then washed with warm saline will yield a positive test with anti-C4 and many broad-spectrum antiglobulin reagents due to complement fixation by anti-H or anti-I (or anti-IH), which has usually eluted from the cells. The same process occurs in a tube of clotted blood stored in the refrigerator. For this reason direct antiglobulin tests are customarily performed on blood samples anticoagulated with EDTA, which binds the free divalent cations necessary for assembling C1 on the surface of sensitized RBC.

Whether immunoglobulins bound to the RBC surface will bring about their accelerated destruction is dependent upon several factors, which will be discussed in detail in Chapter 19. Among these are the amount of bound antibody, its Ig class and subclass, and its ability to bind complement, along with host factors such as the competency of the phagocytic system. Insofar as AHD is concerned, most of the cold autoantibodies are IgM, and their efficiency in binding complement determines 1) whether intravascular hemolysis will occur; 2) whether enough C3b will be bound to cause the cell to be attached to the C3b receptors of the phagocytic reticuloendothelial cells (with possible destruction); or 3) whether sensitization will be too weak to effect any results. Obviously the binding constant of the autoantibody is significant in this connection. In some cases the cell-antibody interaction may be too brief to give time for complement to be activated. In the case of IgG autoantibodies, phagocytes possess a receptor for the C_H3 domain on the Fc portion of the gamma heavy chains of some of the IgG subclasses. Autoantibodies of subclass IgG3 are associated with RBC destruction, IgG1 molecules less so, and IgG2 and IgG4 autoantibodies are generally ineffective in this regard.

Warm-reacting autoantibodies usually produce RBC destruction in the spleen, which, by acting as a filter, increases the chance of interaction between coated RBC and its sinusoidal phagocytes. Splenic sequestration of RBC increases the chances of damage to their surface membrane during the time the cells are bound by the Fc receptors on splenic phagocytes. Even if an RBC is not immediately destroyed, loss of part of its cell membrane results in a change in its shape from a biconcave disc to a sphere, which is rigid and less deformable than is a normal red blood cell and hence more prone to be resequestered.

Autoantibodies reacting at low temperatures apparently do so because RBC membrane alterations in the cold change the configurations of surface molecules to remove steric hindrances or expose antigen-binding sites not accessible at 37 C. Antigen-antibody binding in vivo occurs in blood cooled at the periphery of the body, occasionally resulting in Raynaud's phenomenon, with pain and blanching in fingers and toes due to occlusion of small blood vessels by agglutinated RBC. Complement is bound but often in sublytic amounts. Sequestration in the liver and spleen is effected by the binding sites for C3b on their phagocytic cells. If the red blood cell is not completely ingested and destroyed, it may undergo membrane damage as described above, or its bound C3b may be acted upon by serum C3bINA and cleaved to C3d, for which the phagocyte has no receptor. The cell will then be released, either with membrane damage, in which case its life span will be decreased, or without, in which case it will survive normally, albeit coated with C3d and yielding a positive direct antiglobulin test if an anti-C3d-containing reagent is used.

Harmless warm-reacting autoantibodies are rare findings in healthy persons. Of cases of autoimmune AHD, between 65% and 85% are a result of warm-reacting autoantibodies. The autoantibody is mostly IgG though in a few instances the RBC are also coated with IgA and/or IgM. Cell sensitization with immunoglobulin only occurs in 30% to 40% of cases of warm autoantibody-mediated AHD. Sensitization with immunoglobulin plus complement is found in 40% to 50%, and with complement only in 10% to 20%. Where only complement is found on the red blood cell surface, it is felt that IgG autoantibody is present in concentrations below the threshold of detection, has eluted during the washing step, or is IgM and was not detected by the antiglobulin reagent. Eluates from RBC with only complement demonstrable on the surface will, of course, be unreactive. Little or no free autoantibody is usually found in conventional tests on the serum of patients with AHD caused by warm autoantibodies, but if enzyme-treated RBC are used for testing, autoantibody can be found in up to 80% of cases, in some instances exhibiting hemolytic activity. Apparently the high-affinity autoantibody molecules in the patient's blood are all cell bound and the low-affinity population either not detectable or demonstrable only by the use of enzyme techniques. If the cell-bound autoantibody is IgG, the free autoantibody will also be IgG, but if only complement is detected on the RBC, the free autoantibody will probably be IgM.

The specificity of warm-reacting autoantibodies normally lies in the Rh system, usually in the form of complex, only partially separable reactivity with various normal antigenic determinants and precursors. Three specificities have been designated as : 1) Anti-nl, equivalent to the anti-Hr/Hr_0 alloantibody produced by subjects with Rh-deleted genotypes, reacting as anti-CcEe with normal cells and defining antigens absent from Rh-deleted RBC. 2) Anti-pdl, equivalent to the anti-"total Rh" or anti-RH alloantibody produced by Rh_{null} persons and reacting with antigens absent from Rh_{null} RBC. Anti-LW may be the same as anti-pdl. Anti-U specificity is sometimes found admixed with anti-pdl. 3) Anti-dl, which reacts with Rh precursor substance, variously speculated to be En^a or even Wr^b substance. Simple specificities such as anti-e are often mixed with more complex ones in these sera. Table 15-1 summarizes the concepts outlined. It should be pointed out that not all workers agree with this presentation, denying that autoantibody specificities are the same as identifiable alloantibody specificities. In this view, auto-antibodies are directed against basic RBC structures and only by chance react with Rh determinants.

Blood transfusions to patients with warm autoantibody-mediated AHD do not result in hemolytic transfusion reactions even when crossmatches are incompatible. The transfused cells appear to sur-vive for neither longer nor shorter periods than the patient's own RBC. The blood bank worker however must beware the coexistence of specific alloantibody in the patient's serum, especially if he has been previously transfused.

AHD mediated by cold-reactive autoantibodies is less common than its warm-autoantibody counterpart (15% to 35% of all cases) and occurs in two forms: 1) a usually mild, self-limited disease of acute onset occurring after infection with *Mycoplasma pneumoniae* (atypical pneumonia) or viral pneumonitis; and 2) a chronic occa-sionally idiopathic condition known as cold-agglutinin disease, sometimes occurring in conjunction with lymphoid malignancies. The autoantibody is an IgM, complement-fixing, saline agglutinin optimally reactive at 4 C, and free in the patient's serum in titers of 1,000 or more. In high concentrations the autoantibody may cause saline agglutination in vitro at room temperature but usually not at 37 C. Its reactivity is enhanced in tests employing bovine albumin or enzyme techniques. Cold-reacting autoantibodies usually exhibit anti-I^D plus anti-I^F specificity, though sometimes anti-IH and less

TABLE 15-1

Specificites of Warm Alloantibodies

Antibody Specificity	Produced as Alloantibody in Subjects of Group:	Reactions with RBC Bearing			Similar to or Identical to:
		nl (normal Rh antigens)	pdl (partially deleted Rh antigens)	dl (Rh$_{null}$)	
Anti-dl	? En^a-negative or Wr^b-negative	+	+	+	Anti-precursor (Anti-En^a or −Wr^b)?
Anti-pdl	Rh$_{null}$	+	+	−	Anti-Rh25 (anti-LW) or anti-Rh29 (anti-RH) or anti-U
Anti-nl	Deleted Rh types	+	−	−	Anti-Rh17 or −18 (Anti-Hr$_0$ or −Hr)

An antithetical relationship has been postulated between Rh$_{null}$ and the En^a-negative type. En^a-negative RBC show no En^a, decreased M and N, and increased Rh reactivity; Rh$_{null}$ RBC exhibit increased En^a, M, and N and no mature Rh activity.

commonly IgA anti-Pr (Sp) activity is encountered. The anti-I may be hemolytic at pH 6.8 and is monoclonal with only kappa light chains. Normal low-titered autoanti-I is polyclonal anti-I^D, not hemolytic at pH 6.8, and is neutralized by the I^D substance in saliva and milk, whereas pathologic anti-I^D + I^F is not. Because pathologic cold autoanti-I is in part anti-I^F it may react with cord RBC. The direct antiglobulin test in cases of cold autoantibody-mediated AHD exhibits only bound complement (C4d and C3d), the IgM autoantibody bound at low temperature having eluted.

The presence of large amounts of cold autoantibody in the serum and a positive direct antiglobulin test for bound complement does not necessarily equate with hemolysis or anemia in the patient. The thermal amplitude of the autoantibody is important: complement activity is increased at higher temperatures, but if higher temperatures cause significantly less antibody binding and therefore less complement fixation, hemolysis may not occur. Hemolysis apparently ceases in some patients with cold autoantibodies because of complement depletion. The concentration of C3bINA is important in determining the rate of conversion of C3b to C3d on the cell surface and therefore its ability to attach (or remain attached) to C3b receptors on phagocytes. The binding constant of the antibody is significant in determining whether there will be sufficient time for complement activation before the antibody molecule elutes from a red blood cell. As mentioned above, the functional capacity of the phagocytic system is vital in determining how rapidly RBC destruction can occur. It has been noted that after a time the patient's RBC become resistant to hemolysis, probably because they are coated with C3d and therefore immune to further attack by fresh C3b. Transfusion may result in rapid initial destruction of the new RBC if this is the case. In general, however, hemolytic transfusion reactions are not seen in transfused patients with cold autoantibody-mediated AHD and most of the transfused RBC suvive as well as the patient's own cells.

Patients with infectious mononucleosis sometimes exhibit autoantibodies in their serum including IgM anti-i, IgG anti-i, or IgG anti-i plus IgM anti-IgG. The autoantibody bears no relationship to the Paul-Bunnell antibody and rarely causes significant shortening of the patient's red blood cell lifespan, though occasional cases of frank hemolytic anemia are found. A rare cold autoantibody called the Donath-Landsteiner antibody is produced in patients with paroxysmal cold hemoglobinuria. The subject usually presents with a complaint of hemoglobinuria and sometimes mild jaundice after being chilled and may give a history of antecedent viral illness. The antibody is an IgG, cold-reacting autoanti-P that reacts with the patient's red blood cells at low temperatures. Upon warming, late-reacting complement components are activated and the cells lyse, both in vivo and in vitro. The rate of hemolysis depends on the balance struck between the rate of antibody elution upon warming and the rate of complement activation. An antiglobulin test for bound IgG in the cold would be positive but becomes negative after warming of the cell suspension, with only the anticomplement test now positive. The spacing of the P combining sites on the red blood cell surface is apparently such that much complement is fixed despite the fact that the Donath-Landsteiner antibody is IgG. Rarely, the specificity of the autoantibody in paroxysmal nocturnal hemoglobinuria is anti-IH, anti-I, or anti-i. Screening for the Donath-Landsteiner antibody is accomplished by refrigerating two tubes of clotted blood, warming one of them, and comparing the hemolysis in the two.

It has been observed that in multiple transfused patients there appears to be an unusually high incidence of AHD or at least of patient RBC with positive direct antiglobulin tests unrelated to known alloantibody formation.

Laboratory testing in preparation for transfusion of patients with AHD presents some special problems. In the case of cold autoantibody-mediated AHD blood samples collected in EDTA and rigorously maintained at 37 C from bedside through washing (including washing with warm saline to prevent attachment of blocking anti-I) should be employed for grouping. If the autoantibody is warm-acting and the patient's RBC are coated, gentle elution at 40 C to 47 C for ten minutes may permit valid groupings. Saline typing sera should always be employed: Rh control tests are frequently positive invalidating results obtained using modified tube typing reagents fortified with albumin.

Serum grouping studies, screening tests for alloantibodies, and compatibility testing present special problems in these patients also. Cold-reacting autoantibodies should be absorbed from the patient's serum with aliquots of the patient's own cells collected in EDTA and preferably enzyme treated. Note that this procedure should not be used if the patient has been transfused within three months, for fear of absorbing clinically significant alloantibodies. Alternatively the patient's serum may be warmed to 37 C before testing in an attempt to weaken the reactions of the cold autoantibody, recognizing that alloantibodies nonreactive at 37 C will also be missed. Albumin enhances the reactions of many cold autoantibodies, so that saline screening tests and crossmatches may be necessary. If the cold antibody has anti-Pr (Sp) specificity, enzyme treatment of the test cells will destroy their Pr reactivity.

Patients with warm autoantibody-mediated AHD present some of the same difficulties plus a few special problems. Cell typings require the use of saline-reactive grouping sera and again elution of blocking autoantibody may be required to obtain valid results. Tests for free autoantibody should be conducted with screening cells and if positive, a cell panel should be tested using patient serum in parallel with an eluate from the patient's RBC collected in EDTA (if the IgG antiglobulin test is positive). This is done to determine if the autoantibody has a distinct specificity and to ascertain if alloantibody is present (as well as its specificity). All crossmatches may be incompatible if free autoantibody is present. Autoabsorption is generally unsuccessful in removing such antibody. Dilutions of serum may be used to select the least incompatible blood if transfusion is required.

In cases where AHD is clinically suspected but the routine direct antiglobulin test is negative, performance of the direct antiglobulin test in the cold (with appropriate controls) may enhance the reaction.

DRUG–INDUCED AHD AND POSITIVE DIRECT ANTIGLOBULIN TESTS

The most frequent cause of a positive direct antiglobulin test in hospitalized patients is drug administration. Although hemolytic anemia is mild and uncommon in this situation, the finding of a positive direct antiglobulin test is a source of concern to attending physician and blood bank staff alike and must be elucidated. Immunogens usually have molecular weights in excess of 5,000, and most drugs are simple chemicals with molecular weights of less than 1,000. (Penicillin, for example, has a molecular weight of 320.) For a simple chemical to induce an immune response it must bind to a macromolecule such as a protein. The chemical or one of its metabolites acts as a hapten and the hapten-protein complex can induce antibody formation directed against the chemical.

Four general mechanisms are operative in drug-mediated RBC sensitization:

1) Immune complex adsorption. Drug-anti-drug complexes may attach nonspecifically to the red blood cell membrane and then fix complement. The antigen-antibody complex is weakly bound and may elute to attach elsewhere or be washed off in the process of antiglobulin testing. Free drug-anti-drug complexes can also activate complement, which may subsequently bind to the red blood cell surface. The anti-drug antibody is usually IgM and only the anti-complement (or broad-spectrum) antiglobulin test is positive, but not the anti-IgG reaction. Only small amounts of drug need be taken by the patient to initiate this sequence. Production of this type of positive antiglobulin reaction in vitro requires the simultaneous presence of drug, antibody, and RBC and in practice is usually not successful. Hemolytic anemia as the result of immune complex adsorption is distinctly unusual, but thrombocytopenia occurring on this basis in patients being treated with quinidine is seen rather often. Among the drugs and chemicals reported to result in red blood cell sensitization by the immune complex adsorption mechanism are quinidine, para-aminosalicylic acid, quinine, phenacetin, chlorinated hydrocarbon insecticides, antihistamines, INH, chlorpromazine, pyramidon, dipyrone, phenylalanine mustard, sulfonylurea, insulin, and rifampin.

2) Drug adsorption. A few drugs, notably penicillin, bind firmly to the red blood cell surface. Evidence of the remarkable antigenicity of penicillin and particularly of its major hapten the benzyl penicilloyl group is provided by the fact that over 90% of blood samples from persons in the United States today have been said to contain anti-penicillin antibodies. Most of these are IgM and are readily neutralized by penicillin, but about 13% of people also possess non-neutralizable IgG anti-penicillin antibody. If large doses of penicillin (over 10,000,000 units per day) are administered to a patient with such antibody, a positive direct antiglobulin test can result, and in a few cases there will be accelerated RBC destruction. IgG anti-penicillin antibody does not fix complement and is frequently present in high titer. Cephalosporins may also react in this fashion.

It is possible to elute the anti-penicillin antibody from sensitized

RBC and to test the eluate against cells coated with penicillin in vitro. If an eluate from red blood cells yielding a strongly positive direct antiglobulin test does not react with normal screening cells, the possiblity of drug sensitization should be considered. If the direct antiglobulin test with anti-IgG is positive (and the anti-complement test is negative), an anti-penicillin antibody is a good likelihood. If a history of penicillin administration is obtained, patient serum and the eluate should be tested appropriately. The passive transfer of anti-penicillin antibodies by transfusion can cause febrile reactions in patients being treated with penicillin.

3) Drug modification of the RBC membrane. Red blood cell membranes may be modified by the action of certain drugs such as the cephalosporins in such a way that they non-immunologically adsorb plasma proteins. No antibody formation is involved. A coating of non-immunologically bound albumin, immunoglobulin, complement, fibrinogen, and other plasma proteins is attached firmly enough to the red blood cell surface that it resists being washed away. Direct tests with anti-albumin, anti-fibrinogen, and similar reagents are all positive, as well as those with various antiglobulin sera, including anticomplement sera. The RBC from as many as 3% of patients receiving high doses of cephalosporin drugs may demonstrate this phenomenon. No shortening of RBC lifespan appears to occur. Cephalosporins can also elicit formation of specific antibodies and may cross-react with anti-penicillin antibodies. Normal RBC may be coated with cephalosporins in vitro to test for this possibility.

4) Unknown mechanism. Positive direct antiglobulin tests with anti-IgG and the occasional induction of mild hemolytic anemia serologically indistinguishable from warm autoantibody-mediated AHD may be found in patients treated with alpha-methyldopa (Aldomet). The means by which this comes about is unknown. In contrast to the first three mechanisms described, the drug need not be present for the antibody to attach to the patient's red blood cells: the antibody reacts with determinants on the RBC membrane, not the drug. The induced antibody is IgG, is found both free in the serum and bound to RBC, and has the same range of reactivities as described for idiopathic warm autoantibody-mediated AHD. Up to 15% of patients treated with alpha-methyldopa positive direct antiglobulin tests, though less than 1% develop anemia. The frequency

of occurrence of positive direct antiglobulin tests is dose-dependent; the test does not become positive until after three to six months of treatment and may persist for several months after drug administration is discontinued. The related drug L-dopa also may cause development of positive direct antiglobulin tests on the RBC of up to 10% of treated patients but does not induce hemolytic anemia. Mefenamic acid reportedly can do the same.

LABORATORY INVESTIGATION

The workup in the laboratory of the problem presented by the patient whose RBC yield a positive direct antiglobulin test is directed toward three general goals:

1) Determination of the components on the red blood cell surface as a guide to the type of problem (e.g., drug-induced versus idiopathic AHD).

2) Elimination of the possibility of an alloantibody as the cause of the positive direct antiglobulin test.

3) Ascertainment of the specificity of any antibody present on the cell surface or in the patient' serum.

The first step in investigating the problem should be to obtain a complete and accurate drug and transfusion history as a guide to likely possibilities. Direct antiglobulin testing should be repeated using monospecific antisera, including at least anticomplement and anti-IgG testing. If IgG is present on the patient's red blood cells, an eluate should be prepared and both the patient's serum and the eluate tested using screening cells. If the screening cells react, an RBC panel that includes cord cells and an autocontrol should be tested. Techniques should include saline, albumin, and enzyme tests as indicated by preliminary results, conducted at 37C, room temperature, and/or 4 C. Specially treated (penicillin-coated) RBC are used as required.

The distinction between warm and cold antibody-mediated autoimmune AHD is easily made by the pattern in the monospecific direct antiglobulin tests and the reaction character (especially the thermal amplitude) of any free autoantibody. Distinction between alpha-methyldopa and warm autoantibody-mediated AHD on the one hand and the remainder of the drug-induced conditions characterized by positive direct antiglobulin tests on the other is assisted by recalling that the sera from patients with the former pair of conditions will generally react with enzyme-treated normal RBC, while those from patients with the latter will not react in the absence of the drug. The monospecific direct antiglobulin test pattern is again informative: there is a positive anticomplement test with drug complex adsorption, but the anti-IgG test is usually negative. When drug adsorption alone occurs (penicillin-type) the opposite is the case. When nonspecific drug adsorption has occurred, a multi-specific antiglobulin pattern is present. The presence of high-titered cold agglutinins in the serum will distinguish between positive, direct anticomplement tests in cold autoantibody-mediated AHD and in immune complex adsorption. The distinction between alpha-methyl-dopa-induced and idiopathic warm autoantibody-mediated AHD can be made by history.

Weakly positive direct antiglobulin tests are occasionally encountered on red blood cells from patients with marked reticulo-cytosis or megaloblastic anemia. The explanation for this occurrence is unclear, as pointed out by Mollison. The theory that a reaction takes place between the transferrin normally present on the surface of reticulocytes and anti-transferrin in antiglobulin serum (even if the latter has not been absorbed out by the manufacturer) does not appear to be adequate.

RECOMMENDED READING:

Bell, C.A. and Stroup, M.A.: Autoimmune problems. In: *Transfusion with Crossmatch Incompatible Blood*. Am Assn of Blood Banks. Washington, 1975. p.1

Dodd, B.E. and Lincoln, P.J.: *Blood Group Topics*. Williams and Wilkins. Baltimore, 1975

Garratty, G.: Immune hemolytic anemia. II. Warm and cold antibody auto-immune hemolytic anemia. In: *Advances in Immunohematology*. Vol. 2, No.2. Spectra. Oxnard, Calif., 1973

Garratty, G.: Immune hemolytic anemia. III. Drug-induced hemolytic anemia. In: *Advances in Immunohematology*. Vol. 2, No. 3. Spectra. Oxnard, Calif., 1974

Greenwalt, T.J. and Steane, E.A.: *CRC Handbook Series in Clinical Laboratory Science. Section D: Blood Banking*, Vol. 1. CRC Press. Cleveland, 1977

Issitt, P.D.: Autoimmune hemolytic anemia in patients with a negative

CHAPTER 16

Practical Considerations in Blood Bank Methodology

A variety of factors influences in vitro antigen-antibody reactions and the outcome of blood bank serologic procedures. To avoid false and misleading results, meticulous technique is required, together with an informed awareness of the many variables affecting immunohematologic studies. This chapter discusses some of the practical considerations involved.

Serum rather than plasma is required for the study of reactions between antigens and antibodies in blood banking because so many of them entail complement fixation. In addition, plasma occasionally contains tiny clots that may simulate agglutination. To obtain serum in cases where the patient's blood exhibits a coagulation defect, addition of a drop of thrombin solution may be required to clot the specimen. Care should be taken to prevent bacterial growth in blood specimens to be tested in the blood bank by avoiding gross contamination and by keeping sample tubes under refrigeration when not in actual use. Bacterial contamination of a blood specimen may result in several undesirable consequences: 1) sera may become anticomplementary; 2) sera may become panagglutinating, reacting with all RBC; 3) bacteria or their breakdown products may be adsorbed to RBC and the RBC may be agglutinated by antibacterial antibodies in test serum; and 4) RBC may be T-activated.

Some serum samples contain large amounts of dextran administered as a plasma expander. Sera from patients with diseases such as cirrhosis, sarcoidosis, multiple myeloma, or macroglobulinemia may contain elevated concentrations of globulins, while those from patients with chronic inflammatory disease may also contain large amounts of fibrinogen. Blood samples obtained via a needle through which dextrose solutions have just been administered may be a mixture of blood and dextrose in water. All of these substances cause RBC in vitro to stack like coins (rouleaux formation), and microscopically agglutination may be simulated. Addition of a drop or two of saline to the serum-cell mixture, or replacement of serum with saline after incubation and centrifugation, will usually disperse rouleaux while true agglutination will persist. Fibrinogen is six times as efficient as gamma globulin in producing rouleaux formation. Red blood cell typings employing tube technique and washed cell suspensions are preferable to slide typings using unwashed RBC to avoid this problem as well as the unwanted neutralizing effects of soluble blood group antigens that may be present in the cell donor's serum. Antiglobulin tests are not affected by rouleaux formation, since the washing procedure removes the responsible substances.

The use of hemolyzed blood specimens for cell grouping, serum screening, or compatibility testing should be avoided. Antibody-mediated hemolysis may be masked if the test serum is already hemoglobin-tinged. Although red blood cells from clots may be used, anticoagulated blood is preferable for the preparation of cell suspensions. RBC from clotted blood stored in the refrigerator may exhibit a weakly positive direct antiglobulin test as a result of C4 bound by cold incomplete anti-H or cold agglutinating anti-I or-IH. Blood samples anticoagulated with EDTA avoid this problem because the anticoagulant acts by complexing the divalent cations required as cofactors for complement activity. Clotted or EDTA-anticoagulated blood can be successfully stored for several days at 4 C but if longer storage is contemplated, preservative solutions such as ACD, CPD (see Chapter 23), or Alsever's solution are required or the RBC and serum should be (separately) frozen. Loss of agglutinability of red blood cells stored as clots becomes appreciable after two weeks; and even in preservative solutions, Lewis and MN reactivity is decreased after three weeks of storage. Freezing is particularly useful for long-term preservation of rare RBC samples. Agglutinability remains intact for years after storage in glycerol at –80 C.

The techniques used for blood grouping studies must follow the manufacturer's directions exactly for the use of a given antiserum. Failure to observe this precaution is a common mistake of inexperienced blood bank workers. It cannot be assumed that the testing procedure directed by one manufacturer will be proper for use with a reagent from another, even if the two materials are of the same type. Under no circumstances should antiglobulin testing be used in conjunction with a typing serum unless so specified by the manufacturer: saline agglutinins often contain incomplete antibodies of a second specificity. Antisera should be treated with care to preserve their reactivity. Routine reagents should be refrigerated when not in actual use. Repeated freezing and thawing of little-used antisera will reduce their potency. Care should be taken to mix frozen antisera thoroughly after thawing because of the tendency of thawed sera to layer. Thumbs should not be used for bottle stoppers, especially with antiglobulin sera, which are readily neutralized by desquamated skin cells, body oils, or sweat. When antisera are used from bottles with dropper tops, care must be taken not to interchange the tops. Dropper tips should never be touched to blood, other reagents, or to the skin. Antisera from two bottles should not be pooled. Antisera that have passed their expiration dates are unreliable and should be discarded. Even in-dated reagents may lose their potency, and the practice of using positive and negative controls must be particularly observed when employing little-used or long-preserved reagents. Many antibodies store very poorly, rapidly losing their reactivity even when frozen — a problem that complicates the submission of samples to reference laboratories.

The preservation of complement activity under various storage conditions has been described in Chapter 7. It should be noted that sera stored frozen may become anticomplementary.

Red blood cell antibody and antigen detection techniques as discussed in Chapter 6 are dependent on the proportion of cells to antiserum. Heavy cell suspensions (near 50%) are used for slide tests, weak suspensions (4% to 6%) for tube tests. Considerable care should be used to ensure that cell concentrations are within the prescribed range and that the amount of cell suspension delivered is reasonably uniform in all work. There is reason to question the traditional semiquantitative preparation of RBC test suspensions and the practice of measuring quantities in terms of "drops." Depending on the bore of the pipette, the angle at which it is held, and the viscosity of the fluid being delivered, there may be a difference of fivefold in the amount of fluid in a "drop." Commercial antisera are prepared for use with RBC suspensions of a particular strength. The use of cell suspensions that are too concentrated or the addition of too little antiserum may result in weak or false-negative test results. In general, the sensitivity of red blood cell agglutination reactions is enhanced by increasing the ratio of antiserum to cells. Weak antibodies may require ratios of even 1,000:1 for detection.

The amount of antibody combining with RBC antigens varies with time. Hughes-Jones and his associates found in a study using five volumes of an anti-D serum to one part of Rh-positive RBC that six hours were required for maximum antibody uptake: 25% of the antibody was taken up within 15 minutes, 75% in one hour, and 95% in two hours. The significance of these observations is immediately evident when abbreviated incubations of compatibility tests are requested. Potent antibodies will probably be detected with minimal incubation; weak antibodies may be missed. The assumption that antibodies weakly reactive in vitro are not clinically significant is not always correct. Antibody binding by red blood cells is greatly influenced by temperature: although the association constant of warm-reactive antibodies is not altered at low temperatures, the rate of their uptake is, e.g., anti-D binding may occur 20 times as rapidly at 37 C as at 4 C. In the case of cold agglutinins, the binding constant itself is altered with temperature, and is appreciably higher at 4 C than at 37 C because of temperature-induced conformational changes in antigenic determinants. The presence of bovine albumin also enhances the uptake of many IgG antibodies by red blood cell antigens. IgM uptake is generally not enhanced except for anti-I, the agglutination strength of which may be significantly increased. Low-ionic strength suspending media for RBC greatly increase the speed of uptake of most antibodies, both IgG and IgM, and to a lesser extent, the amount of their uptake. A recently proposed modification of the techniques for antibody screening and compatibility testing using low-ionic strength saline (LISS) permits reduction of incubation times at 37 C from thirty minutes to ten minutes with no loss of sensitivity.

The factors influencing the strength of RBC agglutination reactions are particularly apparent when antiserum strength is determined by titering. The antigenic strength (including storage age) of the red blood cells, the RBC concentration, the duration and temperature of incubation, the nature of the suspending medium, and the technique of producing and reading agglutination all influence the end point. Similar factors influence tests for hemolysis, particularly cell storage age (stored RBC lyse more readily as they age). In addition, the complement concentration in the system affects hemolysis, with more complement required to effect hemolysis as the ratio of antiserum to RBC is decreased. Patient serum is not predictably uniform or reliable as a complement source for serologic work and may occasionally be anticomplementary.

Knowledge of a few special or rare causes of confusing results will facilitate interpretation of routine tests. Important in this regard is the occasional finding of serum antibodies to a variety of passively adsorbed miscellaneous materials on the red blood cell surface, including acriflavine or other dyes, altered albumin, lactose, corticosteroids, and a variety of antibiotics including chloramphenicol, neomycin, streptomycin, and others. Antibodies reactive with yellow dyes such as acriflavine used to color anti-B grouping serum are occasionally encountered. Not unusual are antibodies to bovine albumin stabilized in preparation by the addition of caprylate or other three- to eight-carbon fatty acids that induce conformational changes in its structure. Antibodies to various preservatives as listed above in the suspending media of commercial screening or panel cells may cause reactions that falsely appear to be a result of red blood cell agglutinins. In each situation, fresh RBC without the additive will be nonreactive. So-called albumin autoagglutinins in patient sera may cause errors in slide typing tests using unwashed RBC and anti-D as a consequence of the fact that most slide typing antisera are fortified with albumin. Use of an albumin autocontrol should detect the problem. If, however, the patient's serum contains antibodies to other additives in the typing serum, false-positive tests may still occur that an albumin control in the slide typing test for D will not detect. In consequence of this fact, commercial suppliers now offer Rh control solutions containing the additives but not the anti-D. Note that these control materials are not used to replace albumin in antibody screening or identification tests. The use of washed RBC suspensions in tube typing tests obviates all of the problem but, of course, requires employing an anti-D typing serum that will reliably react in saline tube tests. Occasionally, "albumin autoantibodies" react only in the antiglobulin test. Albumin autoantibodies must be differentiated from examples of albumin-dependent anti-I. It should be noted that commercial albumin preparations differ in their ability to enhance agglutination or sensitization by incomplete blood group antibodies. The action of albumin in this connection is thought to be caused by a contaminant inasmuch highly purified albumin is not effective.

Enzyme testing is widely used in blood banks to enhance weak agglutination reactions. As already noted care must be taken when interpreting tests with enzyme-treated RBC because certain antigens (M, N, S, Fy^a, Fy^b, Tn, Ch^a, Rg^a, Yt^a, and Sp [Pr]) are damaged or destroyed as sialic acid residues are removed from the cell surfaces. Enzyme treatment is not an all-or-none phenomenon, and enhancement of reactions occurs in graded fashion. Overtreatment of red blood cells may cause them to agglutinate spontaneously. Of the commonly used protease enzymes employed in blood bank studies (trypsin, ficin, papain, and bromelin) papain is favored by most workers. Neuraminidase is primarily used for investigative work. It should be recalled that all red blood cell antigen-antibody reactions are not enhanced by enzyme treatment; nonimmune anti-A and anti-B reactions for instance are not typically strengthened. Enzyme solutions are not stable for extended periods, especially when diluted, and should regularly be prepared freshly. Freezing may prolong storage time, but refreezing is not recommended. Different batches of enzyme often vary considerably in potency. Appropriate autocontrols are necessary in all tests using enzyme-treated RBC to rule out misleading positive reactions with cold autoagglutinins. Positive controls should also be used to ensure that RBC enzyme treatment has been effective. It should be observed that RBC already coated with antibody (i.e., cells with a positive IgG antiglobulin test) may react nonspecifically if the one-stage technique is used. Enzyme testing can be carried out as a one-stage procedure with simultaneous combination of RBC, enzyme, and serum, or as a two-stage test in which RBC are pretreated with enzyme solution, washed, and then combined with test serum. Antiglobulin testing may be combined with enzyme treatment of red blood cells to produce a very sensitive test for antibody detection, but caution must be observed in interpreting results: trivial antibodies of no clinical consequence are often detected using this methodology, and much unnecessary effort may be expended in the elucidation of problems of no importance to the patient.

The antiglobulin test when properly performed is one of the most powerful yet trustworthy techniques available in the blood bank to detect antigen-antibody reactions. Methodologic errors, however, may invalidate its results. Inadequate washing of the cell button after exposure to test serum may leave behind traces of globulin that will cause false-negative tests. Prozone phenomena are common with antiglobulin sera, and raw sera are almost always diluted by manufacturers of commercial reagents to eliminate this problem. It should be appreciated that weakly sensitized cell suspensions may still fail to react if the antiglobulin serum is too potent. The dilution optimal for detection of strongly sensitized RBC may not be optimal for detection of weakly sensitized cells or cells sensitized by antibody of a different specificity. The manufacturer's choice of dilution is thus a compromise, albeit usually an acceptable one. It is emphasized that antiglobulin sera vary in their ability to detect antibodies of different specificities, and the antiglobulin serum that reacts crisply with RBC sensitized for example with anti-D may not react as well with cells sensitized with anti-Fy^a, an effect perhaps related to the immunoglobulin subclass of the IgG molecules being detected. Antiglobulin sera purchased commercially are usually pooled products raised in several animals often immunized somewhat differently in an attempt to circumvent this problem. It is not recommended that commercial antiglobulin sera be diluted inasmuch as they are often fortified in such a way that dilution may impair their reactivity. A maneuver occasionally useful in strengthening an equivocally positive direct antiglobulin test on cord red blood cells is to suspend the washed cell button in fresh AB serum for 20 minutes at 37 C, followed by thorough repeat washing and performance of the antiglobulin test. Antiglobulin sera may react more strongly if tests are briefly incubated at 4 C, but like any departure from manufacturer's directions this is done at the user's risk and must be rigidly controlled.

An overall check of the adequacy of an antiglobulin test procedure can be performed by adding a drop of an RBC suspension sensitized by incomplete IgG antibody to negative compatibility tests. The suspension is recentrifuged and re-examined for agglutination. The unreacted antiglobulin serum present at the end of the compatibility test should agglutinate the added presensitized RBC. Suitable suspensions of precoated red blood cells are commercially available or may be readily prepared in the blood bank.

False-positive antiglobulin tests may occur as the consequence of bacterial contamination of serum or RBC, use of tubes with residual detergent from inadequate washing, or the presence in solutions of silica leached from soft glass storage bottles or metals from pipes or stills. Contamination of cord RBC by Wharton's jelly (from the umbilical cord) may cause equivocally false-positive test results. Rarely, antiglobulin sera contain traces of heteroagglutinins (antihuman species antibodies) not completely absorbed out during manufacture. Among the causes of false-negative reactions are the use of glassware with traces of residual serum from past tests, use of too concentrated a cell suspension, inadvertent failure to add antiglobulin serum to the test, or dissociation of the antibody from the RBC during washing or if a prolonged interval supervenes between washing and addition of antiglobulin serum.

In some cases it may be necessary to test sera in which complement activity has decayed or that have become anticomplementary. A two-stage test is recommended under these circumstances. The test serum is first treated with EDTA to bind divalent cations. These are not necessary for antibody binding to the red blood cell suface but are required for the binding of C1, and thus in EDTA-treated serum altered C1 components cannot bind to the cells. Were they to do so, further activation of the complement sequence would be blocked. The EDTA-treated test serum is washed away after it has had an opportunity to react with the test RBC. Fresh AB serum is then added as a source of complement, the mixture reincubated to allow complement fixation, and the antiglobulin test procedure completed. If anti-Lewis antibodies are being sought by this technique, appropriately Lewis-negative AB serum must be used to prevent neutralization of bound antibody by soluble Lewis substance. It should be appreciated that antibodies with low binding constants may dissociate and be lost during the washing steps between the first and second stages of the test.

The saline solution used in blood bank testing deserves more care in its preparation than it sometimes receives. Isotonic saline (0.15 M aqueous NaCl) contains about 0.9% by weight of sodium chloride and has approximately the same osmolality as blood. An appreciably more dilute solution will cause RBC suspended in it to swell or even rupture. Hypertonic solutions (i.e., solutions with osmolalities greater than that of blood) cause red blood cells to shrink and wrinkle (crenate) and may cause bound antibodies to elute. As previously noted, saline must be free from foreign matter: this means that water used in its preparation must be of laboratory reagent grade (sterile, with a pH of about 7.0, and essentially ion-free as measured by a conductance equivalent to less than 4 ppm of dissolved solids). Certain bacteria and fungi will grow in saline, and soft-glass bottles may leach silica into it. These facts require that frequent washing of storage containers and dispensers be carried out. Saline should be prepared in only reasonably small amounts at a time. Many smaller blood banks find it more practical to purchase saline from a commercial supplier than to prepare it.

The effects on RBC antigen-antibody reactions of such variables as temperature and duration of incubation have been discussed previously. It is appropriate to recall that "room temperature" may range from 50 F near a leaky window on a winter's day in the north to 90 F in an antique laboratory in the summer anywhere. Incubation periods should be stated in the laboratory's procedure manual and recommended by the manufacturer for the reagents in use. Foreshortened incubations during compatibility testing or antibody screening give patient antibodies less opportunity to attach to RBC and may cause false-negative test results. It is emphasized, however, that the ultimate responsibility for the care of a patient lies with his attending physician, and that emergency situations may require use of less than optimal testing procedures at his discretion.

Centrifugation is commonly employed with tube testing in American blood banks to speed red blood cell agglutination reactions. It should be appreciated that given enough time such reactions would occur without centrifugation. The amount of centrifugal force (measured in $\times$ G, or number of times the force applied exceeds that of gravity) is determined by the speed of rotation and the radius of the circle through which the tube is spun, according to the formula: relative centrifugal force, or RCF ($\times$ G) = 0.00001118 $\times$ rotating radius (cm) $\times$ speed of rotation (rpm). Nomograms are published in standard manuals, including the "Technical Manual of the American Association of Blood Banks," which facilitate computation of RCF. Forces approaching 1000 $\times$ G are possible in small tabletop centrifuges. Duration of centrifugation is important: short rapid centrifugation may effect agglutination equivalent to that achieved by slower more prolonged spinning. The relationship however is complex and both variables require standardization in the laboratory. Note that the duration and force of centrifugation used in washing cell suspensions is different from that optimal for producing agglutination and that different centrifugation times are used for saline versus antiglobulin tests. Inadequate centrifugation will result in false-negative reactions, while excessive centrifugation may pack even unsensitized red blood cells so tightly that resuspension is difficult and the result misinterpreted as agglutination. The practice of recentrifuging reaction mixtures and performing second readings for agglutination yields unreliable results.

Special testing procedures are used in the blood bank to elucidate particular problems:

1) Inhibition tests are useful for studies involving soluble antigens such as H, A, B, I, i, Sd^a, or Lewis substances in saliva; A, B, i, Lewis, Ch^a, or Rg^a substances in plasma; or Sd^a substance in urine. Inhibition tests are performed by titering an antiserum with equal added amounts of test substance and inert control substance. Positive inhibition requires a fourfold difference in titer (two tubes if doubling dilutions of antiserum are used) to be significant. It is obvious that inhibition tests are insensitive, requiring the neutralization of three fourths of the antibody to be positive. The antiserum used for inhibition tests must be carefully selected: IgM blood group antibodies are generally easily neutralized, but IgG antisera are not. Use of too strong an antiserum means that technical variations may cause false changes, while a weak antiserum may be nonspecifically inhibited.

2) Specific mixed agglutination tests are used for the study of cells either physically not suitable for agglutination tests (e.g., epithelial cells) or diluted in a large volume of nonreactive cells (e.g., a few Rh-positive RBC mixed with large numbers of Rh-negative RBC). The technique involves antibody sensitization of test cells, removal of free antibody, and addition of "indicator" RBC that share the antigen being demonstrated. Thus, in a typical positive test, buccal epithelial cells from a group A subject, treated with anti-A and then washed to remove unbound antibody, would be surrounded by rosettes of group A RBC added to the preparation.

3) Absorption tests are used to demonstrate reduction in the titer of an antiserum by cells that it cannot agglutinate but that nonetheless are capable of antibody uptake. Repeated absorptions may be necessary to demonstrate significant decreases in titer, particularly with antibodies with low binding constants. Several absorptions with small volumes of RBC will remove more antibody than one absorption with a large volume of cells. Put another way, with a serum cell ratio of 5:1, only three times as much antibody will be absorbed as with a ratio of 1:1. Absorption techniques are often used to remove one antibody from a mixture with another to obtain a monospecific

antiserum. Antibody activity of the absorbed specificity may occasionally reappear in time.

4) Elution procedures are much more sensitive than absorption tests: antibody recovery by elution may approach 100% if proper techniques are used. Elution techniques are used to obtain antibodies from sensitized RBC when there is no free antibody or to demonstrate the fact that antibody uptake by weak antigens has occurred. Elution procedures are useful in identifying antibodies in a mixture, in confirming antibody specificity, and in the workup of cases of hemolytic disease of the newborn, hemolytic transfusion reactions, and autoimmune acquired hemolytic disease. In contrast to pure absorption studies, which work best with antisera of high average binding constant, elution procedures are easiest with low-affinity antibodies, which are easily removed from RBC. If the binding constant is very low, however, antibody recovery may be poor, because antibody molecules may dissociate from the red blood cells during preliminary washing and be lost.

The amount of antibody bound to an RBC during absorption studies depends on the ratio of antiserum to cells, the mean binding constant and heterogeneity index of the antiserum, the number of antigen sites per RBC, and whether equilibrium has been reached. The degree of antibody dissociation in elution studies is a consequence of the dissociation constant and the elution technique. When using heat elution methods one should remember that varying degrees of reassociation of eluted antibody with antigen may occur if the cell-eluate mixture cools before separation.

The interpretation of work involving mixtures of antibodies and absorption and/or elution techniques must take into account the Matuhasi-Ogata phenomenon. When an antibody is specifically bound to its corresponding antigen on the surface of a cell a second antibody of different specificity for which the cell lacks the antigen may also be adsorbed. Both antibodies may subsequently be eluted from the cell surface. This phenomenon occurs irrespective of blood group specificity and has been demonstrated with complete and incomplete agglutinins, warm and cold autoantibodies, leukocyte antibodies, and even with antibodies not directed at blood cells. Nonspecific uptake of second antibodies by sensitized RBC explains such phenomena as absorption of anti-A by group O RBC with positive direct antiglobulin tests, or absorption of both anti-A and anti-K from a serum containing both antibodies by D-positive, K-negative RBC.

INTERPRETATION OF SEROLOGIC REACTIONS

The interpretation of the strengths of serological reactions using traditional technics is subjective and open to variation in the hour-to-hour work of a single technologist much less among different technologists on different days in different laboratories. Because so many variables enter into the interpretation of such reactions, minute distinctions (as between $2^1/_2+$ and $3+$ readings) are unreproducible and thus unwarranted. When reading of an agglutination test is performed, the supernatant fluid should first be examined for hemolysis. If the test serum was originally free of hemoglobin, hemolysis constitutes a positive reaction. This also assumes that the test RBC were not unduly fragile because of storage age or other factors and that free hemoglobin was not transferred to the reaction tube with the red blood cells. The latter possibility is another reason for the use of washed RBC suspensions for all blood bank testing.

Detection of agglutination after centrifugation requires that the cell button be dislodged from the bottom of the tube. This is best done by tilting or rolling the slanted tube, or, less desirably, by a minimum of gentle shaking. Gross examination should be conducted in strong light, preferably using a concave mirror or hand lens. Agglutination is graded on the basis of its macroscopic appearance as follows:

4+ – a solid button
3+ – several large clumps
2+ – medium-sized clumps, clear background
1+ – small aggregates, reddish background
Tr (trace) – microscopic aggregates

Microscopic examination should be used to confirm all weak or negative reactions unless the manufacturer of an antiserum states to the contrary for his product. Particular attention should be paid to the character of the agglutination if it is macroscopically weak to ascertain if the aggregation is truly weak, with large numbers of small clumps, or whether it presents a mixed-field pattern, with several large, often loose clumps of cells lying amidst large numbers of free cells. The presence of mixed-field agglutination is a valuable clue to the antigen-antibody reaction occurring. Mixed-field agglutination is seen under the following circumstances: after production of mixtures of RBC in vivo (e.g., after blood transfusion, bone marrow grafting, or fetal-maternal hemorrhage), in chimeras, in polyagglutinable states, in cases where there are reduced numbers of antigen sites on RBC (e.g., RBC from patients with acute leukemia, from elderly patients, or from patients with certain weak variants of A or B), and typically in the reactions of anti-Sd^a and anti-Lu^a.

The application of the Autoanalyzer to blood grouping studies has permitted some very sophisticated research work because of the instrument's extraordinary sensitivity in detecting agglutination. Application to mass routine blood grouping and typing studies in large centers has yielded considerable savings in time and money because of the Autoanalyzer's speed. Figure 16-1 shows a flow diagram of the operation of the instrument as used in RBC antigen-antibody studies. Serum samples are aspirated from sampler cups into plastic tubing where they are mixed with test RBC in isotonic saline or LISS, an enzyme solution (bromelin), and a potentiating agent of agglutination (PVP or polybrene). The controlled introduction of air bubbles between serum samples prevents contamination of each by its predecessor and cleanses the tubing between samples. The mixture is moved in continuous fashion through the system by peristaltic pumps, passing into a mixing coil with a time delay that permits antigen-antibody interaction. Saline is then introduced into the tubing, and the mixture is passed through another coil to disperse rouleaux. After being pumped through a settling coil the partially agglutinated red blood cell suspension next passes to a T-tube where the heavier agglutinates settle out, passing to waste. The remaining unagglutinated cells are then lysed and the hemolysate passed through a colorimeter. Thus, it is the hemoglobin from the unagglutinated RBC that is ultimately measured. The change in optical density from the value obtained using an unagglutinated RBC suspension is proportional to the number of agglutinated cells removed. In other configurations the Autoanalyzer fitted with multiple channels instead of one is used for simultaneous ABO and Rh RBC typing or for antibody screening. Up to 120 blood specimens per hour can be processed. The major disadvantages of the instrument when used for automated typing relate to lack of a positive sample identification system and absence of a printout that interprets reactions. Occa-

sional errors are encountered owing to misinterpretation of weak reactions by the technologist machine operator.

RECOMMENDED READING:

Greenwalt, T.J. and Steane, E.A. (Eds): *CRC Handbook Series in Clinical Laboratory Science. Section D; Blood Banking*, Vol. 1. CRC Press. Cleveland, 1977

Huestis, D.W. et al: *Practical Blood Transfusion*, 2nd ed. Little, Brown and Co. Boston, 1976

Issitt, P.D. and Issitt, C.H.: *Applied Blood Group Serology*, 2nd ed. Spectra. Oxnard, Calif., 1975

Miller, W.V. (Ed): *Technical Manual of the American Association of Blood Banks*. Washington, 1977

Mollison, P.L.: *Blood Transfusion in Clinical Medicine*, 5th ed. Blackwell. Oxford, 1972

Moore, B.P.L. et al: Serological and technical methods: *The Technical Manual of the Canadian Red Cross Blood Transfusion Service*, 7th ed. Canadian Red Cross. Toronto, 1972

Walker, R.H. (Ed): A seminar on problems encountered in pretransfusion tests. Am Assn of Blood Banks. Washington, 1972

CHAPTER 17

Blood Grouping and Compatibility Testing

Because blood transfusion is potentially a hazardous procedure, elaborate safeguards are established to protect the recipient. Chief among these is compatibility testing, or crossmatching. This is essentially a trial transfusion carried out in a test tube to see whether serologic incompatibility that might foreshadow a transfusion reaction in the patient can be detected. Laboratory evidence of incompatibility between the proposed donor's red blood cells and the patient's serum, whether the reaction is hemolysis, agglutination, or sensitization detected by enzyme or antiglobulin testing ordinarily precludes the transfusion of that unit of blood to the patient. Although occasionally this rule is broken intentionally, this is done only on the order of a physician versed in immunohematology and then only reluctantly, for a hemolytic transfusion reaction may result in the death of the recipient.

The first step in selecting blood for transfusion is to determine the patient's ABO blood group and Rh_0 (D) type so that blood of the same type can be selected for compatibility testing. Contrary to popular opinion, clinical situations so emergent that not even a minute can be spared for determining the ABO group of the patient, much less for compatibility testing, and where blood transfusion must be initiated irrespective of potential hazard, simply do not exist. The infusion of crystalloid and/or colloid materials can provide the few minutes of time required for the blood bank to do essential minimum work. The time-honored concept of emergency administration of group O, Rh-negative blood, even with low anti-A and anti-B titers, without doing a compatibility test or at least screening the patient's serum for alloantibodies, is an invitation to disaster. The sera of up

196

to 5% of hospitalized patients bear alloantibodies of potential clinical significance, a large proportion of which will react with random "O-negative" RBC. The emotion surrounding major clinical problems cannot be allowed to interfere with optimal medical care. On the other hand, these comments cannot be used to justify a casual or lackadaisical response on the part of the blood bank to urgent patient-care problems: full cooperation must be extended with all haste consistent with patient safety. What shortcuts or abbreviations of standard procedure are in order is a medical decision, but this must be an informed decision, not an emotional one. If any compromises with standard procedure are made, the reasons for doing so must be fully recorded in the patient's clinical record at once, and complete testing carried out in retrospect. Particularly if the newer compatibility testing procedures are used, employing low-ionic strength saline as described below, two technologists working together can provide a unit of fully crossmatched blood within 15 minutes of receipt of a patient's blood sample.

The usual use of blood permits sufficient time for adequate laboratory testing before transfusion. It is apparent from the preceding chapters that completely compatible blood, identical to that of the patient for all of the dozens of known blood group antigens, cannot be furnished without an identical twin as a donor. Yet we know that random donor RBC bear numerous potent antigens that may be absent from the RBC of the recipient and to which he may become sensitized with antibody production. Such antibodies will present a source of difficulty if subsequent blood transfusions are required (even if a delayed transfusion does not occur) and may result in hemolytic disease of the newborn if a woman later becomes pregnant.

The logistical problems of seeking type-compatible blood for transfusion may be illustrated by an example. If a patient is of group O, approximately two in five random donors will be ABO-compatible. If we require D-compatibility as well and the patient is D-negative, only one in six random donors will be acceptable. Donors who are of group O and D-negative will be only about one in 15. If Kell-compatible blood is also desired, and the patient is of genotype KK (one in 500), the likelihood of a random donor being O-, D-, and K-compatible rises to one in 7,500. If identity for even six or eight antigens is required, the chance of compatibility may become infinitesimally small. Thus, some compromise between risk of sensitization and practicality must be reached, accepting the fact that some hazard is attached to any blood transfusion.

This compromise in usual practice consists of selecting blood identical for the major ABO and D types and screening the patient's serum and that of the donor for clinically significant alloantibodies. The necessity for ABO compatibility is readily apparent in that the isoantibodies reciprocal to the patient's ABO antigens are universally present, and administration of ABO-incompatible blood predictably causes hemolytic transfusion reactions. Group O blood from random donors is not desirable for transfusion to recipients with A and/or B antigens because, although the transfused group O cells provoke no reaction, the isoantibodies in the plasma of a group O donor may be sufficiently potent to destroy the remaining RBC of the patient. The custom of testing for hemolysins or titering the iso-agglutinins in the plasma of group O donors with a view to designating units safe for administration to non-group O recipients is outmoded and should be abandoned. In practice group O red blood cells, preferably washed, and group AB plasma (if required) are given if group-specific whole blood is not available.

Of all other antigens, only compatibility for D is regularly required. This is because D is the most immunogenic of the non-ABO red blood cell antigens and is also statistically likely to produce immunization of a sizable number of people if D-compatibility is not required. Other antigens are potent but rare, or potent but too common to sensitize any large number of random recipients, or too weak to be of clinical concern. It is reasonable to enquire what risk would be run if no crossmatching were performed and only ABO compatibility ensured by testing. Patients can be separated into high- or low-risk groups on the basis of whether they have ever been transfused or pregnant. The low-risk group may still carry naturally occurring antibodies but most of these are weak, not reactive at 37 C, and rarely cause clinically significant problems. Their occurrence in the random population is estimated at less than one per 1,000 hospitalized patients.

As discussed by Sturgeon, the potential for a transfusion problem in the high-risk patient is proportional to the chance that blood group immunization has occurred as the result of previous blood transfusion or pregnancy. In the case of transfused patients this likelihood is the product of the frequency with which a random transfusion contains an incompatible blood group antigen and the frequency with which such exposure induces alloantibody formation. The chance of a transfusion recipient being exposed to an incompatible blood group antigen is the product of the frequency of its occurrence in the population times the frequency of its absence. For example, D-positive persons comprise about 85% of the white population, D-negative persons about 15%. The product of the two values is about 13%. Therefore, if a single blood transfusion from a random donor is administered to a random recipient without regard to D type, 13% of transfusions would result in D-negative recipients receiving D-positive blood.

The immunogenicity of common blood group antigens has been estimated, i.e., the likelihood of antibody production in a patient receiving a single 500 ml transfusion of blood incompatible for a given antigen. Table 17-1 shows the relative chances of such immunization. For D this is 50%. Multiplying 13% by 50% we discover that slightly more than 6% of random recipients transfused with a single random unit of blood would produce anti-D. Since the chance of such recipients receiving D-positive blood on the occasion of a second, later transfusion is 85%, the likelihood of a second transfusion provoking a hemolytic reaction (assuming no crossmatch) is 6% times 85%, or about 5%. Clearly, the occurrence of a transfusion reaction in every twentieth patient receiving blood a second time is unacceptable, and in consequence routine transfusion practice requires not only ABO compatibility and crossmatching but also compatibility for D to prevent sensitization. Contrasting this situation with that found in the case of other blood group antigens (see Table 17-1), we find that only 0.4% of random recipients of a single random unit of blood will produce an antibody to K, the next most immunogenic common blood group antigen after D, and that a later random transfusion, even if it were not crossmatched, would cause a reaction only four times in 10,000. Hence assuring K compatibility is not attempted in usual practice, and donor serum screening for alloantibodies and compatibility testing are relied upon to detect the occasional patient with anti-Kell antibodies in his serum and to prevent administration of incompatible K-positive RBC.

About 1% of recipients of ABO and D-compatible single-unit blood transfusions will become detectably immunized to another blood group antigen. The likelihood of a transfusion reaction in the

TABLE 17-1

Relative Immunogenicity of Common Blood Group Antigens

Antigen	Antigenicity (%)	Percentage of All Recipients Immunized by First Random Transfusion	Percentage of All Recipients with Reaction to Second Random Transfusion
D	50.0	6.4	5.4
K	5.0	0.4	0.036
c	2.0	0.32	0.26
E	1.7	0.36	0.11
k	1.5	0.003	0.003
e	0.6	0.012	0.012
Fy^a	0.2	0.045	0.030
C	0.1	0.020	0.015
Jk^a	0.07	0.012	0.010
S	0.04	0.010	0.005
Jk^b	0.03	0.0059	0.0043
s	0.03	0.0031	0.0028

case of administration of uncrossmatched blood is thus ten times as great in the high-risk group as in low-risk subjects. In the multiply transfused patient the incidence of blood group immunization reaches a plateau value of between 10% and 30%.

A special routine is recommended for use in the case of selected patients whose disease is such that repeated transfusions over a period of years are anticipated necessary, with a high risk of sensitization to multiple blood group antibodies, requiring units of blood so statistically rare as to be almost unobtainable and very expensive to search out. To minimize the development of such situations, as soon as these patients are recognized, extended typing of their red blood cells should be carried out using all commonly available antisera, and those antigens absent from the patient's RBC and potent enough and common enough to make sensitization likely are identified. Blood negative for these antigens is then selected for transfusion insofar as possible.

The routine screening of the sera of both recipients and donors for the presence of alloantibodies is standard practice. The specificity of all unexpected antibodies should be determined before compatibility testing is begun. Units of blood determined by typing tests with potent reagent antisera to be appropriately antigen-negative are then used for crossmatching. The compatibility test should not be used in lieu of this procedure: reliance cannot be placed on the antibody in a patient's serum to detect incompatible RBC in vitro. The serum antibody may be weak and/or the red blood cell antigen weakly expressed, resulting in the incompatibility being missed. Rapid in vivo destruction of the RBC may still occur if the blood is transfused. As discussed in the next chapter, RBC used for screening are specially selected to yield strong reactions with common alloantibodies.

Donor blood is screened for the presence of alloantibodies to prevent their introduction into the recipient's plasma. Although transfused red blood cell alloantibodies rarely cause clinically significant destruction of the patient's RBC, reactions between donor bloods have been reported. Thus, the transfusion of a unit of blood containing potent anti-Kell antibodies into a K-negative recipient would not cause difficulty, but if a second K-positive unit were then immediately administered, antibody-mediated hemolysis of the RBC of the second unit could occur.

ABO GROUPING

ABO grouping employs two sets of tests, one to confirm the other. Red blood cells are grouped with potent anti-A and anti-B (and preferably anti-A,B) typing sera, and the serum is tested for the presence of the reciprocal anti-A and/or anti-B isoantibodies using known group A_1 and group B red blood cells. Serum grouping (or "back-typing") is omitted with specimens from infants under the age of three months for the purposes of determining the baby's ABO group because of the delayed appearance of blood group isoantibodies produced by the baby and the possible persistence of those of maternal origin. ABO grouping of red blood cells is most reliably performed using tube-testing technique with saline suspensions of once-washed RBC. A variety of potential errors and sources of confusion attend the use of slide typing methods as noted below. Slide tests for ABO grouping should not be placed on warming stages: weakened agglutination may result from heating inasmuch as anti-A and anti-B are optimally reactive at low temperatures. The routine

use of O serum (anti-A,B) is recommended to confirm RBC grouping results and to detect some of the weak subgroups of A. Incubation of ABO cell or serum grouping tests at 4 C may be employed to
enhance weak reactions, but care must be taken to employ suitable
controls to guard against nonspecific reactions. Strongly reactive
test RBC must be chosen for use in serum grouping tests to detect
weak patient isoantibodies.

Discrepancies between ABO red blood cell and serum groupings
should be resolved before blood is selected for compatibility testing.
These may be of four types:

1) False-positive RBC grouping reactions may be a result of the
presence in the typing serum of antibodies of another specificity.
Such reactions are unusual if washed RBC are used for grouping
studies unless the cells are already coated, for example, with autoantibody (i.e., yield a positive direct antiglobulin test) in which case
such antibodies as anti-Gm occasionally present in grouping
reagents may agglutinate the RBC. A direct antiglobulin test on the
patient's RBC will identify the problem, and the use of a different
grouping serum will usually circumvent it. If unwashed RBC are
used for grouping, the adherent patient serum may contain antibodies to substances present in typing sera such as the yellow dyes
used to color anti-B (acriflavine, tartrazine yellow #5). The antigen-
antibody complexes formed may attach to RBC and cause false agglutination. Unwashed cord RBC coated with Wharton's jelly may
also give false-positive RBC grouping reactions. Rarely an undetected antibody to a rare, low-incidence blood group antigen is
present in grouping sera and may yield incorrect results, e.g., anti-Bg
activity is occasionally found as are cold agglutinins and unab-
sorbed antibodies of specificities other than that labeled. Routine
quality assurance testing of all lots of reagents will detect some of
these problems.

2) False-negative RBC grouping reactions are rare in the absence
of defective typing sera or technical errors. If unwashed cell suspensions are used, the attached patient serum may occasionally contain
such a large amount of soluble blood group substance (soluble A
and/or B substance) as to neutralize the typing serum and prevent
agglutination. The use of washed RBC suspensions avoids this problem. Weakly reactive RBC reactions also occur in people of subgroups of A or B, in chimeras, and patients with ABO mosaicism, in
patients with, for example, acute leukemia and in newborn infants.

3) False-positive serum groupings are common and have multiple possible causes: cold autoagglutinins (usually anti-I or anti-IH) may agglutinate all RBC. An autocontrol will also give positive test results. Anti-A₁ may be found in the sera of persons with weak subgroups of A or AB. Typing of patient RBC with an anti-A₁ reagent is useful, recalling that anti-A₁ lectin will also react with Tn- and Cad-positive RBC. Anti-H (or anti-IH) may occur in the serum of group A₁ (0.6%) or A₁B (3%) subjects. Routine use of group O RBC in serum grouping reactions will identify this problem. Room-temperature reactive IgM alloantibodies may agglutinate group A or B test cells if they possess the corresponding antigens. Passively acquired alloantibodies may give similar results. Screening tests for alloantibodies will detect these situations. The presence of drugs or chemicals such as antibiotics (e.g., chloromycetin, neomycin, tetracycline), hydrocortisone, sugars, EDTA, stabilized albumin, and other materials used as preservatives in commercial RBC suspensions may cause problems in serum grouping reactions if the patient's own serum contains antibodies to them. The antigen-antibody complexes formed occasionally agglutinate test RBC. Washing of the cells is recommended before preserved RBC are used in any serologic work. If reagent RBC have been contaminated by microorganisms they may become polyagglutinable. Routine quality assurance testing with AB serum should preclude this problem. Rouleaux formation may simulate agglutination and can be dispersed using saline dilution or replacement methods previously described.

4) False-negative serum grouping reactions may occur with sera from patients with hypogammaglobulinemia or other disease states in which the function of the immunologic system is impaired (e.g., advanced Hodgkin's disease or multiple myeloma). Isoantibodies of their own manufacture are, as mentioned, absent from the serum of newborn infants and may be weak in the elderly.

Technical error must be considered a possibility when there is a discrepancy in red blood cell and serum groupings. The use of cell suspensions that are too concentrated, warming of the test, or the use of weak or contaminated reagent RBC, typing sera, patient RBC, or patient sera all may give anomalous results. Occasionally, tests are misread because an optical aid is not used to check for weak agglutination or because hemolysis is interpreted as a negative reaction.

The investigation of ABO grouping problems begins with retesting the patient's RBC using washed cell suspensions and anti-A (plus anti-A₁ if appropriate), anti-B, anti-A,B, and anti-H sera. Repeated serum grouping should include the use of A₁ (and A₂ as indicated) B, O, and cord O red blood cells plus an autocontrol. Incubation periods should be prolonged to 30 minutes at room temperature and at 4 C using proper controls. All apparently negative test results should be examined microscopically. Use of a fresh patient's blood sample for the work is desirable. Screening for alloantibodies may also require repeating. Supplemental work may include absorption-elution studies with the patient's RBC, hemagglutination-inhibition testing for plasma blood group substance, and determination of secretor status. The cause of any mixed-field agglutination seen should be elucidated to ascertain whether it is caused by transfusion, weakened antigens on some cells because of disease, a chimera or mosaicism, or a weak subgroup of A or B.

Rh TYPING

Typing of the patient's red blood cells for the D antigen is customarily carried out simultaneously with ABO grouping. The distinction between pure saline-agglutinating anti-D and the reagents sold for slide typing is becoming blurred inasmuch as most commercial slide-typing sera are also suitable for tube testing of saline-suspended RBC. Anti-D sera labeled for use in saline tube tests may not be suitable for slide typing. If slide typing technique is used, a control test must be performed using a preparation of the diluents and additives included in the anti-D serum by its manufacturer. This precaution ensures against misinterpretation of agglutination of the test cells by, for example, albumin autoagglutinins adherent to the patient's RBC reacting with albumin in the typing serum, or agglutination by one of the additives of patient cells sensitized with AHD antibody. Simple addition of a drop of bovine albumin to patient cells on a slide has been used in the past as a control, but it has been shown that this practice may not detect all false-positive D-typing errors. The use of washed RBC and tube technique for D typing will decrease the problem of false-positive tests. As an aside, it may be remarked that in typing of RBC of partially deleted D phenotypes (e.g., CD-) for antigens other than D, the presence of otherwise insignificant traces of anti-D in the typing sera may result in false-positive test results because of the heightened reactivity of the D antigen on such cells. Thus, traces of anti-D in anti-K typing serum could make Rh-deleted, Kell-negative RBC appear to be K-positive.

Contamination of D typing sera by antibodies of other specificities may also occur. Anti-Bg antibodies may give false-positive test results with rare strongly Bg-positive RBC. If washed RBC suspensions are not used for typing purposes, anti-Gm antibodies in typing sera may react with serum proteins in a cell suspension and the resulting antigen-antibody complex sensitize the red blood cells so that a falsely positive D^u test is obtained.

The improvement in D typing sera in the last decade has reduced the numbers of blood samples not agglutinated by slide anti-D reagents. Before a specimen is accepted as D-negative, however, antiglobulin testing must be carried out on any potentially sensitized cell suspension that has not visibly reacted with the anti-D serum. Red blood cells whose reactions with anti-D are only demonstrable by antiglobulin testing are termed D^u-positive, but are treated as D-positive for both donor and recipient purposes. Unless a direct antiglobulin test on patient RBC is a routine part of a blood bank's pretransfusion testing, one must be performed as a control on all positive D^u tests to rule out false-positive results as a consequence of RBC coating by immunoglobulins prior to D testing. It should be noted that the terms "Rh-positive" and "Rh-negative" as currently used refer to the D antigen only. Specifically, the term Rh-negative does not imply the absence of the antigens C or E as it once did, and CdE red blood cells now qualify as Rh-negative.

The compatibility test or major crossmatch between the prospective donor's RBC and the serum of the patient is conducted to see if a detectable serologic reaction occurs between the two as evidence of the likelihood of an in vivo transfusion reaction. The compatibility test also serves as a check against major errors in ABO grouping and in the screening of the recipient's serum for alloantibodies, although obviously there are circumstances in which the major crossmatch cannot detect mistakes (e.g. group O RBC being crossmatched for a group A patient, D-positive blood being crossmatched for a D-negative recipient lacking anti-D). On the other hand, the major crossmatch may detect incompatibilities not suspected otherwise (e.g., the presence of a serum alloantibody that reacts with a rare antigen absent from the screening cells and therefore missed but present on the donor's RBC). It cannot be emphasized too strongly that good as present blood bank techniques are, they cannot ensure the success or safety of a blood transfusion. Negative compatibility testing does not guarantee normal survival of transfused RBC, does not prove that any alloantibody is present, does not ensure that a hemolytic transfusion reaction, immediate or delayed, will not occur, and cannot prevent immunization of the recipient by donor blood group antigens. There is considerable difference between a test tube and a human subject, and apparently compatible RBC may be rapidly destroyed in some patients. It has been estimated that abnormally short red blood cell survival occurs in up to one of every 20 transfusions despite the absence of demonstrable blood group antibodies, and frank hemolytic transfusion reactions have been seen in their apparent absence. Records of past transfusions should always be consulted before compatibility testing is begun. This is done for two reasons: first, to confirm the patient's ABO group and Rh type (though old records must never be substituted for actual repeat ABO and D testing), and second, to determine if blood group sensitization has ever before been detected. A previously formed antibody may have disappeared and not be demonstrable in the current blood sample, but may reappear in anamnestic fashion if the appropriate antigen is retransfused, with a resulting delayed transfusion reaction. Once a clinically significant blood group antibody has been detected in a patient's serum, all subsequent transfusions must lack the corresponding antigen irrespective of whether the antibody can be demonstrated at a later date.

The procedure for compatibility testing varies somewhat among laboratories, but in general includes mixing a saline suspension of RBC from a prospective donor unit with recipient serum, incubating at room temperature, centrifuging, and reading for hemolysis and/or agglutination. A second tube is similarly prepared with the addition of bovine albumin and incubated at 37 C before centrifugation. Examination is followed by antiglobulin testing. All results should be recorded as they are read. It is obvious that no single test procedure will detect every blood group antibody. The crossmatch in saline at room temperature detects antibodies in the ABO, MN, Lewis, P, Wright, and Lutheran systems, many of which are inhibited at higher temperatures or in the presence of albumin. The test in albumin at 37 C detects Rh antibodies and a few others, and the presence of albumin enhances later antiglobulin testing results.

Antibodies in all systems are detected by the broad-spectrum anti-globulin test, including incomplete IgG antibodies and IgM non-agglutinating antibodies that fix sublytic amounts of complement. Enzyme tests, though not generally a part of routine compatibility testing, supplement the antiglobulin test and detect a few alloanti-bodies (notably examples of anti-E) not found by antiglobulin testing, though missing others as previously noted. Enzyme testing cannot be used in place of the antiglobulin test. It should be appre-ciated that exceptions occur to the above generalities and that a given blood group antibody may react anomalously.

The minor crossmatch, in which donor serum is tested against recipient red blood cells, is now little used and generally thought un-necessary if donor units are screened for the presence of alloanti-bodies. There is little evidence that transfused alloantibodies can cause clinically meaningful harm even if the recipient's RBC bear the corresponding antigen except in extraordinary cases. Recent work suggests that it is feasible to shorten the incubation time at 37 C in compatibility tests from the usual 30 minutes to 10 minutes or less without any sacrifice of sensitivity or specificity if low-ionic strength solutions are used in place of isotonic saline.

A few general comments regarding crossmatching procedures are pertinent. Compatibility testing begins with the drawing of a blood sample from a patient. Positive identification of the patient is essential and must be made by examining the patient's identification wristband, not simply by asking the patient's name. Specimens must be fully labeled at the bedside after being drawn, not beforehand or later, and should bear the patient's full name, hospital identification number, the date and the phlebotomist's initials. Commercial systems that provide multiple pre-numbered identification tabs for requisition, patient specimen, crossmatched unit of blood, and patient records are available. If patient specimens are not properly labeled, they must not be used for testing. Requisitions must agree on all points with specimen labels. Under no circumstances may an improperly labeled or unlabeled patient specimen be returned for "correct" identification or labeling.

Patient blood samples less than 48 hours old are required for compatibility testing to ensure the presence of adequate amounts of complement and to guard against the appearance of a serum allo-antibody in the interim. If serial transfusions are administered, new compatibility tests with a new blood sample from the patient are required every 24 hours because of the increased possibility of allo-antibody production. This means that if several units of blood have been crossmatched at one time but only part of them given to the patient, the remainder must be recrossmatched with a fresh blood specimen if more than 24 hours have elapsed between the first set of transfusions and the second request. Recall that if blood of an ABO group different from that of the patient has been administered, subsequent typing may yield confusing or atypical reaction patterns.

Clotted blood specimens are required to provide serum for compatibility testing. In the case of patients suffering from a coagulation defect a drop of thrombin added to their blood sample will cause rapid clotting. If the patient is receiving heparin, the addition of protamine may be required. It is good practice also to obtain a patient blood specimen collected in EDTA to serve as a source of patient RBC free from complement attached in vitro by cold auto-antibodies. Such a sample is useful in the event that extended RBC typings or a direct antiglobulin test is necessary in the course of elucidating an incompatible crossmatch, a positive antibody screening test, or a transfusion reaction.

Units of blood and blood products should be inspected for hemolysis and/or other evidence of bacterial growth before being released for transfusion. The identification numbers, ABO group and Rh type on the blood unit, and the compatibility certification tag must be collated. The patient name and hospital identification number on the request for blood issue and the compatibility certification tag must be compared. A fully completed compatibility certification tag must be attached to the unit of blood, stating, at a minimum, the patient's name, hospital identification number, the nature and amount of the blood product, its ABO group and Rh type if applicable, the date of testing, a statement of compatibility, the expiration date (and time if applicable), and the initials or signature of the technologist who performed the compatibility test. Many blood banks arrange that this be a two-part form with the first part placed in the patient's clinical record and the second remaining attached to the empty blood bag, to be returned to the blood bank after the transfusion. It is convenient that the second part of this tag contain brief instructions as to procedure to be followed in case of a transfusion reaction and a place where the nature of the reaction can be indicated. The expiration date (and time where applicable) on the bag label should be checked before issue and again before transfusion of any blood product. After a blood transfusion has been administered, donor tubing segments and recipient specimens should be stored at 4 C for seven days for use in case complications occur. The empty blood container should similarly be retained for at least 24 hours. It is emphasized that non-technical errors are the usual causes of hemolytic transfusion reactions: the patient's sample is mislabeled, the wrong unit of blood is issued from the blood bank, or the unit is administered to the wrong patient.

The common causes of incompatible crossmatches are:

1) Clerical error. The patient sample may be misidentified or the wrong patient sample or the wrong segment used for testing.

2) Errors in patient or donor RBC grouping or typing.

3) Presence of a positive direct antiglobulin test on donor RBC.

4) Existence of an alloantibody in the recipient's serum that was not detected during screening. If the screening cells lack a rare antigen, a corresponding patient alloantibody will be missed unless the donor RBC bear the antigen. Red blood cells used for antibody screening tests, even if a mixture of cells from two donors, frequently lack the antigens C^w, Lu^a, Kp^a, Js^a, Di^a, and ce^s.

5) Presence of dextran or paraproteins in patient serum causing rouleaux formation.

6) Existence of cold agglutinins in the patient's serum. These antibodies are the most common causes of problems in compatibility testing. Many cold autoagglutinins are weakly reactive at room temperature and are detected in the saline phase of the compatibility test. These should be removed by autoabsorption if the patient has been given no transfusions within three months. Otherwise it may be necessary to perform a "warm crossmatch."

7) Use of faulty reagents or techniques. Examples of this problem include the contamination of reagents or specimens by such materials as detergents, metallic ions, silica or bacteria; the use of dirty glassware, the use of RBC suspensions that are too concentrated, and overcentrifugation.

8) Presence of antibodies passively derived from a previous transfusion.

Falsely compatible crossmatches may occur if hemolysis is unappreciated, if by error antiglobulin serum is omitted from the test, if inadequate washing precedes the antiglobulin test, if the patient's serum is anticomplementary, or if the antiglobulin serum lacks proper anticomplement activity. A few IgG antibodies, notably

in the Kidd system, and a few IgM antibodies that are not agglutinins at 37 C, mostly in the Lewis system, are detected weakly or
not at all by anti-IgG serum and more strongly by antiglobulin sera
that possess anticomplement activity (specifically, anti-C3b).
Parenthetically, it may be observed that IgM antibodies may be
detected by "anti-IgG" sera if the anti-IgG is not a pure anti-gamma
heavy chain serum but also contains anti-kappa or anti-lambda light
chain activity. Complement-coated RBC are agglutinated by anti-
C4, anti-C3b, anti-C3d and anti-C5, but generally more strongly by
anti-C3b than by anti-C4, as would be expected from the fact that in
the classic complement pathway 100 times as many C3 as C4 molecules are fixed to the red blood cell surface. Potent anti-C4 activity is
actually undesirable in antiglobulin sera used for compatibility
testing inasmuch as RBC sensitized by "normal incomplete cold
antibody" bind principally C4 and less C3. Anti-C3d activity is essential for direct antiglobulin testing but less vital in the antiglobulin serum used for compatibility testing. False-negative antiglobulin tests may rarely occur if the antibody attached to a red
blood cell has a very low binding constant, in which case it may dissociate and neutralize antiglobulin serum without agglutination being produced. This is especially apt to occur if delays intervene
between addition of antiglobulin serum to a cell button and the
centrifugation and reading steps.

The selection of blood for compatibility testing can be simplified
by recalling a simple rule: never administer RBC bearing an ABO
antigen absent from the cells of the recipient. Obviously group-
specific transfusion is most desirable, but limitations of supply sometimes preclude optimal practice. Red blood cells lacking ABO antigens present on recipient RBC can be safely transfused; it is the isoantibody content of the accompanying plasma that occasionally
causes difficulty. Blood should be transfused in such situations as
RBC, preferably washed. If plasma is required, AB plasma may be
added to the RBC or separately administered. Non-group O patients
given large volumes of group O whole blood or even unwashed group
O RBC may receive enough anti-A and/or anti-B to develop weakly
positive direct antiglobulin tests or even exhibit free (transfused) isoantibodies in their serum. The decision as to whether to switch back
to the patient's own ABO group after group O blood has been administered to a non-group O patient is determined by testing for free
isoantibody in the patient's posttransfusion blood sample. In its

absence, crossmatching will yield compatible results with RBC of the patient's own group. If free isoantibody is detected, additional transfusions should be of group O red blood cells until the isoantibody disappears.

Group AB patients requiring large volume transfusions frequently tax the supply of available group AB blood. Group A RBC are reasonably safe to substitute if hemolytic anti-B is absent from the donor's serum. Washed group A cells are preferable. In the selection of blood for group A recipients, the subgroups of A are ignored unless the recipient's serum contains anti-A_1 or anti-H, in which cases A_2 or A_1 RBC are chosen, respectively. Washed group O RBC suspended in AB plasma comprise essentially "universal donor" blood if the recipients' sera contain no alloantibodies.

D-negative blood can be transfused to D-positive recipients without reservation if there are no alloantibodies in the recipient's serum that can react with the transfused cells. The usually short supply of D-negative blood is the only deterrant to this practice. Rather than allow D-negative blood to outdate, it should be given to D-positive recipients. D-positive blood is given to D-negative recipients only under life-threatening circumstances where no alternative is available.

In cases where in vitro serologic incompatibility exists, but there is some question as to its clinical significance and the indication for transfusion is urgent, a small aliquot of RBC from a proposed donor unit can be tagged with the radioactive label ^{51}Cr and administered to the patient without risk. The rate of disappearance from the patient's circulation of the RBC with the radioisotope label can be followed and taken as a clue to the fate of the unit of blood if it were to be transfused.

RECOMMENDED READING:

Beattie, K.: Identifying the causes of weak or "missing" antigens in ABO grouping tests. In: *The Investigation of Typing and Compatibility Problems Caused by Red Blood Cells.* Am Assn of Blood Banks. Washington, 1975. p.15

Greendyke, R.M. and Banzhaf, J.C.: *Blood Bank Policies and Procedures.* Medical Examination Publishing Co., Flushing, N.Y., 1976

Huestis, D.W. et al: *Practical Blood Transfusion,* 2nd ed. Little, Brown and Co. Boston, 1976

212 / Blood Grouping and Compatibility Testing

Issitt, P.D. and Issitt, C.H.: *Applied Blood Group Serology*, 2nd ed. Spectra. Oxnard, Calif., 1975

Mallory, D.M.: Problems in the hemagglutination reaction. In: *A Seminar on Polymorphisms in Human Blood*. Am Assn of Blood Banks. Washington, 1975. p.129

Mallory, D.: ABO blood groups and problems encountered in testing. In: *Blood Group Immunology: Theoretical and Practical Concepts*. Dade. Miami, 1976. p.25

Miller, W.V. (Ed): *Technical Manual of the American Association of Blood Banks*. Am Assn of Blood Banks. Washington, 1977

Mollison, P.L.: *Blood Transfusion in Clinical Medicine*, 5th ed. Blackwell. Oxford, 1972

Walker, R.H. (Ed): *A Seminar on Problems Encountered in Pretransfusion Tests*. Am Assn of Blood Banks. Washington, 1972

CHAPTER 18

Detection and Identification of Alloantibodies

The sera of between 1% and 3% of hospitalized patients contain demonstrable alloantibodies, some of which have been formed as a consequence of pregnancy or transfusion, others of which are non-red blood cell immune. Their presence is generally detected during screening tests conducted prior to compatibility testing or as part of routine antenatal study, but if this screening is not performed or fails to detect the antibody it may later be found as a cause of an incompatible crossmatch, a transfusion reaction or a case of hemolytic disease of the newborn. The routine use of screening tests for alloantibodies on both donor and potential recipient blood specimens is highly desirable: 1) Because the RBC mixtures used for screening are selected to contain most of the common antigens involved in clinically significant reactions, a negative screening test normally ensures the absence of most, though not all, alloantibodies capable of causing transfusion problems. It is emphasized that screening tests of recipient serum do not, however, totally rule out the possible presence of alloantibody. 2) If screening is conducted in advance of the time of actual need for transfusion, an opportunity is afforded to search for rare types or to make other arrangements to secure compatible units of blood. 3) Detection and identification of the specificity of an alloantibody permit specific typing of prospective donor blood before crossmatching, so that incompatibilities will not be missed because the recipient's antibody is weakly reactive. Recall that the minimum number of antibody molecules detectable on the red blood cell surface by conventional testing is greater than the number capable of causing shortened cell survival in the recipient.

213

Weak or even undetected antibodies may thus have biologic significance. 4) The screening procedure detects antibodies in the plasma of donors, which have the theoretical potential to damage recipient RBC or be a source of interdonor reactions. 5) The antibody screen when positive gives an indication of the optimum reaction conditions for further study of the antibody. As a practical aside, if the RBC used for screening are not pooled, they add two more completely typed cell suspensions to the panel used for antibody identification studies.

The choice of RBC to be used for screening is open to some debate, some workers preferring to use a pool of cells from two donors, while others use the same cell suspensions individually. The latter group point out that increased sensitivity is afforded by having whatever antigens are represented in the suspension present on all the cells, not just half of them, which may often be the case when the screening cells are chosen to be complementary to one another in their antigenic makeup, ensuring that clinically significant antigens absent from one screening cell suspension are present on the other. One approach to the selection of screening cells is to begin with paired group O, R^1R^2, and R^2r donors and then make certain that all clinically important antigens with a frequency of occurrence exceeding 8% on the RBC of white subjects are included. At a minimum cells positive for M, N, S, s, Le^a, Le^b, K, Fy^a, Fy^b, Jk^a, and Jk^b must be included. Some antigens such as P$_1$, k, and Lu^b will be found on most cells tested. Antigens commonly missing from RBC used for screening include Lu^a, C^w, Kp^a, Js^a, Wr^a, Di^a, and ce^s, and indeed cell panels used for antibody identification are often similarly deficient. The screening of patient sera for alloantibodies is obviously conducted with individual serum samples, but in the screening of donor sera it is customary in the interest of economy to pool five or even ten sera for testing. This, of course, reduces the sensitivity of the procedure, both because of the dilution factor and the possibility of neutralization of antibody in one serum by soluble blood group substance in another. So-called reagent red blood cells suitable for serum alloantibody screening are widely available commercially and have a shelf-life at 4 C of 14 to 28 days. Because loss of reactivity may occur in time, quality assurance testing must be carried out on these cells upon receipt and as they age. Because the Lewis and MN antigens lose reactivity first, these determinants are the ones most appropriate for testing.

A variety of techniques and temperatures is used in screening inasmuch as no single set of conditions is optimal for detection of all blood group alloantibodies. In general some combination of saline tests at room temperature (occasionally at 18 C) and of albumin-antiglobulin testing and enzyme testing at 37 C is employed. The use of LISS technique is highly recommended. Sera used in alloantibody screening tests ideally are devoid of visible hemoglobin, free from bacterial contamination, and contain complement levels of at least 60% of normal.

The detection of an alloantibody requires that its specificity be identified so that properly antigen-negative blood can be obtained for transfusion. As a preliminary step, a direct antiglobulin test should be performed on the patient's red blood cells to ascertain the possible presence of bound autoantibody or alloantibody. The patient's ABO blood group should be determined: if he is of group A or AB, subtyping for A₁ should be carried out as a clue to possible production of anti-A₁ or anti-H. The patient's fresh serum is then tested with a panel of washed group O red blood cells selected to contain among them as many of the clinically important blood group antigens as possible, and also to lack each of them as well. The RBC types contained in commercially available cell panels are carefully chosen to include cells complementary to one another in different combinations so that identification of the components in antibody mixtures can be made. Some commercial panels are better at this type of discrimination than others. Obviously more than one panel of ten cell types may be necessary to elucidate a difficult problem. Despite all care, commercial cell panels sometimes do not permit positive identification of an antibody; e.g., a homozygous K cell type is often not included, so that certain identification of anti-k may be impossible. Frozen RBC of rare types are stored by larger blood banks for use in such cases. The composition of a typical cell panel is shown in Figure 18-1. An autocontrol and a group O cord RBC suspension should be tested along with every panel; group-compatible A₁, A₂, and/or B cell samples should also be included in the case of sera from non-group O patients.

The patient's serum is allowed to react with the red blood cells of the panel under a variety of test conditions, using the results of the screening tests as a guide; but generally employing tests in saline or LISS at room temperature, albumin-antiglobulin and/or LISS-antiglobulin testing at 37 C and enzyme testing at 37 C with or with-

Test cell	D	C	E	c	e	M	N	S	s	P$_1$	K	k	Le^a	Le^b	Fy^a	Fy^b	Jk^a	Jk^b	Saline RT	Alb 37	AGT 37
1	+	−	−	+	+	+	+	−	+	−	−	+	+	−	−	+	−	+	0	2+	4+
2	+	+	−	−	+	+	+	+	−	+	−	+	−	+	+	+	−	+	0	2+	4+
3	−	−	−	+	+	−	+	−	+	+	−	+	+	−	−	+	+	+	0	0	0
4	+	+	−	−	+	+	+	+	+	+	−	+	+	−	−	+	+	−	0	2+	4+
5	−	−	+	+	+	+	−	+	−	+	+	+	−	+	−	−	−	+	0	0	0
6	+	+	−	−	+	+	+	−	+	+	+	+	−	−	−	+	+	−	0	2+	4+
7	+	+	−	−	+	+	+	+	+	+	−	+	−	+	+	+	+	−	0	2+	4+
8	+	+	+	+	−	+	−	+	+	+	−	+	−	+	+	+	+	−	0	2+	4+
9	−	+	+	+	−	+	+	−	+	+	−	+	−	+	+	+	−	+	0	0	0
10	−	+	−	+	+	+	+	+	+	+	−	+	−	−	−	−	+	+	0	0	0
Cord cell	−	−	−	+	+	+	+	+	+	+	−	+	−	−	−	+	+	+	0	0	0
Patient cell	−	−	−	+	+	+	−	+	+	+	−	+	+	−	+	+	+	+	0	0	0

Figure 18-1. *Reactions of an anti-D serum with a panel of red blood cells of the types shown. A simple way to begin interpretation of such a series of tests is to cross out the antigens listed on the top row across present on test RBC which do not react with the test serum. Antibody or antibodies may be present in the test serum specific for the antigen(s) remaining.*

out subsequent antiglobulin testing. Saline tests may subsequently be reincubated at 4 C and reread. In the study of weakly reactive antisera, increasing the proportion of serum to RBC and/or prolonging incubation times may enhance their reactions.

The interpretation of the reactions given by a cell panel is most easily accomplished by marking off as possible reactants all of the antigens present on those cell suspensions with which the antiserum does *not* react. Ideally all antigens but one are eliminated in this way and a presumptive identification of the antibody specificity accomplished. At this point, the RBC from the patient should be typed to demonstrate the absence of that specificity on his RBC. If not already accomplished by the distribution of the antigen on the red blood cells in the panel, several other RBC specimens known to be both positive and negative for that antigen should be tested with the unknown antiserum to confirm the specificity of the reaction. Table 18-1 shows the levels of confidence that can be attached to antibody identifications based on test results using various combinations of RBC positive or negative for a given antigen.

TABLE 18-1

Number of RBC Samples Bearing the Antigen and Yielding Positive Test Results	Number of RBC Samples Lacking the Antigen and Yielding Negative Test Results	P: The Likelihood of the Reactions Being a Result of Chance
3	2	1:10
4	2	1:15
3	3	1:20
5	2	1:21
4	3	1:35
5	3	1:56
4	4	1:70
7	3	1:120
5	4	1:126
5	5	1:252
7	6	1:1716

The statistical likelihood that a given antibody identification is correct and not a result of chance is shown in the situations above, where various combinations of correctly predicted test results are obtained using RBC of known antigenic type. The numbers in the first and second columns may be interchanged without affecting the p value. Acceptable certainty is usually taken to be present when p values are less than 1 in 20.

Various other criteria must also be met before the blood group specificity of an antiserum is considered to be established. Positive reactions should be obtained with all cell samples in the panel bearing the appropriate antigen. Note, however, that RBC from heterozygous donors or with weakly expressed antigens may not react with weak antisera. RBC from heterozygous C, M, and Fy^a subjects in particular may not react with weak examples of their corresponding antibodies. The antigens P$_1$, Sd^a, Ch^a, and Bg antigens are also widely variable in reactivity and may be weakly expressed on red blood cells listed as "positive" in the key accompanying a commercial cell panel. When antibody specificity is being determined, the reactions demonstrated should be characteristic of antisera of that specificity with regard to suspending medium (e.g., saline vs. albumin), optimal reaction temperature (4 C, room temperature, 37 C), type of reaction (hemolysis, agglutination, need for antiglobulin test), dosage characteristics, ability to fix complement, and effects of enzyme testing (enhancement, no effect, abolition of reaction). Atypical reactions admittedly occur, but are suspect and require confirmation. If numerous crossmatches have been performed, some idea of the possible specificity of the antibody present in a patient's serum can be obtained from a consideration of the number of random units found compatible. Tables 18-2 and 18-3 give data useful in such a situation. Classically, immediate agglutination in saline characterizes the reactions of IgM alloantibodies with homozygous RBC; room temperature incubation enhances their reactions and permits agglutination of RBC from heterozygous donors. Reincubation at 4 C will increase the strength of most IgM antibody reactions, accentuate dosage effects, and detect antibodies unreactive at room temperature such as anti-P$_1$ or normal autoanti-I. IgM saline agglutinating antibodies reactive at 37 C are usually anti-D, rarely anti-K or anti-C. Saline agglutinins at room temperature are usually anti-M, -N, -Le^a, Le^b, -P$_1$ or -I (or -IH) though other specificities are found, including anti-C^w, -Lu^a, -Wr^a, -S, -Sd^a, and -Lu^b. Antibodies reacting immediately in albumin are either antibodies in the Rh system, the reactions of which are enhanced after incubation at 37 C, or cold autoanti-I, which is inhibited at 37 C. In interpreting antiglobulin tests it should be recalled that agglutination may persist from the albumin phase of the test. If an antibody reacts only by antiglobulin testing, it is usually IgG and immune.

Use of a variety of special techniques may assist in confirming

TABLE 18-2

Frequency of Compatible Blood from White Donors with Patient Sera Containing Selected Blood Group Alloantibodies

If a Serum Contains:	The Frequency of Incompatible White Blood Donors will Be (%)	Usual Temperature (C) and Technique for Demonstration	Remarks
Anti-k	99.8	AGT:37	Rare, immune
Anti-Lu^b	99.8	Sal:22, AGT:37	Rare, naturally occurring or immune
Anti-e	98	Alb, AGT or Enz:37	Occurs in R^{2}R^2 subjects with anti-C, or patients with warm autoantibody AHD
Anti-s	89	AGT:37	Usually immune
Anti-D	85	Sal, Alb, AGT, Enz:37	Immune. Most common alloantibody
Anti-G	85	Sal, Alb, AGT, Enz:37	Immune. Present in anti-C and/or D sera
Anti-c	81	Alb, AGT, Enz:37	Immune. Occurs in R^{1}R^1 subjects with anti-E
Anti-Fy^b	80	AGT:37	Immune. Antigen destroyed by enzymes
Anti-M	78	Sal:22 or AGT:37	Naturally occurring, rarely immune. Antigen destroyed by enzymes
Anti-P$_1$	78	Sal, Enz:4-22	Naturally occurring
Anti-Jk^a	76	AGT, Enz + AGT:37	Immune. Enzyme enhanced
Anti-Jk^b	74	AGT, Enz + AGT:37	Immune. Enzyme enhanced
Anti-Le^b	73	Sal:4-22; AGT, Enz:37	Naturally occurring. Often with anti-Le^a
Anti-N	72	Sal:22	Rare. Naturally occurring. Antigen destroyed by enzymes
Anti-ce	67	Alb, AGT, Enz:37	Immune. Present in many anti-c and anti-e sera
Anti-C	68	Alb, AGT, Enz:37	Immune. Found with anti-D
Anti-Fy^a	66	AGT:37	Immune. Antigen destroyed by enzymes

(Continued)

TABLE 18-2 (Cont'd)

Frequency of Compatible Blood from White Donors with Patient Sera Containing Selected Blood Group Alloantibodies

If a Serum Contains:	The Frequency of Incompatible White Blood Donors will Be (%)	Usual Temperature (C) and Technique for Demonstration	Remarks
Anti-S	55	Sal:22, AGT:37	Naturally occurring or immune. Antigen destroyed by enzymes
Anti-E	29	Sal:22; Alb, AGT, Enz:37	Naturally occurring or immune. Often with anti-C
Anti-Le[a]	23	Sal:4-22; AGT, Enz:37	Naturally occurring or immune. May be hemolytic. Often reacts only by enzyme
Anti-K	9	AGT:37	Immune
Anti-Lu[a]	8	Sal:22	Immune, weak
Anti-C[w]	2	Sal:4-22; Alb, AGT, Enz:37	Naturally occurring or immune. Often with anti-C
Anti-Wr[a]	0.1	Sal:22; AGT, Enz:37	Naturally occurring or immune. Common in AHD sera

TABLE 18-3

Frequency of Reaction with Random White Donors of Antibodies of Different Specificities, Classified According to Optimal Reaction Conditions

Optimum Technique for Demonstration	Temperature Optimum	Percent Frequency of Positive Reactions with Random Donors				
		0–10	10–50	50–75	75–90	90–100
Saline	4–22	Lu^a I	Le^a	Le^b	P M, N	I, H
Saline	22–37	C^w Lu^a Wr^a	E Le^a S	C Le^b	D c s	e Lu^b Vel Sd^a
Antiglobulin test	37	C K, Kp^a Lu^a Di^a Yt^b Wr^a	E Le^a S Js^a	C Le^b Fy^a Jk^b Do^a Xg^a	D c Fy^b s Jk^a Au	e k, Kp^b Lu^b Vel Di^b U Ge Yt^a Js^b Sd^a
Enzyme	37	C	E Le^a	C Le^b	D c	e
Saline (hemolysis)	37		Le^a	Le^b Jk^b	Jk^a	Vel
All	All		Le^a			Tj^a

(Adapted from *Technical Methods of the American Association of Blood Banks*, 6th ed., p. 107.)

the probable specificity of an antibody. Anti-M, -N, -S, -Fy^a, -Fy^b, -Ch^a, -Yt^a, -Tn, and -Pr (Sp) may no longer be demonstrable after enzyme treatment of RBC, whereas the reactions of anti-Le^a, -Le^b, -Jk^a, -Jk^b, -I, and -E may be enhanced. Anti-M activity may be increased by acidification of serum to pH 6.5. Anti-P_1 activity may be neutralized by hydatid cyst fluid, anti-Ch^a and -Rg^a by serum from antigen-positive donors, anti-Sd^a by urine from an Sd^a-positive subject, anti-I^D by saliva or milk, and anti-Le^a or -Le^b by saliva from appropriate donors. The characteristic mixed-field agglutination produced by anti-Lu^a and anti-Sd^a is a useful clue. The enhancement of agglutination by antiglobulin sera containing anti-C3b as opposed to that caused by anti-IgG serum indicates complement fixation, suggesting antibodies in the Lewis, Kidd, or occasionally Duffy system, and almost rules out antibodies in the Rh system. Hemolysis is a clue to the presence of possible Lewis antibodies or the rare anti-Tj^a. Kidd antibodies may hemolyze enzyme-treated RBC. Serum may be treated with 2-mercaptoethanol or dithiothreitol to destroy IgM antibody activity. Recall that cord blood is a good source of RBC with weakly reactive or absent antigens having a high incidence in adults, including Le^a, Le^b, I, Sd^a, Yt^a, and Ch^a.

Agglutination of all of the red blood cell specimens in a panel as well as the patient's own cells suggests the presence of a cold-reacting autoantibody, discussed below, or a panagglutinin. If all cells but the autocontrol react, a mixture of alloantibodies or an antibody to a high-incidence antigen is suggested. In the latter case it is useful if RBC samples from siblings can be tested, inasmuch as blood relatives may ultimately prove to be the only compatible donors for the patient. A clue to the specificity of an antibody to high-frequency antigens may be gained by typing the patient's RBC with antisera (as available, to such antigens as k, Lu^b, Vel, U, Yt^a, Sd^a, Kp^b, Js^b, and Di^b plus some of the shared WBC-RBC antigens. If the patient's RBC lack one of these very common antigens, the antibody may be of that specificity. Though relatively rare, these antisera are more easily acquired than are samples of the correspondingly negative cells for use in testing. Alternatively the patient's cells may be typed for the presence of low-incidence antigens such as Yt^b, Kp^a, Js^a, Di^a, and even K and Lu^a for hints, inasmuch as such subjects may conceivably be homozygous and capable therefore of making antibody to common high-frequency antigens. If all cells react, but weakly, the possibility of anti-Sd^a, anti-Ch^a, or anti-Rg^a should be considered. The recognition of these antibodies has been discussed above. Ch^a-positive RBC lose their reactivity upon storage.

Compatibility testing data should not be forgotten when attempting to solve the problem of the cell panel in which all cells but the autocontrol react. If crossmatches are compatible and the panel cells all react, anti-H is suspect. Inclusion of group A_1, A_2, and B RBC along with test panels is useful in such cases. The opposite situation, with an incompatible crossmatch and a negative antibody screening test cell panel suggests anti-A_1 in the subject with a weak subgroup of A, an antibody to a low-incidence antigen, or an antibody that reacts only with RBC from homozygous donors. Mixtures of antibodies should be suspected if the RBC in the panel do not react uniformly or if not all cells react and no pattern is apparent. Ideally such mixtures can be distinguished by the use of additional RBC samples that are positive and negative for the antigens corresponding to the antibodies suspected. Occasionally absorption and elution techniques may be required to separate and identify mixtures of antibodies. One antibody of a suspected pair may be absorbed with RBC bearing only one of the corresponding antigens, leaving behind the second specificity in relatively pure form for identification. The first antibody may be eluted and its specificity likewise confirmed. Various combinations of RBC and absorption and elution procedures can be tailored to fit the problem. Occurrence of the Matuhasi-Ogata phenomenon must always be recalled, however, when planning and interpreting such work. Usable eluates can generally be made from even weakly sensitized RBC by concentration procedures that reduce their water content while leaving behind the antibody molecules. Failures under such circumstances are usually the consequence of antibody loss during preliminary washing of the sensitized RBC. Note that eluates are unstable on storage and freeze poorly.

Cold autoantibodies often interfere in screening and identification tests for alloantibodies. Although rarely of clinical significance, cold autoagglutinins may mask the presence of an alloantibody that is of potential importance. If a transfusion has not been administered within three months, cold autoagglutinins should be absorbed from patient sera at 4 C with aliquots of enzyme-treated patient cells and the absorbed serum used for antibody screening tests, testing with cell panels as indicated, and compatibility testing. Recent transfusion makes autoabsorption undesirable because of the danger of removing alloantibodies that might otherwise be detected.

The exact identification of the specificity of cold autoantibodies is not usually necessary in practice, but if desired it can be accomplished using a scheme similar to that shown in Table 18-4.

TABLE 18-4

Differential Reactions of Common Cold Agglutinins in H, I, and Sp Systems

	Anti-IH	Anti-H	Anti-I	Anti-i	Anti-Sp
ABO group of serum donor	A, A₁ B, B	A, A₁ B, B	All	All	All
Reactions with RBC of group					
OI (adult)	++++	++++	++++	±	++++
A₁I (adult)	+	±	++++	±	++++
A₂I (adult)	++++	++	++++	±	++++
Oi (cord)	±	++++	±	++++	++++
A₁i (cord)	−	++++	−	++++	++++
Effect of enzyme treatment of RBC on agglutination	Inc.	−	Inc.	−	Abolished

Inc. = increased.

Many examples of anti-I react with cord RBC as well as adult cells and may require dilution before their specificity becomes apparent. The Pr (Sp) antigens are found on all human RBC. Occasional cold autoantibodies have anti-Pr specificity, and anti-Pr may be found in cold-agglutinin disease. The Pr antigens are found on cord RBC as well as adult cells and are inactivated by enzyme treatment.

RECOMMENDED READING:

Allen, F.H. et al: Further observations on the Matuhasi-Ogata phenomenon. *Vox Sang* 16:47, 1969

Greendyke, R.M. and Banzhaf, J.C.: *Blood Bank Policies and Procedures.* Medical Examination Publishing Co. Flushing, N.Y., 1976

Huestis, D.W. et al: *Practical Blood Transfusion*, 2nd ed. Little, Brown and Co. Boston, 1976

Issitt, P.D. and Issitt, C.H.: *Applied Blood Group Serology*, 2nd ed. Spectra. Oxnard, Calif., 1975

Kaczmarski, G. and Wilson, J.: Antibody identification. In: *Blood Group Immunology: Theoretical and Practical Concepts.* Dade. Miami, 1976

Miller, W.V. (Ed): *Technical Manual of the American Association of Blood Banks*. Am Assn of Blood Banks. Washington, 1977

Mollison, P.L.: *Blood Transfusion in Clinical Medicine*, 5th ed. Blackwell. Oxford, 1972

Moore, B.P.L. et al: Serological and technical methods: *The Technical Manual of the Canadian Red Cross Blood Transfusion Service*, 7th ed. Canadian Red Cross. Toronto, 1972

Race, R.R. and Sanger, R.: *Blood Groups in Man*, 6th ed. Blackwell. Oxford, 1975

Walker, R.H. (Ed): *A Seminar on Problems Encountered in Pretransfusion Tests*. Am Assn of Blood Banks. Washington, 1972

CHAPTER 19

Immunologic Complications of Blood Transfusion

Despite the sophistication brought to bear in the laboratory, blood transfusion remains a clinical experiment. A safe outcome can generally be anticipated, but unexpected reactions occur despite all precautions, and no guarantees can be offered. A wide variety of complications may be experienced by a patient being transfused, ranging in severity from negligible to fatal and including such phenomena as lytic, febrile, or allergic reactions to RBC, WBC, platelets or plasma proteins, anticoagulant-related intoxications, disturbances of the coagulation mechanism, transfusion-transmitted infectious disease, mechanical problems such as circulatory overload or embolization, problems caused by defective function or transfused cells, iron overloading, and, of course, blood group sensitization. These problems will be discussed in this and the succeeding chapter.

HEMOLYTIC TRANSFUSION REACTIONS

The accelerated destruction of incompatible RBC mediated by blood group antibodies may range from an asymptomatic slight shortening of survival of transfused cells to a catastrophe characterized by massive intravascular hemolysis and death. A wide variety of factors determines whether a hemolytic transfusion reaction will occur as well as the nature and extent of the process. Among these are 1) the antibody concentration; 2) its Ig class and subclass; 3) the ability of the antibody to activate complement; 4) the mean binding constant of the antibody; 5) the thermal amplitude and optimum of the antibody; 6) the number of antibody-combining sites per RBC; 7) the number of RBC transfused; and 8) the functional state of the reticuloendothelial (phagocytic) system of the recipient. The sum of these factors determines the severity of a transfusion reaction, and in light of their multiplicity it is not possible to predict with confidence the outcome in a given case. In general there is reasonably close correlation between in vitro test results and in vivo red blood cell survival. Thus, antibodies hemolytic in the test tube are apt to produce intravascular hemolysis, although antibodies such as anti-D, which are not hemolysins in vitro, can still cause hemoglobinemia if proper conditions obtain in the patient. A few milliliters of incompatible RBC may not provoke a clinical reaction whereas 200 or 300 ml may do so. As little as 25 to 50 ml of incompatible blood may cause a frank hemolytic transfusion reaction, although in other cases several incompatible units have been given without incident. Large volumes of incompatible RBC are generally eliminated more slowly than small volumes because of the binding of fewer antibody molecules per cell and because of the limited capabilities of the reticuloendothelial system to clear sensitized cells. The effect of increased numbers of antigen sites per RBC is illustrated in the more rapid clearance of incompatible group A_1 than group A_2 cells and the accelerated clearance of incompatible homozygous M or Jk^a RBC as opposed to heterozygous [MN or Jk(a+b+)] cells. Weak antibodies in low concentrations and/or with low binding constants are less apt to cause reactions than are potent antibodies. Warm-acting antibodies are much more likely to cause pathologic effects than those reactive only at lower temperatures. Of greatest importance, however, seems to be the amount of antibody fixed to a given RBC, a function of antibody concentration and binding constant plus antigen site density, the latter in turn combining with the Ig class and subclass to determine complement binding.

Antibody-mediated red blood cell destruction is thought to occur by four mechanisms: 1) intravascular hemolysis; 2) phagocytic destruction following adherence of cells coated with C3b to C3b receptors on phagocytes; 3) phagocytosis following adherence of cells sensitized by IgG antibodies to Fc receptors on phagocytes; and 4) metabolic damage secondary to agglutination.

RBC with C4b/C3b fixed to their surfaces may be engulfed by phagocytes and destroyed at once, or may have a cytotoxic lesion induced on their surfaces in the form of membrane loss without being phagocytized immediately. In activators of C4b and C3b may split the bound "b" complement components leaving only attached C4d/C3d, for which the phagocyte has no receptor. In consequence the RBC are released back into the circulation where they survive for hours to days as spherocytes unduly susceptible to splenic trapping and destruction. Alternatively, they may circulate as essentially normally shaped cells, but coated with C4d/C3d, and live out a normal lifespan immune to further attack by fresh complement. The number of C4/C3 molecules initially bound to the RBC suface plus the capabilities of the macrophages of the reticuloendothelial system control which of these outcomes will predominate in a given situation. IgM antibodies probably act by this mechanism in cases where antibody attachment to RBC activates complement in vitro but does not cause lysis. Only IgG antibodies of subclasses 3 or 1 are able to bring about complement-mediated RBC damage, and the fact that pure IgG4 and perhaps IgG2 molecules induce only slow or minor degrees of red blood cell destruction probably is related to this observation. Noncomplement fixing IgG antibodies cause sensitized RBC to be entrapped in the spleen by virtue of the presence of phagocytic receptors for the Fc portion of their gamma H chains, but the process is much slower and less effective than that accomplished through complement fixation. IgG1 and IgG3 molecules appear to be more efficient than IgG4 or IgG2 molecules in this regard also. Each macrophage has about 10^5 IgG receptors, and this number can increase with persistent stimulation of the cell. There is a general correlation between the amount of alloantibody IgG fixed to the RBC surface and the speed and completeness of cell destruction: this observation is not necessarily true in the case of autoantibodies. IgM antibodies that do not bring about RBC destruction through complement fixation or hemolysis can still cause intravascular agglutination, with filtration of the RBC primarily in the liver and destruction secondary to metabolic damage.

We have seen how the complement cascade can be activated by immune complexes not involving blood group antigens, with attachment of complexes and C3 or attachment of free C3b to innocent bystander RBC. Subsequent destruction by macrophages or even lysis may occur, or as noted above, C4bINA activity may leave C3d-coated RBC that may survive normally. Complement fixation to a cell in the absence of specific antibody attachment can be beneficial, e.g., activated free C3b can fix to bacteria, sensitizing them for attachment to C3b receptors on macrophages even in the absence of specific antibody sensitization, and thereby greatly multiplying the effects of even small numbers of antibacterial antibody molecules. On the other hand, this phenomenon can be harmful if the activated complement attaches for example to a platelet or neutrophil and causes its premature destruction. This mechanism may be operative in the thrombocytopenia occasionally occurring after incompatible RBC transfusion (if complement activation occurs). It may also cause destruction of a patient's own platelets after antiplatelet antibodies react with incompatible transfused platelets. Similarly a patient's RBC may be destroyed after antileukocyte antibodies react with incompatible transfused WBC or transfused antileukocyte antibodies react with the patient's own WBC. It has been shown that complement activation occurring in the course of a hemolytic transfusion reaction owing to RBC antigen-antibody interaction may result in destruction of the patient's own RBC.

Though intravascular hemolysis as the result of complement activation may occur in paroxysmal cold hemoglobinuria or cold agglutin disease, it is rare in warm autoantibody-mediated AHD. The puzzle as to why such variation occurs in the rate of red blood cell destruction in the latter disease is at least partially explained by the observation that although IgG3 AHD antibodies sensitize RBC to accelerated destruction, IgG1 autoantibodies may or may not do so and those of subclass IgG2 (and probably IgG4) rarely if ever cause damage. According to Engelfriet, most warm-reacting autoantibodies are of subclass IgG1, and only a few include IgG2 and IgG3, while IgG4 is rare.

In the absence of hemoglobinemia and hemoglobinuria, the rapid disappearance of incompatible red blood cells suggests sequestration in the liver, whereas a slower rate indicates splenic removal. The spleen is 100 times more efficient on a weight basis than the liver in removing sensitized RBC but is only one tenth as large and receives only one tenth the blood flow. If the in vitro serological properties and immunoglobulin class of blood group antibodies are related to the pattern of RBC destruction which they cause, it may be generally said that:

1) Antibodies strongly hemolytic in vitro (e.g., anti-A, anti-B, anti-Tj[a]) cause intravascular RBC destruction, are complement fixing and IgM and/or IgG.

2) Antibodies weakly hemolytic in vitro (e.g., weak anti-A or

anti-B, anti-Le^a) produce principally extravascular destruction in the liver, are incompletely or weakly complement-fixing and IgM.

3) Agglutinating antibodies without the potential to fix complement (e.g., saline-agglutinating anti-D) cause hepatic destruction and are IgM.

4) Non-agglutinating, complement-fixing antibodies (e.g., anti-Jk^a, a few examples of anti-Fy^a) result in RBC destruction in the liver and are IgG.

5) Non-agglutinating, noncomplement fixing antibodies (e.g., incomplete anti-D, anti-C, most examples of anti-Fy^a and anti-K) effect cell destruction in the spleen and are IgG.

IgG antibodies which fix complement and IgM antibodies irrespective of complement-fixing ability, if not potent, produce destruction of incompatible RBC, which is described by a two-component curve. This occurs as a consequence of the presence of unagglutinable cells, uneven distribution of antigen among cells, varying cell susceptibility with age (older cells are more vulnerable to destruction), resistance to damage due to coating with C3d, exhaustion of antibody, and, in the case of Le^a and Le^b antigens, elution of antigen. Unless complement is fixed, IgM blood group antibodies are less effective, molecule for molecule, than their IgG counterparts in bringing about RBC destruction.

To fix complement, IgG molecules must form doublets, whereas attachment of only a single IgM molecule is required. On an RBC with for example 800,000 A sites, only 1,000 IgG molecules need attach before two would be close enough to form a doublet and activate complement. The same cell could carry only 10,000 to 30,000 D sites, thus essentially precluding the possibility of two IgG anti-D molecules attaching closely enough to form a doublet. Rarely is the rate of cell destruction limited by the amount of complement available. On the other hand, the speed with which the macrophages of the reticuloendothelial system can remove sensitized cells from the circulation and break them down is often a rate-limiting factor. The reticuloendothelial system of a 70 kg subject cannot clear more than about 420 ml of incompatible RBC or about two units of blood per 24 hours.

The rate and extent of the intravascular destruction of large volume transfusions of incompatible RBC by antibodies such as anti-A or anti-B is limited only by the supply of antibody. Only part of the anti-A or anti-B, however, will bind complement, and some is usually IgG. The relationship between the amount of antibody and the amount of hemolysis is therefore variable. If an isoantibody is potent, destruction of an entire 450 ml unit of blood may occur in less than an hour. A low-titer antibody may all be absorbed and the incompatible RBC survive for days or even weeks. As noted, the supply of complement is not a limiting factor except in the case of potent autoanti-I where hemolysis may deplete the supply, in which case transfusion may supply complement and aggravate RBC destruction. In contrast to the situation in the ABO system, a potent Rh antibody may only destroy 200 to 300 ml of RBC per day. Free antibody persists because of the limited numbers of Rh sites per cell. If over 400 ml of cells are given some may remain even after 24 hours. If the antibody is initially weak, incompatible cells may persist for four or five days, following which a marked increase in anti-D titer occurs with rapid cell destruction and clearing of the Rh-positive RBC within a week. In the case of primary immunization by transfusion, the appearance of anti-D may be delayed, with sudden red blood cell destruction concomitant with antibody production occurring after 20 to 30 days. Survival of the incompatible cells in this situation is described by a "collapse curve." It is apparent that the immediate danger of an incompatible transfusion in the presence of a weak antibody is usually, though not always, small and that a delayed reaction represents the principal threat. Although usually not so, a delayed transfusion reaction may be as serious as an immediate one.

The threat posed by most Lewis-incompatible blood transfusions is at least partially limited by the presence of soluble Lewis substances in incompatible plasma. Neutralization of IgM antibodies by soluble blood group substance is effective, and therapeutic use of this fact is occasionally made if Lewis-incompatible blood transfusions must be given by first administering plasma from Lewis-incompatible donors to neutralize the antibody. Lewis antigens are eluted from incompatible RBC after transfusion, thus minimizing their susceptibility to damage by antibody produced in response to transfusion.

Accelerated destruction of transfused RBC may occur in the absence of serologically demonstrable antibody, although antibody may (but not always) appear later. The disappearance of the donor RBC may be slow or rapid, and undefined differences among donors play a part in determining this occurrence. Mollison states that in low-volume ostensibly compatible transfusions, abnormally rapid cell destruction may occur in up to 30% of cases. Repeat transfusions may elicit several responses: 1) cell destruction may be rapid from the outset, with production of demonstrable antibody in two to four weeks; 2) the same situation may obtain, without antibody ever becoming detectable; or 3) normal or near-normal RBC survival may occur. The possibility of acquired tolerance arises in the last case.

Red blood cell destruction may uncommonly result from transfusion of group O plasma containing potent isoantibodies to non-group O recipients. Rare but severe hemolytic reactions have been reported. The practice of transfusing substantial volumes of group O plasma with platelet or leukocyte preparations to non-group O recipients may cause mild reactions and frequently results in the recipient RBC becoming positive in direct antiglobulin tests. Transfused alloantibodies rarely cause clinically apparent problems, though reactions are potentially possible. The usual absence of reaction probably is caused by the considerable antibody dilution that occurs in the recipient's plasma and the distribution of antibody over a large cell mass, resulting in the attachment of but few antibody molecules per RBC. Since the degree of sensitization bears strongly upon the effect of an antibody on cell survival, little result would be anticipated. Exceptions might occur with massive transfusion or the administration of very potent antibodies. The same sorts of considerations apply to the problem of interdonor incompatibility when antibodies are transfused. It should be noted that despite a $T^1/_2$ for IgG of 22 to 26 days, passively acquired blood group antibodies may be demonstrable up to four months after their transfusion.

The term hemolytic transfusion reaction is used to describe the clinical syndrome caused by, and including, accelerated red blood cell destruction as a result of RBC antigen-antibody reaction. The expression is not limited to reactions occurring as a consequence of immediate intravascular hemolysis. The signs and symptoms of a hemolytic transfusion reaction may vary from absent to catastrophic. In the case of intravascular hemolysis, the patient may complain of none, some, or all of a constellation that includes a burning sensation along the vein being used for transfusion, headache, nausea, backache, dizziness, faintness, a constricting sensation in the chest, or shortness of breath. He may be febrile or exhibit a shaking chill, with signs of shock, including tachycardia, tachypnea, pallor, cold perspiration, and hypotension, and ultimately he may lapse into unconsciousness. Anuria sometimes occurs, and in severe cases a generalized bleeding diathesis is often present. Depending on the rapidity, extent, and site of RBC destruction, free hemoglobin may be present in the plasma and urine. Urinary output may cease, and in most severe cases death may ensue within hours. More often than not recovery occurs, but sometimes only after a period of several days of anuria that may require hemodialysis to sustain life until renal function returns. In less severe cases, the symptoms are milder and kidney function may not cease. In some instances, the first sign of a hemolytic transfusion reaction may be the excretion of red or dark reddish-brown urine filled with hemoglobin and its break-down products. The clinical signs and symptoms of a hemolytic transfusion reaction are principally the result of complement activation, either by initiation of the classic pathway by the antigen-antibody reaction, or as a consequence of liberated thromboplastic substances from destroyed RBC activating thrombin, plasmin, Factor XII, and the alternate complement pathway. The anaphylotoxin fragments (C3a, C5a) freed in the course of complement activation interact with a variety of cells to liberate the vasoactive materials responsible for the clinical picture. Disseminated intravascular coagulation may occur when stromal lipid from RBC hemolyzed intravascularly triggers the blood coagulation system. DIC is rare as a complication of extravascular RBC destruction, even if hemoglobinuria occurs.

A feared complication of intravascular antibody-mediated hemolysis is acute renal failure due to tubular damage. Tubular damage occurs with a spectrum of severity ranging from transient functional alterations through acute tubular necrosis to renal cortical necrosis. The latter is almost inevitably fatal, while even with modern treatment acute renal tubular necrosis carries a mortality rate of up to 50%. The pathogenesis of these changes does not involve anatomic obstruction of the tubule and is not a simple consequence of hemoglobin release, inasmuch as free hemoglobin alone causes no renal toxicity. Rather the renal damage is due to tubular ischemia and decreased glomerular filtration as a consequence of decreased renal cortical blood flow, DIC, and disturbances in vasomotor control targeting on the kidney. These abnormalities occur as a consequence of activation of the coagulation and complement cascades by intravascular blood group antigen-antibody reactions culminating in RBC lysis. The preferential effect of the DIC with localization of fibrin in the glomerular tuft and arterioles is mediated chiefly by norepinephrine. Thus the hemolytic transfusion reaction has two major effects: 1) the activation of coagulation, and 2) the production of hemodynamic effects via a) serotonin release from platelets, b) activation of Hageman factor with subsequent activation of kallikrein and production of bradykinin, c) complement activation with release of anaphylotoxins that act on mast cells to cause release of histamine, and d) norepinephrine release from the adrenal medulla. The traditional mannitol-induced diuresis for the treatment of the renal failure of a hemolytic transfusion reaction is neither theoretically sound nor clinically effective because it does not increase blood flow but only urine flow. Furosemide or ethacrynic acid treatment has been recommended as has the use of the alpha-adrenergic blocking agent phentolamine. Anticoagulation with heparin is highly effective if employed before DIC occurs, but is of little value in reversing established DIC.

When intravascular hemolysis occurs, hemoglobin released into the plasma is either converted from its original tetramer to a dimer and/or its iron is oxidized to the ferric state to form methemoglobin. The hemoglobin dimer is bound by a carrier protein called haptoglobin. The haptoglobin in 100 ml of plasma can bind about 100 mg of hemoglobin dimer. The hemoglobin-haptoglobin complex is cleared by the reticuloendothelial system, predominantly in the liver. Small amounts of the hemoglobin-haptoglobin complex are removed with a $T^1/2$ of 20 minutes; if totally saturated, the plasma haptoglobin is cleared at a rate of about 13 mg of hemoglobin per 100 ml of plasma per hour. Haptoglobin regeneration is rather slow, approximating 50% of normal within 36 hours. Total replacement requires seven to nine days. As hemoglobin catabolism proceeds, bilirubin is formed. An increase in unconjugated serum bilirubin of 0.5 mg/dl occurs for each 15 to 20 gm of hemoglobin acutely released, the peak value occurring three to six hours after acute RBC destruction. If the binding capacity of haptoglobin is exceeded, free hemoglobin circulates in the plasma. When concentrations of free plasma hemoglobin exceed 25 mg/dl, hemoglobin begins to appear in the urine, although frank hemoglobinuria does not occur until plasma hemoglobin values exceed 150 mg/dl. The methemoglobin formed is broken down to globin and heme, the latter binding to albumin to form methemalbumin or alternatively binding to a beta globulin called hemopexin. These complexes are probably removed by the reticuloendothelial system. Shumm's test for serum methemalbumin becomes positive after the rapid destruction of RBC containing about 14 gm of hemoglobin or the equivalent of roughly 100 ml of blood. Methemalbumin may appear in the plasma within five hours of acute red blood cell destruction and persists for 24 hours or longer. When large amounts of hemoglobin are rapidly released into the plasma, about one third is excreted in the urine. Plasma hemoglobin levels of 40 to 60 mg/dl are cleared in about five hours. Hemoglobin in the glomerular filtrate is partially reabsorbed by the renal tubular epilthelium and converted into the iron-containing pigment hemosiderin. Exfoliated tubular epithelial cells containing stainable granules of hemosiderin may be demonstrated for several days in the urine sediments of patients in whom hemoglobinuria has occured, i.e., those in whom plasma hemoglobin concentrations have exceeded 25 mg/dl. Most of the hemoglobin released from destroyed RBC is converted by the liver to bilirubin and excreted in the bile – the amount excreted by this route being inversely proportional to the rate of RBC destruction. If RBC breakdown is primarily extravascular, the slower pace of the process usually does not exceed the ability of bodily mechanisms to cope with it and there is little or no hemoglobinemia and no hemoglobinuria, although, depending on the amount and rate of RBC destruction, there may be some transient, mild increase in unconjugated serum bilirubin concentrations.

Antibodies that are hemolytic in vitro (e.g., anti-A, anti-B, anti-Tj[a]) produce intravascular hemolysis in vivo. More than 90% of a small volume of ABO-incompatible RBC may undergo intravascular hemolysis, though only half of a large transfusion may do so. In the patient with a weakly hemolytic antibody (e.g., anti-Le[a]) incompatible RBC may be cleared by the reticuloendothelial system before intravascular lysis can occur, but if the volume of incompatible cells given is sufficiently large that the reticuloendothelial system is overloaded, hemolysis may occur in the bloodstream. Antibodies that hemolyze only enzyme-treated red blood cells in vitro may cause intravasular hemolysis in vivo, but probably only after reticuloendothelial system damage to sensitized RBC has taken place. Even antibodies that are not hemolytic in vitro (e.g., anti-D) may cause some intravascular hemolysis by this mechanism. Whether hemoglobin-uria occurs in the last situation depends at least in part on the plasma haptoglobin concentration.

The laboratory findings in a patient experiencing an acute hemo-lytic transfusion reaction vary according to its severity, ranging from a simple failure to observe the expected increase in hematocrit to the entire constellation produced by hemolysis, acute renal failure, and DIC. In major hemolytic reactions, free hemoglobin is found in the plasma an shortly thereafter in the urine, together with RBC, albumin, and casts. Plasma haptoglobin will be absent. Peripheral blood smears will exhibit spherocytosis and fragmentation of remaining transfused RBC, plus nucleated patient RBC and numerous reticulocytes. A positive direct antiglobulin test will usual-ly be found unless all of the incompatible red blood cells have been destroyed. Free serum alloantibody may be present or absent. If the incompatibility is in the ABO system, isoantibody is rarely com-pletely absorbed. Either leukopenia or leukocytosis may be found. If DIC is present, the blood may be incoagulable and demonstrate pro-longed thrombin, prothrombin, and partial thromboplastin times, thrombocytopenia, increased concentrations of fibrin split products, and a decreased Factor VIII concentration. Breakdown of the hemo-globin of destroyed cells will cause hyperbilirubinemia and occa-sionally visible jaundice. Delayed hemolytic transfusion reactions may cause a similar but less abnormal set of laboratory findings. DIC is unusual as a result of a delayed reaction.

NON–HEMOLYTIC TRANSFUSION REACTIONS

A second and much more common type of response to blood transfusion is the febrile or non-hemolytic reaction. Most febrile episodes are a result of reactivity of antibodies in the patient's plasma with donor leukocytes, while a few are caused by anti-platelet or anti-serum protein antibodies, and a few are un-explained. The opposite situation may also obtain, in which reac-tions are caused by non-red blood cell antibodies in donor plasma reacting with various constituents of the recipient's blood. Although febrile transfusion reactions are usually mild and characterized only by low-grade fever and chills, a more severe picture suggestive of a hemolytic reaction may occur, with malaise, high fever, chills, hypo-tension, cyanosis, leukopenia, headache, and tachycardia. Release of leukocyte pyrogens and lysosomal enzymes plus complement activation are thought to cause the clinical symptom complex. The onset of the reaction may occur within minutes after the transfusion is begun, but may not appear until as much as two to four hours after it is completed. Symptoms may persist for several hours but are generally transient.

A particularly severe type of leukocyte reaction occasionally takes place when donor plasma contains anti-granulocyte antibodies reactive with the recipient's leukocytes or vice versa. Within a few minutes after the start of the transfusion, the patient may experience acute pulmonary edema, with fever, chills, dyspnea, cyanosis, cough, and pulmonary infiltrates demonstrable on roentgenographic study. Treatment consists of the administration of epinephrine and corticosteroids and the use of washed RBC for subsequent transfusions.

One study of 74,000 transfusion reported reactions in 1.8%, of which three fourths were febrile. Of these, 44% were associated with leukoagglutinins. In studies employing cytotoxicity testing for leukocyte antibodies, considerably higher figures are found. The interpretation of reactions thought to be caused by platelet antibodies is complicated by the facts that leukocyte antibodies are almost always present and that WBC almost always contaminate platelet preparations.

The antigens most strongly expressed on leukocytes and platelets are HLA antigens (see Chapter 22), which are common to most body cells. Advantage is taken of their presence on lymphocytes to type donors and recipients for organ-graft compatibility. Other antigens unique to neutrophils and platelets also exist. As noted previously, leukocytes and platelets also bear certain RBC antigens in small amounts, including ABH, Ii, MN, and P antigens, though not those of the Rh system. Autoanti-I and -i as well as many anti-Le^a sera have been shown to be lymphocytotoxic. The transfusion of blood from which at least 90% of leukocytes have been removed, preferably as washed RBC, usually prevents febrile reactions.

Another "minor" variety of transfusion reaction is the allergic response or immediate hypersensitivity dermal reaction. Allergic reactions are considered to be the result of the presence of foreign immunoglobulins in transfused blood to which the recipient has been sensitized or vice versa. The urticarial reaction is caused by the liberation of histamine and perhaps serotonin from mast cells that are found throughout the body, especially in the skin. The release of these vasoactive principles may be triggered directly by the antigen-antibody reaction or by complement. Blood group antigen-antibody reactions do not appear to cause allergic responses. Characteristically, the patient experiencing an allergic reaction to blood transfusion develops wheals (hives), erythema, itching, occasionally facial swelling, and rarely tachycardia. The clinical picture usually appears within minutes after the start of the transfusion. Such reactions are common, occurring in about 3% of transfusions. Transfusions causing allergic reactions should be interrupted but may be resumed at the discretion of the attending physician. Antihistamines usually are effective in treating allergic transfusion reactions, but under no circumstances should they be mixed with the blood. The transfusion of washed RBC prevents this type of reaction.

Two additional and serious types of transfusion reaction also occur as the result of interaction of patient antibodies with transfused immunoglobulins. One variety is indistinguishable from classic serum sickness as seen in patients with antibodies to heterologous serum proteins (e.g., horse serum). One to five days after transfusion the clinical syndrome appears, with rash, malaise, myalgia, fever, arthritis, pericarditis, pleural effusion, vomiting, and abdominal and back pain. The symptoms may last for several days and are treated with adrenal corticosteroids. The transfusion of washed RBC prevents recurrence.

Anaphylactoid response may occur within minutes after the start of a transfusion in a small group of patients who exhibit class-specific absence of serum IgA and who have produced anti-IgA, either "spontaneously" or as a result of pregnancy or globulin infusion or injection. More usually, however, there is little or no quantitative IgA deficiency demonstrable. The antibody is immune and reactive only with a particular IgA allotype, under which circumstances the reaction is less severe. Rarely anti-Gm antibodies have caused anaphylactoid reactions. The full-blown attack includes wheezing, dyspnea, flushing, cyanosis, laryngeal edema, nausea, abdominal, back, and chest pain, and shock. Anaphylactoid reactions may be fatal in minutes if not immediately treated. Therapy inludes administration of epinephrine, adrenal corticosteroids, oxygen, and fluids. Similar reactions can occur after intramuscular injection of gamma globulin into patients with hypogammaglobulinemia. IgA deficiency is relatively common, occurring in up to one in 700 persons. Such patients should receive only washed RBC and/or IgA-deficient plasma. Fortunately, anaphylactoid reactions are rare, occurring only once per 20,000 transfusions.

The type of anti-immunoglobulin reaction occurring in a patient depends on whether the antibody is free or bound. Its distribution is a function of the class of the immunoglobulin antigen. Thus, anti-IgE complexes bound to mast cells will cause histamine release and urticaria, whereas anti-IgG complexes may precipitate in joints and cause arthritis. It should be emphasized, however, that the usual anti-IgG antibodies cause little clinical problem. Anti-IgG antibodies are generally directed against a group of polymorphic antigenic determinants situated on the gamma H-chains of the IgG molecule and known as the Gm antigens. Because they exist in multiple different forms, Gm antigens can elicit antibody formation during pregnancy, after transfusion, or after immunoglobulin injections. Repeated exposure is usually required. Anti-Gm antibodies are often found as autoantibodies in patients with rheumatoid arthritis. In patients with infectious mononucleosis with IgG anti-i, IgM anti-IgG may be found as a cause of hemolytic anemia. Anti-IgM antibodies are occasionally encountered after repeated transfusions as are antibodies to kappa-chain determinants known as Km (Inv) groups.

LABORATORY STUDY OF TRANSFUSION REACTIONS

When the signs and symptoms of a possible hemolytic transfusion reaction appear, the transfusion, if in progress, should be stopped at once. Fresh blood samples, both clotted and in EDTA, a urine sample if available, and the remainder of the untransfused blood should be sent to the blood bank immediately together with a description of the clinical reaction. Upon receipt of these samples, the technologist should carry out the following:

1) Check for clerical error. This includes confirming donor and recipient identification data as recorded on the blood bag label, the compatibility certification tag, the labels on both the pretransfusion and posttransfusion patient blood specimens and the worksheet on which the compatibility testing results were recorded. He should also compare patient name, donor identification number, patient hospital identification number, patient age, sex, location, physician, ABO group, Rh type, and any data regarding alloantibodies listed on the various records.

2) Examine the posttransfusion patient serum for visible hemolysis. Hemoglobin in serum is usually detectable visually in a column 1 cm in diameter when the concentration exceeds 20 mg/dl. Recall that the presence of hemoglobin in the plasma or urine has causes other than antibody-mediated hemolysis, and its presence after a transfusion does not necessarily indicate a transfusion reaction. Traumatic specimen collection may be misleading in this regard. Faulty blood storage may cause red blood cell damage and in vitro hemolysis as a consequence of freezing, heating to temperatures over 50 C, or simply prolonging storage past the expiration date of the blood, with resultant hemoglobinemia. The transfusion of large numbers of nonviable RBC without blood group antigen-antibody interaction does not produce symptoms of renal damage, though an increase in serum bilirubin may result from the excessive hemoglobin load presented to the liver to catabolize.

Faulty transfusion technique may also be to blame. Drugs or other substances may have been added to the blood. The blood may have been infused concurrently with glucose in water: glucose rapidly enters RBC, followed by water, and the cell bursts. Sometimes blood is transfused through small-bore needles or under excessive pressure, and this results in mechanical hemolysis. Donor abnormalities such as red blood cell glucose-6-phosphate dehydrogenase deficiency may result in rapid RBC destruction if the cells are transfused to a patient with a drug such as a synthetic antimalarial or a sulfonamide in his plasma. A whole host of patient abnormalities may cause nonimmunologic hemolysis of host and donor RBC, including such entities as faulty mechanical heart valves or urinary bladder irrigation with distilled water.

3) Examine the returned bag of blood for visible hemolysis, clotting, discoloration, or other evidence of cell destruction, including signs of overheating, freezing, or bacterial contamination. If the latter is suspect, make a gram-stained smear of the blood and examine it microscopically for the presence of microorganisms.

4) Perform a direct antiglobulin test on the pre- and posttransfusion patient RBC and on the donor RBC. The direct antiglobulin test on the posttransfusion patient RBC sample should be examined microscopically to detect mixed-field agglutination. Incompatible transfused RBC may form agglutinates on a background of free patient cells. If almost all of the cell supension is agglutinated, one of

two possibilities obtains: the patient may have AHD or incompatible plasma may have been administered, which has reacted with the patient's RBC. An eluate should be made from RBC yielding a positive anti-IgG test and the antibody specificity determined.

5) Repeat the ABO grouping and Rh typing on the blood from the returned container and on the patient's pre- and posttransfusion RBC specimens.

6) Repeat the compatibility tests, performing both major and minor crossmatches with both the pre- and posttransfusion patient blood samples. The major crossmatch may include the use of enzyme-treated RBC, prolonged incubation, and testing at 18 C.

7) Call the attending physician with a preliminary report of the test results; emphasize positive findings. Early recognition and prompt treatment of a hemolytic transfusion may abort a potentially fatal outcome. All test results, to whom reported and when, should be recorded at once on the Transfusion Reaction Investigation form for inclusion in the patient's clinical records.

At the time of the preliminary report, inquiries should be made, if the information is not already known, as to:

a) Whether anything was added to the blood before or during the transfusion.

b) Whether the transfusion was begun immediately upon receipt of the blood on the floor or whether it was delayed. If the transfusion was delayed, ascertain where the blood was stored and for how long.

c) Whether and how the blood was warmed before administration.

d) What drugs or other infusions (e.g., dextrose in water) the patient might have been simultaneously receiving, and in general what medications are being administered.

After the completion and reporting of the initial phase of the investigation, further study may proceed in a more ordered fashion.

8) Repeat the screening tests for alloantibodies on the pre- and posttransfusion patient samples and on the donor blood. If negative, the tests may be repeated using enzyme-treated red blood cells, prolonged incubation periods, and testing at 18 C. Negative results must be examined microscopically, with a particular search made for mixed-field agglutination. The specificity of any antibody detected should be identified.

9) If an antibody specificity is determined, the retained segment from all units of blood that the patient has received should be typed for the corresponding antigen.

10) Test the urine specimen chemically for hemoglobin. The urine sediment should be examined microscopically for RBC and casts.

11) A stained peripheral blood smear should be examined for RBC fragmentation, spherocytosis, nucleated RBC, reticulocytosis, and thrombocytopenia.

12) A workup for DIC should be initiated if there is any evidence of intravascular hemolysis as the result of red blood cell antigen-antibody reaction.

Additional procedures that may be useful, depending on the circumstances of the reaction and the elapsed time since its occurrence, include:

1) Culture of the blood remaining in the transfusion container. Both aerobic and anaerobic microorganisms, including bacteria and fungi, should be sought. Culturing should be carried out both at room temperature and 37 C.

2) A search for leukoagglutinins and lymphocytotoxic antibodies in both the pretransfusion patient serum and in the donor plasma. Antibodies to platelet and granulocyte antigens may be sought under some circumstances.

3) Quantitation of serum IgA levels in the recipient's pretransfusion serum. A search for anti-Gm or anti-IgA allotypes may be indicated.

4) Comparison of serum hemoglobin, methamalbumin and haptoglobin concentrations in pre- and posttransfusion patient sera.

5) Comparison of hemolytic complement titers and C3 and/or C4 concentrations in pre- and posttransfusion patient sera. A shift in mobility of C3 and C4 on immunoelectrophoresis may indicate complement activation.

6) Determination of serum bilirubin concentrations in patient samples obtained immediately after the reaction and at three, six, and nine hours later.

7) A search for hemosiderin granules in urine sediments from samples obtained 24 to 48 hours after the reaction.

8) Comparison of anti-A and/or anti-B titers in the pretransfusion patient serum and in samples obtained seven to ten days later.

9) Repeat screening for serum alloantibodies in patient serum seven to ten days after the reaction.

10) Screening of patient pretransfusion serum with RBC bearing low-incidence antigens.

11) Infusion of a very small amount of fresh RBC from the original donor tagged with ^{51}Cr, with determination of their rate of disappearance. This may be particularly necessary if additional transfusions are contemplated.

If a possible transfusion reaction is not reported for many hours or even days after it is alleged to have occurred, all of the above may no longer be possible. Abnormalities to be sought several days after the fact are principally confined to the appearance of alloantibodies previously undetected or in the case of an ABO-incompatible transfusion, an appreciable increase in anti-A or anti-B titer. In the absence of other explanations, a failure of the expected increase in hemoglobin, hematocrit, or red blood cell count 24 to 48 hours after transfusion suggests the possibility of accelerated RBC destruction. Frequently, it is possible in the case of single-unit transfusions to find an antigen in the transfused unit absent from the donor's cells. Treatment of an RBC suspension prepared from a posttransfusion blood sample with appropriate antiserum should produce mixed-field agglutination involving 10% or more of the sample. Absence of agglutination indicates substantial loss of transfused RBC.

There is evidence that if D-positive RBC are transfused inadvertently or by dint of circumstances to a D-negative recipient, immunization to the D antigen can frequently be prevented by the immediate administration in the form of commercially available Rh immune globulin of 20 to 25 μg of a potent IgG anti-D per ml of RBC given. The use of such preparations in the prevention of maternal Rh sensitization is discussed in Chapter 21.

RECOMMENDED READING:

Dodd, B.E. and Lincoln, P.J.: *Blood Group Topics.* Williams & Wilkins, Baltimore, 1975

Engelfriet, C.P.: C4 and C3 on red cells coated in vivo and in vitro. In: *An International Symposium on the Nature and Significance of Complement Activation.* Ortho Raritan, N.J., 1976. p. 69

Garratty, G.: Antibody-mediated cell destruction. In: *Advances in Immunohematology.* Spectra. Oxnard, Calif, N.D

Goldfinger, D.: Complications of hemolytic transfusion reactions, pathogenesis and treatment. In: *New Approaches of Tranfusion Reactions*. Am Assn of Blood Banks. Washington, 1974, p.15

Greendyke, R.M. and Banzhaf, J.C.: *Blood Bank Policies and Procedures*. Medical Examination Publishing Co., Garden City, N.Y., 1976

Grumet, F.C. and Yankee, R.A.: Non-red cell reactions. In: *New Approaches to Transfusion Reactions*. Am Assn of Blood Banks. Washington, 1974, p.39

Huestis, D.W. et al: *Practical Blood Transfusion*, 2nd ed. Little, Brown and Co., Boston, 1976

Issitt, P.D. and Issitt, C.H.: *Applied Blood Group Serology*, 2nd ed. Spectra. Oxnard, Calif., 1975

Miller, W.V.: Transfusion reactions. In: *Blood Group Immunology: Theoretical and Practical Concepts*. Dade, Miami, 1976. p. 125

Miller, W.V. (Ed): *Technical Manual of the American Association of Blood Banks*. Am Assn of Blood Banks. Washington, 1977

Mollison, P.L.: *Blood Transfusion in Clinical Medicine,* 5th ed. Blackwell, Oxford, 1972

transfusion is still required to provide RBC, several measures have been found helpful. Warming the patient will encourage peripheral pooling of blood and lessen the volume that can accumulate in the lungs. Transfusing the patient in the sitting position accomplishes the same purpose. Administration of a rapidly acting diuretic to such patients before transfusion has also been suggested. In patients with established congestive heart failure it may be necessary to remove blood from one vein while administering RBC through another.

Discussion of the metabolic problems potentially associated with large volume transfusions must begin with an understanding of the alterations occurring in blood upon storage. It is obvious that the artificial environment in which blood is preserved is a poor substitute for the circulation. The dextrose in the preservative solution provides a source of energy for cell metabolism, but the red blood cell membrane still gradually loses its functional integrity with the passage of time, and the cell becomes increasingly fragile. Sodium leaks into the cell and potassium escapes. Lactic acid is produced as a result of RBC glycolysis, and the pH of the plasma falls. These changes are reversible in most red blood cells during the first few days of storage, but as the "storage lesion" becomes more severe, increasing numbers of RBC die, with escape of hemoglobin into the plasma. By the time that three weeks of storage in CPD preservative have elapsed (or four weeks in CPD-adenine), up to 30% of the RBC are nonviable and are rapidly removed by the reticuloendothelial system of the recipient when transfused. Some of the alterations in the composition and characterisitics of blood refrigerated in CPD for various periods of time are shown in Table 20-1. It will be noted that depletion of red blood cell adenosine triphosphate (ATP) and 2,3-diphosphoglycerate (2,3-DPG) occurs on storage. These enzymes are vitally concerned with energy transfer and energy-producing reactions in RBC. Depletion of red blood cell ATP is associated with a change in shape of stored cells from biconcave discs to spheres, loss of membrane lipid, decreased critical hemolytic volume, and increased rigidity, all of which contribute to increased cell fragility. Depletion of red blood cell 2,3-DPG causes a shift in the oxygen dissociation curve of blood (which relates P_{O_2} to percent oxygen saturation), indicating decreased ability to release oxygen. The "storage lesion" is reversible and viable RBC return to biochemical normality within hours to a few days after being transfused. The pathogenesis of the storage lesion appears to be related to

TABLE 20-1

Composition and Characteristics of Blood Stored in CPD Preservative
Solution at 4 C for Various Periods of Time

Component	Duration of Storage (Days)			
	0	7	14	21
Percent viable RBC 24 hours after transfusion	100	98	85	70–80
Plasma pH (37 C)	7.20	7.00	6.89	6.84
ATP (% of initial value)	100	96	88	86
2, 3-DPG (% of initial value)	100	99	80	44
P_{50} (mm Hg)	23.5	23	20	17
Plasma Na (mEq/l)	168	166	163	156
Plasma K (mEq/l)	3.9	11.9	17.2	21.0
Plasma hemoglobin (mg/dl)	1.7	7.8	12.5	19.1
Plasma dextrose (mg/dl)	345	312	282	231
Hematocrit	36	36	36	35

the glycolytic metabolism of the red blood cell. Despite the fact that glycolysis proceeds in RBC stored at 4 C only one fortieth as rapidly as it does at body temperature, the accumulation of lactic and other organic acids upon storage and the resultant fall in pH interfere with the function of hexokinase and other enzymes involved in energy production in RBC. As glycolysis slows, ATP concentrations decrease, and by the time RBC ATP falls to a third of normal, cell viability has been reduced by half.

Considerable attention has been paid to the depletion of 2,3-DPG in stored RBC because of the increased affinity for oxygen exhibited by such cells. Cells deficient in 2,3-DPG exhibit decreased ability to release oxygen to the tissues when in circulation. In this connection, however, several facts need to be recalled: there is almost no red blood cell loss of 2,3-DPG during the first week of storage in usual preservative solutions, and only a 20% loss at the end of two weeks. Reduced RBC concentrations of 2,3-DPG are 50% restored within four hours after transfusion and are normal within 24 hours. Total replacement of blood volume by transfusion even twice within 24 hours has not been shown to reduce the blood P_{50} (the oxygen tension at which hemoglobin is half saturated) below a physiologically acceptable value (20 mm of Hg). The concentration of red blood cell

2,3-DPG is only one of several factors affecting the oxygen affinity of blood. Chief among these is blood pH, which has a major effect on the position of the oxygen dissociation curve. A decrease in blood pH of 0.3 exerts a countereffect on oxygen dissociation equal to the consequences of total 2,3-DPG depletion. Hence, in the case of transfusion of 2,3-DPG depleted blood, tissue anoxia and lactic acidosis shift the oxygen dissociation curve back to normal. The harmful effects of alkalosis in this situation are obvious. It is also emphasized that increased cardiac output is a major compensation brought to bear by the body when oxygen unloading is, for some reason, compromised. Similarly, the increase in A-V oxygen difference occurring in the tissues may be large enough to increase oxygen delivery to adequate levels. It thus appears that only when the compensatory mechanisms of the body are exhausted does the 2,3-DPG concentration in transfused RBC become critical. Multiple transfusions may impair oxygen delivery to the tissues by virtue of the metabolic alkalosis that results from the metabolism of administered citrate, from the increased oxygen affinity of blood during hypothermia caused by shock, the transfusion of cold blood and/or hypothermia intentionally induced during anesthesia, and by the traditional blood bank practice of dispensing older units of blood first. Alkalosis, hypothermia, and reduced 2,3-DPG concentrations in transfused blood have an additive effect in increasing hemoglobin affinity for oxygen.

In patients experiencing prolonged shock, suffering fixed cardiac output, or undergoing coronary artery bypass procedures, the transfusion of RBC with high concentrations of 2,3-DPG may be advantageous. In the case, however, of transfusions of even multiple units to normal persons with the usual compensatory mechanisms operative, attention to 2,3-DPG levels is not considered necessary.

The participation of blood transfusion in the acid-base inbalance seen in severely injured patients is complex. Stored blood has an appreciable acid load from its citrate anticoagulant content and the lactic acid produced by red blood cell glycolysis. Most patients who require large blood transfusions already exhibit varying degrees of metabolic acidosis associated with hypovolemia and incipient or frank shock. Transfused citrate and lactate are, however, normally rapidly metabolized in the liver, and the systemic acidosis is improved by restoring adequate circulating blood volume by transfusion. Patients who are not in shock and have normal hepatic function manage the acid load of transfusion readily, and alkalinization is unnecessary.

The interrelationship between the citrate load in blood transfusions and the recipient's ionized serum calcium levels is also of concern. The effects of transfusion in this connection are influenced by the rate of citrate administration in blood and the rate of its catabolism by the liver, by the rate of calcium mobilization from skeletal stores (which may be considerable) and by the effects of abnormal pH values on calcium and citrate metabolism. Ionized calcium levels are affected to a lesser degree by the binding effects of phosphate and lactate administered in stored blood. Increased potassium ion concentrations (found in the sera of patients with tissue damage or shock and in stored blood) may have an additive effect in producing hypocalcemia. Calcium mobilization is reduced in shock. Alkalosis increases the binding of ionized calcium by plasma proteins and decreases total serum calcium levels.

The problem of hypocalcemia due to citrate administration can be put in proper perspective by appreciating that to produce hypocalcemia in a normal adult, blood transfusions must be given at a rate exceeding 15 units (7.5 liters) per hour. In a 3 kg infant, hypocalcemia may result if more than one unit of blood per hour is exchanged. The citrate load in exchange transfusions in infants, using CPD-preserved blood, can be reduced from 4.7 mMol per unit of whole blood with a hematocrit of about 36 to 1.2 mMol if blood with a hematocrit of 65 is used, and to 0.3 mMol if the blood has a hematocrit of 85, under which circumstances the risk of citrate intoxication except in cases of severe liver disease is negligible. It should be noted that if exchange transfusion in an infant is carried out using whole blood, the baby may receive up to 600 mg of citrate per kg and plasma citrate concentrations may reach the toxic level (100 mg/dl) at which muscle tremors and electrocardiographic changes can occur. These effects are not caused by hypocalcemia solely but are aggravated by acidosis and hyperkalemia.

Whereas normal RBC contain about 100 mEq of potassium per liter, normal plasma levels are of the order of 4 to 5 mEq, increasing with storage in CPD up to 9 to 17 mEq after 21 days at 4 C. In infant exchange transfusions, the use of blood stored over a week can raise serum potassium levels to 8 mEq/l or more, and death is almost certain if concentrations exceed 10 mEq/l. On the other hand, in considering transfusions to adults it should be recalled that even at a plasma concentration of 25 mEq/l, a liter of stored blood contains only about 12 mEq of potassium in excess of normal plasma levels – a negligible amount. Hypokalemia is a common occurrence in massively transfused patients as a result of mixed respiratory and metabolic (citrate) alkalosis, though balanced to various degrees by the hyperkalemia of shock and metabolic (lactate) acidosis. The additive effects of elevated potassium and citrate concentrations have been noted above.

Miscellaneous metabolites that accumulate in stored blood include ammonia and phosphate, but these are generally of little clinical significance. The blood ammonia levels in blood stored in ACD solution may reach 700 μg/dl after 21 days, but these amounts are very small in comparison to the total ammonia content of the body water. Similarly, phosphate is present in CPD preservative solutions and increases in stored blood with time, but the amount of phosphate administered in a unit of blood is again small in relation to the total body stores.

In summarizing the metabolic effects of blood transfusion to adults one cannot improve upon Collins: "An intact circulation is a very good defense against the metabolic problems of massive transfusion." In the patient with massive hemorrhage, the more blood used early, the less the overall impact of a large transfusion will be. Many of the undesirable effects attributed to the massive transfusion of stored blood appear to be due to giving too little too late.

Coagulation defects are traditionally mentioned in discussions of the complications of blood transfusion but are uncommon in practice. Postsurgical bleeding may be caused by a number of factors, including inadequate or excessive neutralization of heparin with protamine, inadequate mechanical hemostasis (i.e., severed blood vessels that have not been tied off), and disseminated intravascular coagulation triggered by tissue trauma. Dilution of procoagulants by massive transfusion of stored blood deficient in labile coagulation factors (platelets, Factor VIII and Factor V) is theoretically possible and conceptually logical but rarely causes coagulation problems if the patient's coagulation mechanism was normal and intact before the transfusions. The amounts of Factor V required for adequate hemostasis are of the order of 5% of normal, and the Factor V content of blood stored for 14 days averages 50% of normal, so that Factor V dilution by transfusion of stored blood is indeed unlikely. The situation with Factor VIII is different inasmuch as Factor VIII levels of 30% are necessary for surgical hemostasis, and Factor VIII levels in stored blood decrease rather rapidly, falling by an average of 20% after 24 hours and 40% after 48 hours. Replacement of Factor VIII by the body of a bleeding patient, however, occurs relatively rapidly, so that in the absence of DIC, bleeding due to Factor VIII dilution by stored blood, though possible, is distinctly unusual. Dilutional thrombocytopenia, however, does occur, albeit rarely, owing to the fact that platelets remain viable in blood stored at 4 C for only a few hours, and in blood stored more than 24 hours they are almost absent. In subjects without splenomegaly, the spleen sequesters a quantity of platelets equal only to about 20% of the circulating platelet pool. In patients operated upon with the use of pump oxygenators, thrombocytopenia occurs routinely and may persist for several days, but in the absence of complications rarely causes bleeding.

Hemosiderosis, the widespread deposition of iron-containing hemosiderin pigment in the tissues of the body, is a predictable complication of chronic transfusion therapy. One liter of blood contains about 500 mg of iron, essentially all of which is retained when the RBC in which it was contained are destroyed. Body iron loss in the male averages only about 1 mg/day. Although hemosiderosis of considerable degree may cause no organ dysfunction, cardiac malfunction and cirrhosis related to hemosiderosis have been reported.

The transfusion of large amounts of cold blood may induce hypothermia, and the infusion of over 3000 ml/hr may decrease the core temperature of the recipient sufficiently that cardiac arrhythmia or standstill may result. Even without this complication, it has been calculated by Collins that the warming of 10 liters of blood from 4 C to 37 C requires about 300 kilocalories of heat energy. If the transfusion is given over the space of two hours, 150 kilocalories of extra heat energy are required per hour or twice the normal resting expenditure. Put another way, 300 kilocalories represent the energy requirement for an hour's moderate work, and the consumption of about 62 liters of extra oxygen to metabolize completely the amount of glucose necessary to provide this amount of heat. This added requirement obviously occurs at the worst possible time for patient whose respiratory reserve frequently is already compromised. Hypothermia also slows hepatic catabolism of citrate and lactate, which leads to acidosis and increases the chance of hypocalcemia. Hypothermia also increases the affinity of hemoglobin for oxygen, impairs blood clotting, and aggravates potassium leakage from tissue cells already losing potassium as a consequence of acidosis. Blood warmers that lack most of the objectionable features of early microwave types are now available, and their use is almost mandatory in rapid massive transfusions, including exchange transfusions in infants and in transfusions to patients sufficiently ill to require the use of intensive care facilities.

Whenever blood is transfused the possibility exists of small clots making their way from the blood container into the patient's circulation and lodging in the capillary bed of the lungs. To prevent this occurrence, blood is passed through a filter as it is transfused. The standard blood filter has a pore size of 170 μ, which is sufficient to remove gross clots and larger particles of debris comprised of fibrin strands and aggregates of platelets and leukocytes. Smaller clumps, however, begin to form in blood stored for 24 hours and are numerous after ten days. These clumps escape through the usual filter and may lodge in substantial quantities in the lungs. It has been postulated that such microemboli may obstruct pulmonary blood flow with release of vasoactive substances that can cause capillary damage and lead to pulmonary insuffiency. Up to 90% of microemboli are removed from blood by washing or by the use of one of several commercially available microaggregate filters made of Dacron or having graded pore sizes. Some problems are encountered in the use of these filters when very rapid administration of blood is desired because of their tendency to clog after three or four units of blood have been passed through them. The indications for the use of microaggregate filters are still debated, but many anesthesiologists feel that they should be used for transfusions during surgical procedures involving pulmonary bypass, because blood is damaged by the pump oxygenator and the cerebral circulation is vulnerable. The occurrence of progressive pulmonary insufficiency in the massively transfused patient is frequently seen but has multiple causes other than microembolism, the most important of which are sepsis, shock with DIC, and left ventricular failure.

A very important consideration in the transfusion therapy of patients with anemia or who are undergoing surgery is the concept of blood sludge or the aggregation of RBC in the microcirculation. The formation of blood sludge is a consequence of several diseases but also influences their course. Sludging occurs in any situation where blood viscosity and the tendency to RBC aggregation in vivo is increased and is aggravated by slow blood flow. Sludge impairs the microcirculation and leads to tissue anoxia, acidosis, and cell necrosis. Anemia is interpreted as a physiologic defense in combating the formation of blood sludge by decreasing blood viscosity, increasing flow rates, and thereby decreasing RBC aggregation. By this view, hemodilution is physiologically advantageous in many disease states. Blood sludging due to sluggish blood flow occurs in patients in shock, with congestive heart failure, or with venous occlusion and is aggravated by the increased serum concentrations of fibrinogen and alpha-2 macroglobulin that occurs in patients with such diseases as dysproteinemias, diabetes mellitus, and rheumatic disease. In the normal circulation in vivo (as opposed to the in vitro situation discussed under forces influencing antibody-mediated RBC agglutination) RBC are kept separated by the hemodynamic forces of flowing blood. In sludged blood, shear forces do not keep cells dispersed, either because the shear force is decreased or the adhesive forces of plasma proteins are increased. At slow rates of flow, one factor enhances the other. The blood hematocrit determines the consequences of these two factors: at a hematocrit of 40 to 45, low shear stresses permit aggregation of RBC by normal concentrations of plasma proteins, but at hematocrits below 35, even abnormally increased plasma protein concentrations do not appreciably increase aggregation if blood flow is slowed. On the other hand, at hematocrit values of more than 55, marked sludging occurs even when shear forces are not decreased by diminished flow. In vivo, anemia is associated with decreased RBC aggregation. What aggregation does occur has a minor effect on blood viscosity. Anemia is thus beneficial to the patient in combating blood sludging and its consequences whenever clinical situations characterized by decreased blood flow occur. Intentional induction of anemia or hemodilution, is often practiced at surgery to take advantage of this fact.

TRANSMISSION OF INFECTIOUS DISEASE

A number of infectious diseases can be transmitted by blood transfusion, of which the most important is viral hepatitis. This disease is produced by several different viruses, the clinically most severe form being hepatitis B. In this disease, the Dane particle, a 20-nm spherical virus-like mass containing DNA-polymerase (a virus-specific enzyme) is produced in the nuclei of infected hepatocytes.

This particle is known as hepatitis B core antigen (HB_CAg) and represents the core of the hepatitis B virus. Cores are released into the cytoplasm of infected hepatocytes where they are coated by hepatitis B surface antigen (HB_SAg) to form complete hepatitis B virus. A great excess of surface antigen is produced and released unassembled into the blood. Various subtypes of HB_SAg have been described.

The incubation period of hepatitis B varies from 50 to 160 days after the transfusion of blood containing demonstrable HB_SAg. Antigenemia occurs within three to 13 weeks, followed shortly thereafter by clinical disease. HB_SAg may appear in the blood in detectable amounts a few days before or simultaneously with increased concentrations of serum aspartate aminotransferase (SGOT). The serum HB_SAg concentration peaks as symptoms begin and in uncomplicated cases disappears within six to 12 weeks, at which time anti-HB_S appears. As many as 10% of persons with hepatitis B become chronic carriers of the virus. Many are asymptomatic and are said to have latent hepatitis, but a few continue to have active symptomatic liver disease that may vary in severity from the condition known as chronic persistent hepatitis to unrelenting, progressive chronic active hepatitis. Chronic hepatitis may evolve into one form of cirrhosis of the liver or cause hepatic failure before cirrhosis develops. Anti-HB_C is found in the serum of most patients with chronic hepatitis B and its presence correlates well with persistence of replicating virus. The hepatitis B virus has also been implicated in the pathogenesis of primary hepatocellular carcinoma. Another antigen called "e" is found in the serum of patients with chronic hepatitis B and may well be a host antibody directed against virus-modified hepatic cell membranes. Anti-e (not to be confused with blood group anti-e) appears to be an anti-antibody that reacts with modified "e" now recognized as antigenic. The e system is thought to be a marker for chronic hepatitis B with continuing liver cell damage.

Transmission of hepatitis B occurs by several routes of exposure, including needle injection into the skin or bloodstream, transfer through skin abrasions or cuts, or introduction through mucous membranes (e.g., eye, mouth) of infected blood or serum. The disease can also be transmitted by introduction of known infectious secretions such as saliva, urine, or seminal fluid onto mucosal surfaces, or by indirect transfer of virus via insect vectors or inanimate surfaces. Airborne transmission and infection via the intestinal route do not occur. The onset of hepatitis B is usually gradual; the symptoms and signs consist of some combination of anorexia, nausea, malaise, abdominal pain, jaundice, and arthralgia. The severity of the disease is related to the dose of virus and the age of the patient, older patients faring less well.

Prophylaxis of hepatitis B with hepatitis B immune globin is effective, though expensive, and appears to be indicated for use in patients in hemodialysis units where hepatitis B is endemic. It is also recommended for postexposure prophylaxis in medical personnel following needle sticks with HB_SAg contamination, in spouses of patients with acute hepatitis B, and in infants born of mothers with positive serologic tests for HB_SAg.

Two major steps have contributed to a reduction in the once considerable incidence of posttransfusion hepatitis B in the United States. The first of these was the introduction of mandatory testing of all donor blood for HB_SAg by radioimmunoassay or an equally sensitive procedure. The incidence of positive tests in a clinically well, volunteer donor population is about 1/1000 people. The second step, and probably the more important, has been to eliminate the practice of obtaining blood from paid donors. It has been shown that the likelihood of transfusion-induced hepatitis in recipients of blood obtained from commercial sources is ten times or more higher than it is when volunteer donors are used. Although the screening of blood for HB_SAg has reduced the incidence of posttransfusion hepatitis B by half or more, there remain cases where blood negative to testing remains infectious, probably because the dose of virus capable of causing disease remains below the threshold of sensitivity of the current assays.

The radioimmunoassay procedure that has become standard procedure in most blood banks is a solid-phase test. Unlabeled antibody to HB_SAg of animal origin is fixed to a solid support such as a bead or the wall of a polystyrene test tube. Test serum is added and the test incubated. Antigen if present is fixed to the antibody. Unfixed protein is removed by washing, and ^{125}I-labeled anti-HB_S is added, forming a sandwich with the antigen if HB_SAg was fixed in the previous step. Free anti-HB_S is washed away, and the radioactivity of the preparation counted. Specificity is assured by repeating positive tests and adding unlabeled anti-HB$_S$ before introduction of radioactive anti-HB$_S$, thereby blocking specific uptake of the labeled antibody.

Even after the elimination of cases of hepatitis caused by the hepatitis A and B viruses, the cytomegalovirus (CMV), and the Epstein-Barr virus (see below) there remains a large group of cases of posttransfusion hepatitis, currently listed as a result of "non-A, non-B" hepatitis virus or viruses. The disease caused by this group of agents is generally less severe than hepatitis B, but may progress to chronic hepatitis. There is no currently known way to detect the agent(s) of this disease, but it has been found that the change from paid to volunteer blood donors has reduced its prevalence somewhat. Some 70% to 90% of posttransfusion hepatitis in the United States is now of the non-A, non-B type.

Subjects with anti-HB$_S$ do not transmit hepatitis B. All blood products but gamma globulin, albumin, and purified protein fraction can transmit posttransfusion hepatitis, though washed RBC have a much reduced likelihood of doing so. There is an obviously increased risk of infection from products prepared from pools of serum or plasma.

The "post-perfusion" syndrome, so named because of its initial recognition after coronary bypass procedures were introduced, can occur after any blood transfusion, but is particularly common after the administration of fresh blood in large amounts. In 3% to 11% of such cases, two to seven weeks after transfusion the patient develops a disease resembling infectious mononucleosis, with fever, lymphadenopathy, hepatosplenomegaly, skin rash, and the presence of atypical lymphocytes in the peripheral blood. Two viruses of the herpes group are causative, of which the cytomegalovirus is more often implicated than the Epstein-Barr virus. Up to 12% of blood donors have leukocytes infected with CMV, and 50% to 65% have serum complement-fixing antibodies for CMV. The viruses may persist for years without clinical manifestation. Disease in the blood recipient is usually a reinfection and is generally subclinical. Some 20% of recipients of more than one transfusion whose serum was originally negative on testing form antibodies to CMV.

Syphilis may also be transmitted by blood transfusion, although present-day precautions all but preclude the possibility. Routine serologic tests for syphilis have traditionally been performed on all units of blood, though the need for this in the United States is questioned. Patients with primary syphilis may be seronegative.

Seropositive blood may be transfused if treatment has rendered the donor noninfectious. Storage of blood at 4 C for four days kills the spirochetes of syphilis. Transfusion-transmitted syphilis has an incubation period of four weeks to four months, averaging nine to ten weeks, and presents with the skin eruption of the secondary disease.

Transfusion-transmitted malaria remains a problem in some parts of the world. All species of plasmodia infectious for man survive for weeks in blood stored at 4 C. Blood donor histories must include questions about residence or recent travel in known malarious areas.

Blood when drawn from a donor is not bacteriologically sterile in about 2% of cases, despite the use of meticulous technic in collection. The defense mechanisms present in blood (bacterial antibodies, complement, phagocytes) and refrigeration of the unit usually keep bacteria in check, and within four days almost all units are sterile, but if blood is allowed to remain at room temperature for several hours, massive bacterial growth may, on rare occasions, take place. Blood that has been warmed or out of refrigeration long enough to reach a temperature of 10 C (about 30 minutes under most circumstances) is not considered safe for subsequent transfusion and should not be returned to stock by the blood bank. Gram-negative bacteria, usually *Pseudomonas* species or members of the *Escherichia-Aerogenes* group, may grow slowly in blood at 4 C without a log-growth phase, but if the blood is warmed log growth may occur in six hours. Transfusion of as little as 50 ml of blood heavily contaminated by such bacteria can produce, within 30 minutes or less, a clinical picture characterized by flushed dry skin, fever, abdominal pain, vomiting, shock, collapse, and frequently death. It should be appreciated that blood heavily contaminated by bacteria need not necessarily be hemolyzed. The usefulness of stained smears to detect bacterial contamination is limited by two facts: Debris in the blood makes bacterial identification difficult, and more than 100,000 organisms per ml are generally necessary for detection. In passing it may be noted that pyrogenic bacterial products may remain after sterilization in equipment or supplies through which blood passes.

RECOMMENDED READING:

Alter, H.J.: Radioimmunoassay tests for hepatitis B surface antigen. In: *A Seminar on Current Technical Topics*. Am Assn of Blood Banks. Washington, 1974, p. 1

Alter, H.J.: How frequent is post-transfusion hepatitis after the introduction of third generation screening for hepatitis B? *Vox Sand* 32:346, 1977

Bergentz, S.E. et al: What is the significance of blood sludge today – cause or effect of disease? *Vox Sang* 32:250, 1977

Bredenberg, C.E. et al: Does a relationship exist between massive blood transfusion and the adult respiratory distress syndrome? *Vox Sang* 32:311, 1977

Collins, J.A.: Problems associated with the massive transfusion of stored blood. *Surg* 75:274, 1974

Greenwalt, T.J. (Ed): *General Principles of Blood Transfusion*. Am Med Assn Chicago, 1977

Grindon, A.J. and Wallas, C.H.: Non-immunologic complications of blood transfusion. In: *New Approaches to Transfusion Reactions*. Am Assn of Blood Banks. Washington, 1974, p. 63

Huestis, D.W. et al: *Practical Blood Transfusion*, 2nd ed. Little, Brown and Co., Boston, 1976

Immune globulins for protection against viral hepatitis. *Morbidity and Mortality Weekly Report*. U.S. Public Health Service. Atlanta, Vol. 26, No. 52, Dec. 30, 1977

Mollison, P.L.: *Blood Transfusion in Clinical Medicine*, 5th ed. Blackwell, Oxford, 1972

Solis, R.T.: Microembolization and blood transfusion. In: *A Seminar on Current Technical Topics*. Am Assn of Blood Banks. Washington, 1974, p. 31

Spurling, C.L.: Transmissible disease and blood transfusion. In: *New Approaches to Transfusion Reactions*. Am Assn of Blood Banks. Washington, 1974, p. 53

CHAPTER 21

Hemolytic Disease of the Newborn

Hemolytic disease of the newborn (HDN), or erythroblastosis fetalis, is a hemolytic anemia caused by the transplacental transfer of maternal blood group antibody that reacts with an antigen present on fetal red blood cells and causes their premature destruction. Accelerated fetal RBC destruction may begin as early as the fourth month of gestation. Most maternal antibody transfer is beneficial to the fetus inasmuch as the immunologic system of the newborn infant is not fully functional for up to 18 months, but HDN represents an example of a harmful immunologic response. HDN occurs in a spectrum of severity. Less than 0.5% of all infants born are affected at a clinical level, though subclinical HDN can affect up to 15% to 20%. In clinical HDN, the unborn infant becomes anemic. Compensatory increases in red blood cell production in the liver, spleen, and elsewhere may be considerable. If anemia becomes sufficiently severe, congestive heart failure occurs, and the fetus becomes edematous (hydrops fetalis). Death may occur by the twentieth week of gestation, and the stillborn rate in HDN due to anti-D may reach 12%.

If the infant is born alive, he can frequently be saved, although severe anemis is a poor prognostic sign. Jaundice (icterus gravis) appears within a few hours after birth as a consequence of the continuing destruction of the infant's antibody-sensitized RBC and the inability of his immature liver to metabolize the excessive load of blood pigment. Jaundice does not occur antepartum because fetal hemoglobin breakdown products enter the maternal circulation and are excreted by the mother's liver. The hyperbilirubinemia in the infant progresses in severity during the hours following birth, reaching a peak in the term infant within 48 to 96 hours, but often later in premature babies. Hyperbilirubinemia, if sufficiently severe, causes staining and degenerative changes in the basal ganglia of the brain, a condition known as kernicterus, or bilirubin encephalopathy. Kernicterus is caused by the toxic effects of unconjugated bilirubin when dissociated from the serum albumin to which it is normally bound. The affected infant exhibits lethargy, poor feeding, opisthotonos, and respiratory irregularity, which may culminate in death. Surviving infants often exhibit permanent brain damage.

Infants with moderately severe HDN who are not given blood transfusions may become severely anemic. Usual newborn red blood cell production is depressed by the relatively high oxygen tension associated with the transition to respiration, and the hemoglobin concentration normally decreases during the first two months of life. In premature babies this trend is enhanced so that blood hemoglobin concentrations at age 60 days average 9.5 gm/dl. In babies with HDN, this sequence of events is aggravated by continuing destruction of newly formed RBC by residual antibody, so that hemoglobin values may fall to 6 gm/dl or even less.

The best criterion of the severity of HDN is the cord blood hemoglobin, and not the hemoglobin concentration of a blood sample obtained later from the baby. In the case of a 3,500-gm infant with a blood volume of 270 ml, there will be up to an additional 150 ml of blood in the placenta. If the umbilical cord is not clamped for five minutes after birth there will occur a "transfusion" of this blood, averaging 100 ml, from the placenta into the baby. Seventy milliliters of plasma can leave the infant's circulation in 30 minutes, and in three to four hours, the plasma loss may exceed the total volume of the placental transfusion. The net result is that the infant's blood hemoglobin concentration may be increased by as much as 6 gm/dl, thereby masking all but the most severe anemia. Only half of babies with significant HDN have cord hemoglobin concentrations in excess of 14.5 gm/dl. In one series of untreated infants with HDN, kernicterus occurred in 46% of those with cord hemoglobin concentrations below 10 gm/dl but in only 5% of babies in whom cord hemoglobin exceeded 16 gm/dl. There is a less-reliable correlation between cord bilirubin values and severity of HDN, although values exceeding 4 mg/dl have been used as an indication for exchange transfusion.

Blood group sensitization of a pregnant woman is possible whenever the red blood cells of her fetus bear an antigen (determined by a paternal gene) that she lacks. The factors determining whether HDN can occur in a given pregnancy include 1) the statistical likelihood that the fetus has inherited a gene producing an antigen absent in the mother, 2) the immunogenicity of that antigen, 3) the mother's ability to produce the corresponding antibody, and 4) the ability of the antibody to be transported across the placenta. About one in ten pregnancies resulting from matings of white persons result in a D-positive baby being born to a D-negative mother. If two D-positive pregnancies in a D-negative woman always led to sensitization and HDN, half of all D-negative women pregnant a second time would theoretically have an affected baby. In actuality the figure, was only an eighth of this or about 6%, even before the use of Rh immune globulin became common. Less than 10% of D-negative women bearing children by D-positive men become immunized: 1) The man may be heterozygous for the D gene and, therefore, there is an even chance that the fetus will be D-negative; 2) sufficient numbers of D-positive fetal RBC may not reach the maternal circulation to induce sensitization; and 3) 30% of women do not respond immunologically to the D antigen. Only IgG antibodies are transferred across the placenta, though all subclasses are included. The process is one of active transport involving a specific domain on the Fc portion of the gamma heavy chain of the antibody molecule. IgG transfer begins by the tenth week of gestation, and at birth fetal serum IgG concentrations are greater than those of the mother.

The first pregnancy of an untransfused woman rarely results in HDN due to blood group alloantibodies, and when this does occur, a previous abortion is suspect. ABO erythroblastosis, on the other hand, can occur in first-born babies. The magnitude of the problem of HDN is indicated by the fact that prior to the advent of suppression therapy one infant of every 180 born to white parents had HDN as a consequence of maternal Rh sensitization. If we exclude HDN due to antibodies in the ABO system, 99% of cases of HDN in the past have been caused by anti-D, although almost every blood group antibody that exists in an IgG form has been implicated, including antibodies to C, C^w, c, E, e, K, k, Kp^a, M, S, s, Fy^a, Fy^b, Jk^a, Jk^b, Di^a, Di^b, Wr^a, and others, though not to the Lewis or P antigens. Since the introduction of Rh immune globulin to prevent maternal sensitization to fetal D antigen, the number of cases of HDN has been reduced sharply. Inasmuch as Rh prophylaxis is over 90% effective, it is possible to reduce the incidence of Rh-caused HDN to one in 2,000 births. Current data indicate that 93% of non-ABO HDN in the United States is still due to anti-D or anti-CD, 6% to other Rh antibodies, and 1% to antibodies in other blood group systems.

Maternal sensitization by fetal RBC occurs most commonly at delivery, at which time small amounts of the infant's blood often gain access to the maternal circulation, but may occur less frequently during the last trimester of pregnancy. Antenatal fetal-maternal hemorrhage occurs in 10% to 20% of pregnancies, usually in amounts less than 0.1 ml. Fetal-maternal hemorrhage occurs at the time of delivery in 20% to 50% of women. Postpartum, 1% of women have 3 ml of fetal RBC in their circulation and 0.3% have more than 10 ml. An increased risk of fetal-maternal hemorrhage is present with abortion (2% to 6% of cases), ectopic pregnancy, amniocentesis (up to 11% of cases), external version, abruptio placentae, forceps delivery, manual extraction of the placenta (up to 23% of cases), and Cesarean section. Between 0.8% and 2.3% of D-negative women with ABO-compatible D-positive fetuses develop anti-D before the end of their first pregnancy, but if suppressive treatment with Rh immune globulin is not given, about 7% will have demonstrable anti-D in their serum six months postpartum. A total of about 17% will have been sensitized as evidenced by the appearance of anti-D before 20 weeks of gestation with a second D-incompatible pregnancy. The liklihood of anti-D appearing for the first time in succeeding pregnancies is very small.

A volume of 0.1 ml of D-positive RBC appears to be the optimal dose for primary immunization when given intravenously. Postpartum, about 20% of women exhibit this amount of fetal RBC in their circulation. On the other hand, there is evidence that larger single doses of ABO-compatible, D-positive RBC are more effective than small doses in evoking anti-D production in some patients. In one study of D-negative women bearing their first D-positive infants, if only rare fetal RBC were detectable in their circulation postpartum, only 2% to 3% produced detectable anti-D; if the fetal-maternal hemorrhage was less than 0.1 ml, 7% made anti-D; if 0.1 to 1.0 ml, 15% to 20% made the antibody; and if 1 to 10 ml, 20% to 60% produced it. D-positive RBC with larger numbers of D determinants such as the R^2r phenotype are somewhat more effective in sensitizing to D than are those with fewer D sites (e.g., R^1r phenotypes). Pregnancy with a group A or B, D-positive baby is less likely to result in maternal immunization to D if the mother is of group O than if her baby is ABO-compatible with her. Sensitization to all blood group antigens, not simply D, is prevented. It is felt that ABO-compatible D-positive fetal RBC in the mother's bloodstream are slowly destroyed over a long period of time as they reach the end of their life span, thereby providing a protracted stimulus to the mother's immunologic system. ABO-incompatible RBC, in the process of being destroyed rapidly, would provide a larger but single stimulus.

Up to 20% of the anti-D antibodies appearing postpartum are detectable only with enzyme tests and may not appear until up to six months after delivery. Some women in the process of making anti-D make an antibody that reacts only in enzyme tests with either D-positive or D-negative but not Rh_{null} RBC. Issitt has suggested that this may be anti-LW similar to that made by individuals of weak LW phenotypes, recalling that the expression of LW on maternal RBCs is often weakened during pregnancy. Later antibody will have usual anti-D specificity and is frequently first found primarily as an IgM saline agglutinin, although some IgG molecules are usually present. As the pregnancy progresses, IgG antibody predominates, and IgM anti-D may essentially disappear.

It is emphasized that all maternal alloantibody produced in response to pregnancy does not necessarily produce harmful effects in an incompatible fetus. IgM antibodies are not transported across the placenta. Even if the antibody does reach the fetal circulation, its binding constant may be too low to sensitize fetal RBC sufficiently strong enough to bring about accelerated destruction. Alternatively, weak expression of the antigen on the fetal RBC may effect a similar result. In the case of antigens such as A or B, almost all body cells, not just RBC, absorb antibody, diluting its effects on the infant's red blood cells.

The prenatal considerations with regard to the liklihood of HDN occurring in the offspring of a pregnant woman may be summarized as follows: If the mother has never been transfused or previously pregnant the likelihood of HDN is very low; it is essentially zero if she is of group A, B, or AB, and less than one in 150 for even mild ABO HDN if she is of group O and the father is not. If the mother has not been transfused, has no demonstrable blood group alloantibody and has borne a previous child without jaundice or anemia, the chances of a significant problem with HDN are low, though primary sensitization may occur and can rarely present difficulties. If a previous infant has been affected with HDN caused by an alloantibody, a subsequent fetus will be affected if it bears the antigen in question at least as severely as the last affected infant. If the last infant was stillborn owing to alloantibody-induced HDN, the chances are two in three that a subsequent pregnancy will also eventuate in a stillbirth.

On the occasion of the first visit of a pregnant woman to her physician, a blood sample should be obtained for determination of her ABO group and D type and for screening for the presence of serum alloantibodies. The specificity of any alloantibodies detected should be determined and a sample of the father's blood obtained to determine his ABO group, to ascertain whether his RBC bear the antigen corresponding to any maternal alloantibody, and, if possible, to find out whether he is homozygous or heterozygous for the responsible gene. In babies with HDN due to anti-D the ratio of homozygous to heterozygous fathers is 4:1. The reason for the interest in the father's and mother's ABO groups is first to determine whether it is possible for ABO erythroblastosis to occur but more importantly because HDN does occur almost exclusively in ABO-compatible pregnancies, i.e., the baby's RBC bear no ABO antigen absent in the mother. A suggested scheme for repeat testing of the mother's serum for alloantibodies is given in Figure 21-1. Note that all pregnant women should have serum screened for alloantibodies, not just D-negative mothers. If there is a history of a stillbirth but no alloantibody is detected in the mother's serum on routine screening, repeat testing should be conducted against her husband's RBC if the two are ABO-compatible.

The estimation of the outcome of pregnancy in a D-negative woman with a D-positive husband is uncertain, but a few general guidelines are useful. The baby is probably D-positive if anti-D first develops during the pregnancy, if the anti-D rises in titer as the pregnancy progresses, if the father is probably homozygous for the D gene, or if anti-D can be demonstrated in the amniotic fluid. The situation is less certain if the husband is probably heterozygous or the antibody titer remains stable throughout pregnancy. Prediction of the severity of HDN is very important as a guide to treatment. If the anti-D titer is less than 32, and there is no history of stillbirth, infant mortality is less than 2% and half of the infants do not require exchange transfusion. If the maternal anti-D titer is greater than 32, amniocentesis is generally indicated.

Whenever maternal alloantibody is detected, its titer should be determined as an indication of the degree of immunization of the mother, although it must be emphasized that maternal titers do not correlate reliably with the severity of fetal disease. However, a few generalities are useful: The pregnancy in which the antibody first oc-

curs is rarely severely affected unless the mother has had previous exposure to antigen by transfusion. Maternal antibody titers of 8 or less seldom are associated with severe HDN. A rising titer indicates that the fetus is potentially affected, but a stable titer does not ensure that the fetus is D-negative or not severely affected. Titers are, in general, of most value in the first affected pregnancy. Increases in titer are rare in D-negative pregnancies. If there is no previous history of stillbirth, the chances of stillbirth are four times as great when the maternal anti-D titer is 64 or higher as when it is less than 64. There is little to be gained by repeating titers more frequently than once every two weeks. Serum should be frozen for comparison purposes when serial antibody titers are to be determined. Titers are meaningful only when antiglobulin technique is used: only IgG antibody is of physiologic concern, and antibodies detected in saline, albumin, or enzyme tests may be IgM. Titrations should always be conducted with RBC of the same genotype. Enzyme testing may be useful, however, in screening tests because this technique may demonstrate antibody before it is found using other methods.

Because intrauterine transfusion or early delivery of a baby with severe HDN may be lifesaving, it is essential to be able to predict the severity of the condition in more reliable fashion than the titering of maternal serum alloantibodies can accomplish. Bilirubin estimation on fluid obtained by amniocentesis is effective in this regard and is used when the past obstetric history and/or titers are indicative of possible severe disease. Because the turbidity of amniotic fluid interferes with conventional chemical estimation of bilirubin content, scanning spectrophotometry between 350 and 650 nm is conducted on the fluid to determine its optical density in that portion of the absorption spectrum where bilirubin exerts its effect (450 to 460 nm). If a straight line is drawn connecting the absorbance tracing at 365 and 550 nm, the height of the peak above the baseline at 450 nm is a measure of bilirubin content. Good correlation exists between this value and the severity of HDN. Normally the absorbance of amniotic fluid decreases as pregnancy progresses, and a stable absorbance reading on serial testing indicates increasing severity of HDN. A peak height (difference in optical density from the baseline to the peak at 450 nm) of less than 0.2 indicates, in the case of possible HDN due to anti-D, a D-negative or an unaffected or mildly affected D-positive fetus. If the peak height is 0.2 to 0.34, the fetus is D-positive and probably affected; if it is between 0.34 and 0.7, the fetus is severely affected; and if it is greater than 0.7 the fetus is hydropic and moribund. Any fetal RBC aspirated during amniocentesis should be subjected to a direct antiglobulin test, ABO grouping, and D or other typings. Amniocentiesis is not without hazard, occasionally causing fetal damage, placental hemorrhage or fetal-maternal hemorrhage with increased maternal sensitizatiion. Rh immune globulin is normally administered after amniocentesis to D-negative mothers at risk.

Occasionally intrauterine transfusion of blood into the abdominal cavity of the unborn infant is performed if the baby is too immature to be delivered, and amniotic fluid studies indicate severe HDN. Indications include an amniotic fluid absorption peak greater than 0.3 before 33 weeks of gestation, or a peak greater than 0.2 and rising, or a previous early fetal death due to HDN. Roentgenographic evidence of fetal hydrops is a contraindication. Fresh (one-to-two day old) group O, leukocyte-poor RBC suspended in fresh group AB plasma to a hematocrit of 85% to 90% are used. Frozen or washed RBC are desirable for their decreased lymphocyte content and almost absent risk of transmitting hepatitis B. The RBC must be compatible with the mother's serum. The blood is warmed before administration. Suggested transfusion volume is 35 to 40 ml to fetuses of gestational ages of 26 weeks and 100 to 110 ml at 32 weeks.

HDN due to ABO incompatibility is quite different from its Rh counterpart: ABO-HDN may occur in first pregnancies, it is generally a very mild disease, its severity is not predictable from maternal isoantibody titers, and successive pregnancies at risk are not equally affected. HDN caused by anti-A and anti-B occurs almost exclusively in ABO-incompatible infants of group O mothers, whose IgG isoantibodies can cross the placenta in contrast to the predominantly IgM anti-A or anti-B of group B or group A mothers, which cannot. Although 20% of the infants of white parents are ABO-incompatible with their mothers, less than one in 30 of these infants shows any detectable evidence of hemolysis, less than one in 150 exhibits jaundice, and only one in 3,000 requires exchange transfusion. The mild nature of HDN due to ABO incompatibility is thought to be the result of the weak expression of the A and B antigens on infant RBC. The condition is found only in group A^1 and not group A^2 infants. Intrauterine death due to ABO-HDN does not occur, amniocentesis is not indicated, and premature induction of labor is not required for infant salvage.

The laboratory diagnosis of HDN due to ABO incompatibility requires demonstration of clinical disease, appropriate infant and maternal ABO groups and the presence of anti-A or anti-B in an eluate from cord RBC. Free isoantibody in cord serum is presumptive evidence only. The direct antiglobulin test on cord RBC will be weakly positive or occasionally negative. Routine laboratory testing should document anemia (in the cord sample), spherocytosis, and increased numbers of reticulocytes and peripheral blood normoblasts if the diagnosis of jaundice due to isoantibody-induced HDN is to be sustained.

A few general comments are appropriate on the subject of laboratory testing in cases of HDN of all types. The strength of a positive direct antiglobulin test cannot be taken as a guide to the severity of infant disease. Forty percent of infants born with a positive direct antiglobulin test on cord RBC require no treatment. False-positive direct antiglobulin tests may occur with cord RBC contaminated with Wharton's jelly from the umbilical cord, if washing is not thorough and repeated. Cord RBC from infants with alloantibody-induced HDN who have received intrauterine transfusions may yield negative direct antiglobulin tests. D-typings on cord cells heavily coated by "blocking" anti-D may give false-negative results. On the other hand, fortifying agents in typing sera may cause sensitized cord cells to agglutinate, leading to false-positive results. Typing serum diluent and not albumin must be used in control tests. As noted previously, cord and not infant peripheral blood hemoglobin determinations are essential in the evaluation of anemia in the newborn. Normal cord hemoglobin values are in excess of 17 gm/dl, and values of 15 gm/dl indicate anemia. Cord serum bilirubin values in excess of 4 mg/dl indicate severe disease, as does an increase in concentration exceeding 0.5 mg/dl/hr. Normal infant peripheral blood reticulocyte counts are 6% to 7% on the first day of life and fall to 2% by the fourth day.

All neonatal jaundice is not caused by HDN. The immature liver of the newborn has a limited capacity to conjugate bilirubin, a deficiency that is aggravated in premature infants. The list of non-hematological causes of infant jaundice includes "physiologic jaundice" (especially in premature babies), meconium ileus, maternal diabetes, overdosage with vitamin K analogues, G-6PD deficiency, cytomegalic inclusion disease, disseminated herpesvirus infection, toxoplasmosis, syphilis, bacterial sepsis, galactosemia, hepatitis, congenital anemias such as hereditary spherocytosis, hereditary deficiency of hepatic glucuronyl transferase, hematomas, poly-cythemia, intestinal obstruction, hepatic obstruction, the respiratory distress syndrome, and a number of drug effects. Free unconjugated bilirubin of whatever cause is toxic to the brain of the newborn. It is traditionally thought that serum bilirubin levels below 20 mg/dl do not result in brain damage, but this concept requires refinement, inasmuch as it is the concentration of bilirubin not bound to serum albumin that is significant. The capacity of serum to bind bilirubin is related to the amount of albumin present and to the concentration of substances such as aspirin, sulfonamides, cephalothin, and oxacillin, which compete with bilirubin for albumin-binding sites. The low serum albumin concentrations of premature infants render them susceptible to brain damage at bilirubin levels tolerated by term babies. The ability of the albumin to bind bilirubin is also affected by plasma pH, and is decreased in acidosis such as occurs with hypothermia or hypoxia. The damaging effect of acidosis does not end when blood pH is returned to normal because the increased concentrations of serum fatty acids occurring in acidosis persist, and these, too, compete with bilirubin for binding to albumin. Hypoglycemia increases serum free fatty acid concentrations and may aggravate the problem.

Transfusion therapy for HDN is aimed at reducing the mortality and morbidity that occur at each of three stages: 1) Anemia present within 24 hours of birth. Death occurs as the result of cardiac failure due to anoxemia. Exchange transfusion in this situation provides oxygen-carrying capacity to the infant's circulation. 2) Anemia with hyperbilirubinemia occurring 36 to 96 hours after birth. Death occurs as the result of kernicterus. Exchange transfusion is aimed at removing infant RBCs that would otherwise be hemolyzed, correcting anemia, reducing serum bilirubin levels, decreasing antibody levels, and increasing albumin concentration. 3) Anemia after the first week of life. Of infants with positive cord RBC direct antiglobulin tests and hemoglobin concentrations in excess of 15 gm/dl, one in 20 requires transfusion for anemia. If exchange transfusion is performed on an infant, the final blood hemoglobin concentration should be at least 17 gm/dl.

The process of exchange transfusion is quite safe in capable hands, with a mortality of less than 1%. As rules of thumb, exchange transfusion of newborn infants with HDN should be considered when the cord hemoglobin concentration is less than 12 gm/dl, the cord serum bilirubin is greater than 5 mg/dl, or the reticulocyte count is more than 8%. Exchange transfusion should be considered at lower values if the infant suffers from prematurity, acidosis, hypoalbuminemia, hypoglycemia, respiratory distress, or hypothermia, or if the mother has received drugs that bind to serum albumin. The technique of exchange transfusion involves performance of multiple small phlebotomies with continuous or intermittent transfusion. The efficiency of exchange transfusion is given by the formula:

$$R = (\frac{V\text{-}S}{V})\, n$$

where R is the proportion of the baby's blood remaining, V is the baby's blood volume in ml, S is the syringe size employed (in milliliters) and n is the number of syringes full of blood removed and replaced. An infant's blood volume in milliliters is equivalent to approximately 10% of its body weight in grams. An exchange transfusion of an infant employing a full unit of blood (500 ml) gives an almost 90% replacement of the baby's blood. Mollison cites the example of an infant with a hemoglobin concentration of 6 gm/dl and a RBC life span of two to three days. In this situation 500 mg of bilirubin would be produced per day, and a 90% exchange would remove a potential 450 mg of bilirubin. If exchange transfusion is carried out when the bilirubin concentration is 10 mg/dl, a 300-ml plasma exchange will remove less than 30 mg of bilirubin. The relative ineffectiveness of a second exchange transfusion is also pointed out: If only 0.5 gm/dl of the infant's own RBC remain, the second exchange will remove a potential 50 mg of bilirubin. If the serum bilirubin is now 18 mg/dl, about 50 mg of actual bilirubin is also removed. As a general rule it may be expected that an exchange transfusion of 500 ml will reduce the infant's plasma bilirubin concentration to 65% of its original value at its conclusion but it should be recalled that a "rebound" will occur as extravascular bilirubin diffuses into the bloodstream. Exchange transfusion is generally not required in the full-term infant if the serum bilirubin concentrations remain below 10 mg/dl for the first 24 hours of life, below 14 mg/dl during the second 24 hours, and below 17 mg/dl during the next 24 to 48 hours.

The choice of blood for exchange transfusion depends on the antibody present, the ABO groups of the mother and infant, and the D type of the infant. In general, blood of the baby's own ABO and D type is used if the blood is compatible with the mother's serum. This means that if the baby is, for example, of group A, and the mother is of group O, blood of the baby's own ABO group cannot be used. In the last edition of this book a lengthy table of preferred and acceptable choices of blood for exchange transfusion was presented. The author currently recommends as logistically easier and less prone to error the choice of washed group O, D-negative RBC, suspended in fresh AB plasma for all exchange transfusions, with the further notation that consideration must be given to other antigens reactive with maternal alloantibodies. Compatibility testing for a first exchange transfusion should always be conducted with the mother's serum, not the baby's. If repeat exchanges are required, both should be used. Only if for some exceptional reason maternal blood cannot be obtained should the baby's blood alone be used for crossmatching, and even then an eluate prepared from cord RBC should be used in addition to the infant's serum. If compatible donor blood cannot be found because of the presence in the mother's serum of some unusual antibody, washed maternal RBC suspended in fresh AB plasma can be employed.

Blood for exchange transfusion should be less than five days in storage to minimize the possibility of potassium toxicity, provide RBC of maximal viability, and ensure maximal RBC content of 2,3-DPG. Washed RBC contain reduced numbers of leukocytes, and frozen RBC may be desirable from this viewpoint. The hematocrit of the unit should be adjusted to approximately 65% to correct for any anemia present and to leave a sufficiently high hemoglobin value at the conclusion of the exchange. Blood for exchange transfusion must be warmed before administration. Small amounts of albumin (e.g., 4 ml/kg of 25% albumin) are sometimes transfused to an infant before exchange transfusion to increase bilirubin binding.

Mild neonatal jaundice is profitably treated by exposure of the infant to strong light at the blue end of the spectrum, which decomposes bilirubin to relatively nontoxic products. Phototherapy alone is not adequate for treatment of significant cases of HDN. Induction of increased activity of hepatic glucuronidase enzymes involved in bilirubin metabolism has been accomplished by treating pregnant women or their erythroblastotic infants with certain drugs, notably phenobarbital. Simple transfusions to correct anemia in babies with HDN may be required for as long as three months. Maternal antibody may persist in the baby's circulation this long and continue to destroy new infant RBC. It should be remembered that exchange transfusion depresses erythropoiesis in the infant.

Because of the serious consequences of HDN, intensive efforts have been made in recent years to develop effective prophylaxis, at least for that major portion of cases caused by Rh incompatibility. The success of the treatment has been gratifying and has markedly reduced the incidence of significant HDN. The material used is immune globulin made from potent IgG anti-D sera selected to have a high mean binding constant. Obviously Rh immune globulin is of value only in preventing maternal sensitization to the D antigen and is considered of no value once maternal anti-D has been produced. Rh immune globulin is administered intramuscularly in a standard dose of $300\mu g$ to D-negative mothers (who have not made demonstrable anti-D) within 72 hours of delivering a D-positive infant. Maternal plasma anti-D levels reach 70% of their maximum within 24 hours and peak at 48 hours. Rh immune globulin is cleared from the injection site at a rate of about 35% per day and distributed in a space slightly greater than twice the plasma volume. Passively acquired anti-D, administered to the mother as Rh immune globulin, is detectable in serum in almost all patients six weeks postpartum and in half of the patients at three months, though it is rarely found at five months and is gone by six months.

The mechanism by which Rh immune globulin is thought to prevent sensitization of the mother has been discussed in Chapter 6. Rh immune globulin is administered only to mothers demonstrated to be D^e (and D^u) negative, who have no anti-B detectable in their serum postpartum, and whose infants are D-positive. As an extra precaution, a crossmatch is conducted in the laboratory between the maternal RBC and a diluted sample of the Rh immune globulin to ensure compatibility. Retyping of the maternal blood sample should be carried out postpartum and the results of both this typing and the Rh immune globulin crossmatch examined microscopically to detect typing errors, a positive maternal direct antiglobulin test (weak but uniform agglutination), or a massive fetal-maternal hemorrhage (mixed-field agglutination). In the case of the latter occurrence, the standard 300 μg dose of Rh immune globulin, sufficient to prevent sensitization by up to 15 ml of D-positive RBC, may be inadequate. Means of accurately measuring the size of a fetal-maternal hemorrhage are not available. The Kleihauer-Betke test carries with it an error of up to 100%, due to the fact that the test detects RBC with a high content of fetal hemoglobin. In the last trimester of pregnancy, maternal RBC contain increased amounts of F hemoglobin, nonuniformly distributed, so that some maternal RBC may be mistaken for fetal cells. A few women also have congenitally high RBC levels of F hemoglobin. More than the standard dose of Rh-immune globulin should be administered if the fetal-maternal hemorrhage exceeds 30 ml of fetal blood (15 ml of RBC). A hemorrhage of this size is usually detectable by virtue of the mixed-field agglutination it causes in the retyping of the mother's RBC from the postpartum blood sample and/or in the crossmatch with the Rh immune globulin. It is now recommended that Rh immune globulin also be given to Rh-negative women undergoing abortion (unless the fetus is shown to be D-negative) and amniocentesis. In both cases reduced doses are given.

Failure of Rh immune globulin to prevent sensitization to the D antigen may occur as the result of:1) Primary immunization during pregnancy as a consequence of antenatal fetal-maternal hemorrhage; 2) previous abortion or amniocentesis; 3) a delay in administration beyond the recommended 72-hour limit after delivery; or 4) a large inadequately treated fetal-maternal hemorrhage. The failure rate of prophylaxis is about 0.5% as judged by the presence of detectable serum anti-D produced within six months of delivery, but 2% as judged by the appearance of anti-D in a second D-positive pregnancy, as opposed to 17% without treatment.

RECOMMENDED READING:

Dodd, B.E. and Lincoln, P.J.: *Blood Group Topics.* Williams & Wilkins, Baltimore, 1975

Greenwalt, T.J. et al (Ed): *General Principles of Blood Transfusion* 2nd ed. Am Med Assn Chicago, 1977

Huestis, D.W. et al: *Practical Blood Transfusion* 2nd ed. Little, Brown and Co. Boston, 1976

Issitt, P.D. and Issitt, C.H.: *Applied Blood Group Serology* 2nd ed. Spectra. Oxnard, Calif., 1975

Mollison, P.L.: *Blood Transfusion in Clinical Medicine*, 5th ed. Blackwell, Oxford, 1972

Moore, B.P.L. et al: Serological and technical methods: *The Technical Manual of the Canadian Red Cross Blood Transfusion Service.* 7th ed. Canadian Red Cross, Toronto, 1972

CHAPTER 22

Histocompatibility Testing
Leukocyte and Platelet Antigens

The histocompatibility locus antigen (HLA) system is a complex of at least four closely linked loci, each with multiple alleles, situated in close proximity on chromosome number 6. The HLA genes behave as autosomal codominants. Three loci named A, B, and C have been defined using serologic techniques, while the fourth, D, is demonstrated using the mixed-lymphocyte reaction described below. In a system such as HLA one would expect the various possible gene pairs to occur in random assortment; that is to say the system would be in a state of genetic equilibrium. This is not the case for the HLA genes: certain combinations are found more frequently than would be predicted by chance. Thus, the combination of HLA-A1 and B8 occurs unusually often, as does HLA-A3 and B7. This situation is known as genetic disequilibrium.

Up to eight different HLA genes can be represented in a single genotype, one at each of four loci on each of the two number 6 chromosomes. Nineteen alleles are known at the A locus, 20 at the B locus, five at the C locus, and six at the D locus. Several hundred thousand combinations are thus possible, and the likelihood of finding two random persons who are not identical twins with the same genotype is almost nil. The HLA antigens are expressed on the surface of all cells of the body, though for practical reasons lymphocytes are customarily used for testing. A problem in HLA typing arises from the difficulty of obtaining monospecific antisera. Most sera containing HLA antibodies are mixtures of various specificities, particularly if the antigenic stimulus has been prolonged, as in pregnancy. There is considerable overlapping of specificities and cross-reactivity among antisera so that a given serum may react with an antigen, a portion of that antigen, or a shared portion of another antigen. Some antisera appear to recognize compound antigens, and a few exhibit dosage effects. These characteristics of HLA antisera plus the existence of multiple alleles complicate HLA typing to the point where much of the original investigative work was done with the aid of computers to sort out the data. Monospecific typing sera are just becoming commercially available; their rarity and expense require that microtechniques be used for HLA testing.

It was noted in the discussion of immunologic complications of blood transfusion that multiple blood transfusions may give rise to the formation of antibodies reactive with antigens on leukocytes and platelets, among which HLA antibodies are important. It has been conclusively shown that the preexistence of antibodies in the serum of a tissue- or organ-graft recipient reactive with HLA antigens on the engrafted tissue can cause its prompt rejection. Such antibodies may also develop later in response to HLA antigens present in the grafted tissue and cause its delayed rejection. In the case of grafted kidneys, this rejection is associated with lymphocyte infiltration of the organ, changes in its arteries and glomeruli, and cessation of function with death of the tissue. The rejected graft must then be surgically removed. Two approaches are made clinically to reduce the chance of graft rejection. One is to suppress the immunologic system of the graft recipient by the use of irradiation, chemotherapy, or antilymphocyte antisera, which impair the host's ability to react to the transplant. The second is to minimize the number of HLA antigens present on a donor graft which are absent in the recipient and to which antibodies might be formed. A great deal remains to be learned about which antigens and even which loci are more important in such reactions. It is statistically true that the better the match between donor and recipient HLA types, the better the graft survival in patients not preimmunized to HLA antigens found on the graft, but so many exceptions occur that an HLA mismatch usually does not deter organ grafting operations. Although most HLA antigens are poor immunogens, some are apparently weaker than others. Survival of grafts between identical twins is excellent; relatively good results can be anticipated if only one "mismatch" is present, especially if the graft is obtained from a blood relative. Less satisfactory outcomes are more common if multiple incompatibilities exist. Some of the exceptions that occur are probably related to the antibody-forming ability of the graft recipient. It is possible that unrecognized factors are of equal or greater importance than HLA compatibility in determining whether graft survival will occur. Recent work suggests that "enhancing antibodies" may be produced in response to exposure of a graft recipient to small numbers of foreign leukocytes, and that patients who have received small amounts of WBC during transfusions may tolerate grafted organs better than do nontransfused hosts. ABO antigen compatibility is also necessary to optimal survival of organ grafts; it will be recalled that ABO antigens are present on almost all body cells and not solely on RBC.

The presence of preformed host antibodies to HLA antigens present in an organ graft usually ensures its prompt rejection. In consequence most centers try to minimize the exposure of potential graft recipients to foreign HLA antigens by administering leukocyte-poor blood to such patients if they require transfusion. It has been suggested that part of the "enhancing effect" of blood transfusion noted above may be in its selection of nonresponders to foreign HLA antigens. Before grafting is done, a compatibility test is carried out using recipient serum and lymphocytes from the organ donor in an attempt to detect preformed recipient antibodies reactive with donor HLA antigens.

HLA testing is conducted primarily in the following situations:

1) To establish the HLA types of donors and recipients of organ or tissue grafts, including visceral organs, skin, platelets, and leukocytes.

2) To detect relationships between HLA antigens and disease.

3) To assist in the elucidation of transfusion reactions.

Although several types of serologic tests have been used, those most commonly employed are:

1) A test for leukoagglutinins, in which test lymphocytes suspended in buffered saline plus EDTA are agglutinated by HLA antibodies.

2) A lymphocyte cytotoxicity test in which live lymphocytes are killed by complement after incubation with cytotoxic antibody. Death of the lymphocytes is recognized by their inability to resist staining by dilute eosin or other dyes.

In light of the multiplicity of HLA antigens, lymphocytes from multiple donors must be used to ensure the presence of even the common HLA antigens in screening tests. Another technique for determining histocompatibility, and the only way of testing for antigens at the D locus, is the mixed lymphocyte culture. This test is based on the fact that mixtures of lymphocytes from persons unlike with regard to HLA-D antigens will stimulate one another as evidenced by "blast" transformation in tissue culture. The donor's lymphocytes are generally rendered immunologically unreactive by prior addition of mitomycin C or a similar agent. The usefulness of the test is limited by the amount of time required for its completion.

An extensive series of associations between HLA antigens and a variety of disease states has been documented. It has been suggested that these associations may be a consequence of particular dangerous genes existing in genetic disequilibrium with certain HLA genes. The risk of developing certain diseases is greatly increased in people of certain HLA types, as reviewed by Touey. The most striking association is that between the presence of the gene determining HLA-B27 and ankylosing spondylitis. Associations are also common between HLA-B27 and some eye diseases, especially uveitis; between HLA-B13 and some skin diseases, particularly psoriasis; between HLA-B8 and endocrine diseases including diabetes mellitus, Grave's disease, and Addison's disease; between HLA-B8 and gastrointestinal diseases including celiac disease and chronic active hepatitis; and between HLA-B8 and myasthenia gravis and HLA-DW2 and multiple sclerosis. In most of the above cases and in others as well associations exist with HLA antigens of more than one series. It has been speculated that a particular HLA antigen may resemble a given virus so closely that the immunologic system of a carrier of the antigen may not recognize the virus as foreign and therefore not mount an adequate defense. Alternatively, HLA antigens may act as receptors for certain infectious agents, thereby increasing host susceptibility to them. Apart from the case of the patient with possible ankylosing spondylitis, HLA typing is not generally considered of diagnostic value at this time.

Antibodies to leukocyte antigens are the most common cause of febrile transfusion reactions, and the reactions they provoke may be severe. In one study of 274 febrile transfusion reactions, approximately half of the patient sera contained leukoagglutinins. Half bore lymphocytotoxins, a fifth exhibited platelet agglutinins and a fifth demonstrated complement-fixing platelet antibodies. Leukoagglutinins are commonly found in the sera of massively transfused subjects: the sera of 15% of one series of patients who had undergone coronary bypass procedures contained such antibodies. In a study of the sera of parous women, 2% were found to contain leuko-agglutinins following one pregnancy, 10% after two. Lymphocyto-toxic antibodies have been demonstrated in the sera of 25% of women after one pregnancy and 55% after three. Febrile reactions to blood transfusion in patients sensitized to leukocyte antigens can be minimized or eliminated by the administration of washed, leuko-cyte-poor RBC.

The recognition of platelet-specific antigens dates from 1958. Antibodies to platelet antigens are detected by agglutination and complement-fixation tests, and are generally immune in nature, aris-ing after pregnancy, blood transfusion, skin grafting, organ trans-plantation, or platelet and/or leukocyte administration. Antibodies to platelets were found in one study in 5% of immunologically com-petent recipients of one to ten blood transfusions, 24% of patients who had received 25 to 50 transfusions, 80% of persons given more than 100 transfusions. Antibodies to platelet-specific antigens are frequently multispecific mixtures and are generally found in sera containing HLA antibodies. Platelet antigens are of three types: 1) platelet-specific antigens, of which seven are known, including three sets of alleles (Table 22-1); 2) HLA antigens; and 3) antigens shared with RBC, of which only A and B have any potential clinical sig-nificance. Of the three types, antigens specific to platelets are of least importance in the development of a refractory state to platelet transfusion. HLA antigens, on the other hand, appear to be of considerable importance in this regard. In immunologically compe-tent recipients, a refractory state to platelet transfusion may develop within the space of as little as one week of repeated platelet trans-fusion, with subsequent platelet administration causing febrile reac-

---

TABLE 22-1

Frequency Distribution of Common Platelet Antigens in White Subjects

Antigen	Frequency in White Subjects (%)
Pl^{a1}	97
Pl^{a2}	26
Pl^{e1}	99
Pl^{e2}	5
Ko^a	14
Ko^b	99

tions but no sustained increase in platelet count or hemostatic effect. Administration of HLA-matched platelets to such patients may still produce good results; as the number of HLA mismatches increases, the benefits of platelet transfusion decreases. Some HLA antigens such as B8 and B12 are poorly expressed on platelets. Incompatibility for such antigens is less important clinically than it is in the case of other platelet antigens. Cross-reactivity occurs among HLA antigens and may in some cases permit good responses to platelet transfusion despite mismatches. The significance of ABO compatibility in determining the survival of transfused platelets is disputed. Red blood cells, however, should be removed from platelet preparations given to ABO-incompatible recipients so that the transfused (or patient) platelets are not destroyed as innocent bystanders in RBC reactions. Granulocytopenia with a decrease in recipient peripheral blood WBC of up to 70% and lasting up to three days may occur as a complication of HLA-incompatible platelet transfusion. Again the mechanism is thought to be sensitization of recipient granulocytes by circulating immune complexes and/or activated complement components. Posttransfusion thrombocytopenia is a rare complication that may develop a few days after blood or platelet transfusion. Anti-Pl[a] is found in the recipient's serum, reactive with donor but not recipient platelets. Antigen-antibody complex formation as above is considered responsible. Neonatal thrombocytopenia, analogous to HDN, occurs about once in 10,000 births as a consequence of transplacental passage of maternal antibody reactive with fetal platelet antigens. Free antibody is found in the mother's serum though not in the baby's, and the mother is not thrombocytopenic. Although 10% to 20% of pregnant women produce HLA antibodies, clinically recognizable effects in their infants are rare. Very rarely neonatal neutropenia may be seen as a result of the transplacental transport of maternal antineutrophil antibodies.

On occasion, drug-induced immune thrombocytopenia is found. The mechanism of the development of this condition is similar to that described for some types of drug-induced cases of RBC sensitization. Antidrug antibodies form immune complexes that activate complement, and the immune complex and/or complement attaches to platelets and effects their premature destruction. Drugs commonly implicated in this type of thrombocytopenia include quinine, quinidine, sedormid, and chlorothiazides.

Even though most of the blood used in a hospital may come from a central source, some larger institutions find it desirable to maintain a file of emergency donors and/or donors of special blood types who may be called upon under special circumstances. Extra care should be taken by the blood bank staff to cultivate the good will of these people and to take note of the inconvenience to which sudden blood bank needs may put them. Some institutions have organized "blood clubs" with meetings at which outstanding efforts by donors are acknowledged with suitable publicity. Care in explaining to such donors the particular value of their donation, perhaps giving them some deeper insight into how and why their blood is being used will repay the effort many times. Although the blood bank administration is primarily responsible, the technical staff can be profitably involved in the area of donor recruitment through personal efforts.

Care must be exercised in the selection of blood donors for the protection of both donor and recipient. These safeguards include obtaining a medical history from the donor, a brief physical evaluation, and certain laboratory tests, all performed on the occasion of each donation. To protect the donor against potential harmful effects of the loss of a pint of blood, screening procedures require that he be of a certain age and body weight, meet a minimal level of hemoglobin concentration, be mentally competent, in good health, not pregnant, not subject to unusual hazard immediately after donation, and not have donated blood within a specified time. To protect the recipient of the donation, efforts are made to eliminate donors who are potentially carriers of various disease-producing organisms or whose blood may be a source of problem to the recipient.

Formal written records are required to document all phases of blood collection and processing. The blood bank procedure manual must specify in detail each step to be taken. Donor identification forms must include the full name of the donor, home and business address and telephone, date of birth, sex, the date of collection, and, if there is no objection, the donor's social security number as a final proof of identity. Blood donors should be between the ages of 21 and 65 years, although donors 17 to 21 years of age may be accepted if local law permits. Older donors may be accepted if they present written physician authorization not over two weeks old and meet the other donor criteria. Donations are limited to five per 12-month period and should be at least eight weeks apart. A signed consent and release form authorizing the blood bank to draw and use blood from a prospective donor must be obtained upon the occasion of each donation. The procedure followed in drawing blood and the possible complications of the procedure, including fainting, vomiting, and convulsions must be clearly explained to the donor in lay terms. The donor must be asked if he has questions about the procedure and given an opportunity to refuse before signing the form. The form may also contain a statement releasing the blood bank from legal liability for complications of the donation.

Useful information to be obtained from prospective donors includes the following:

1) Time and nature of last food intake by the donor. Fasting is not desirable, and the incidence of reactions appears to be increased in fasting donors. Refreshments should be offered to such persons before blood is collected.

2) The donor's hobbies and occupation. People predictably engaged in activities in which fainting could be unduly hazardous to themselves or others should be appropriately cautioned. A 12-hour interval is considered a safe margin after blood donation, although aircraft operators are considered to be at risk for 72 hours.

3) Racial origin of the donor. A search for specific blood types may be greatly facilitated by this knowledge.

A detailed medical history must be obtained from the donor on the occasion of each visit. Privacy should be ensured when the history is taken. Specific medical diagnostic terms are best avoided or carefully explained in lay language. Answers must be recorded as obtained, together with any explanatory notes. The interviewer should refer to the responsible blood bank physician any uncertainties. The following areas must be specifically enquired about:

1) The donor's general health, including whether he is under a physician's care, has ever had a major illness, has had surgery in the past six months, tooth extraction in the past 72 hours, or recent unexplained weight loss. Specific questions should be addressed to the presence of heart, lung, gastrointestinal, liver, kidney, or neurologic disease, and cancer. Questions about symptoms and signs such as chest pain, shortness of breath, cough, blood in sputum, vomitus, stool or urine, fainting, and convulsions, and additional questions about specific diagnoses such as hypertension, congestive heart failure, valvular heart disease, active tuberculosis, cirrhosis, nephritis, epilepsy, and diabetes mellitus, all of which disqualify a prospective donor and should be included in the interview.

2) Evidence of acute illness. Acute respiratory or gastro-intestinal disease including such symptoms as cough, sore throat, severe headache, nausea, or diarrhea are cause for rejection of the donor until symptoms are gone.

3) General evidence of disease, including previous rejections as a blood donor and current intake of medications. Use of contraceptives, salicylates, tranquilizers, or vitamins does not per se disqualify a donor, but the reason for treatment with more potent medications must be ascertained.

4) Evidence of specific disqualifying conditions, such as pregnancy within the past six weeks or blood donation within eight weeks.

5) Evidence of specific diseases, including asthma, convulsive disorders, untreated syphilis, a hemorrhagic diathesis, malaria, or viral hepatitis. Persons who have had malaria, visitors from malarious areas as defined on a World Health Organization map, or travelers who have taken malarial prophylaxis are rejected for three years. Travelers to malarious areas who have not taken antimalarial drugs are rejected for six months.

Because of the possibility of posttransfusion hepatitis transmitted by blood or blood products, a very careful series of questions must be asked to eliminate as blood donors possible carriers of the hepatitis viruses. In addition to specific questioning about jaundice or hepatitis, the interviewer must ask about exposure to people with hepatitis, receipt of blood or blood products, ear piercing, acupuncture, tattooing, and injections of any type, as well as drug addiction or use of illegal drugs. Donors are rejected permanently if there is a history of viral hepatitis (but not the hepatitis of infectious mononucleosis), a positive test for HB_SAg, drug addiction, or proof of a previous blood donation having caused viral hepatitis in a recipient. Rejection for six months is required after various skin-puncturing procedures and household contact or exposure to hepatitis in an endemic situation (e.g., a renal dialysis unit).

6) Recent immunization. Persons vaccinated against smallpox are rejected until the scab is lost or for two weeks after an immune reaction. A two-week waiting period is imposed after immunization against rubeola, mumps, yellow fever, and poliomyelitis (oral vaccine) or with tetanus antitoxin; the interval is increased to two months after rubella vaccination, and one year after rabies vaccination.

If evidence of any of the various conditions listed above is uncovered, specific details as to the timing, severity, and nature of the condition must be obtained and recorded. If there is question or doubt, the blood bank director may wish to consult with the donor's personal physician. Patients with mental disease and specifically those who are institutionalized should not be accepted as blood donors: consent forms may be voidable and the blood bank held legally liable.

The general physical state of the donor must be evaluated to ensure that he appears to be in good health. Donors under the influence of alcohol or drugs are rejected. Both arms should be examined for evidence of needle punctures, thrombophlebitis, and scars possibly as a result of drug injection. The phlebotomy site should be free from skin lesions. In addition, the following donor criteria must be met:

1) Weight. Donors weighing 50 kg (110 lb) may give 450±45 ml of blood, plus not more than 30 ml for processing requirements. Smaller donors may give less blood collected into proportionately reduced amounts of anticoagulant.

2) Temperature. The oral temperature should not be greater than 37.5 C. Recent smoking or drinking by the donor may cause false values.

3) Pulse. The pulse should be between 50 and 100 per minute, without irregularity.

4) Blood pressure. The blood pressure should be between 90 and 180 mm Hg sytolic and 50 to 100 mm Hg diastolic, without an abnormally wide pulse pressure.

5) Hemoglobin or hematocrit. The hemoglobin concentration should be at least 12.5 gm/dl for female donors, 13.5 gm/dl for males. Alternatively the hematocrit values should be 38 and 41, respectively.

The technique for preparation of the phlebotomy site and collection of blood are set forth in the *Technical Manual of the American Association of Blood Banks*, seventh edition, 1977, to which the reader is referred for details.

Significant donor reactions during or after properly performed blood collection are relatively uncommon, but the blood bank should be prepared to cope with them: 1) Phlebotomists should be thoroughly versed in the treatment of minor reactions. 2) A list of instructions for emergency first aid in case of donor reaction should be posted in the donor room. 3) A physician must be readily available when blood collection is in progress. 4) An appropriate kit of in-dated materials for treatment of donor reactions should be kept in the donor room.

Both psychologic and physiologic factors may play a role in pre-cipitating donor reactions. Obvious apprehension in a donor should be a warning to the phlebotomist, as should a history of previous reactions. Experience suggests that donors who have not eaten or slept for long periods may be unusually prone to fainting episodes. Symptoms and signs of a donor reaction usually include some com-bination of the following: dizziness, weakness, sweating, pallor, chills, a tingling sensation, nausea, fainting, tremors, loss of consciousness, convulsions, and incontinence. Rapid loss of blood volume may partially account for this picture, as may hyperventila-tion with excessive respiratory loss of carbon dioxide and resultant alkalosis. If the donor fails to rest the recommended ten minutes after blood collection or rapidly stands upright, circulatory adjust-ments may not be rapid enough to maintain cerebral blood flow and the donor may faint. Donors should be continuously observed during and immediately after blood collection so that reactions may be anti-cipated and treated at once, particularly from the viewpoint of pre-venting injury in falls.

If a donor reaction occurs while phlebotomy is in progress, the tourniquet and needle should be removed at once. Usual first aid measures are generally all that are required. The donor's head should not be administered under these circumstances. If the donor loosened and cold compresses applied to the forehead. If vomiting occurs, the donor's head should be turned to prevent aspiration of vomitus. If the donor is hyperventilating, instructing him to re-breathe in a paper bag may alleviate symptoms of alkalosis. Oxygen should not be administered 7nder these circumstances. If the donor feels faint, aromatic spirits of ammonia may be administered by in-halation. Convulsions are rare, but if they occur, medical aid should be summoned at once if not already at hand. The donor should be gently restrained and prevented from injuring himself, especially by falling. A tongue blade inserted between the teeth will prevent biting of the tongue. Loose dentures should, if possible, be removed to pre-vent their aspiration. Pulse, respiration, and blood pressure should be recorded at intervals until recovery is complete, and a detailed signed record made of the nature and treatment of the reaction.

It is recommended that an oral iron supplement be prescribed for all people who donate blood regularly to replace iron stores depleted by increased erythropoiesis. Normally, a blood donor will exhibit a reticulocyte peak about nine days after phlebotomy. The hemoglobin concentration will reach its lowest value about a week after blood donation and usually returns to normal within three to four weeks. Biologic false-positive reactions in serologic tests for syphilis frequently occur after repeated blood donations.

The special requirents of therapeutic bleedings, plasmapheresis, and plateletpheresis are discussed in the *Technical Manual of the American Association of Blood Banks*, to which the reader is referred.

A variety of anticoagulant materials has been used in blood preservative solutions, but the one most commonly used is citrate. Citrate acts by binding the ionized calcium required for blood to coagulate. EDTA has not proved satisfactory in this connection. Heparin is useful under certain conditions, but blood can be stored for only 48 hours in heparin anticoagulant. Blood collected into conventional anticoagulant-preservative solutions such as CPD (see below) is usually heparinized and recalcified before use in pump oxygenators. In coronary bypass procedures the patient's entire circulation is heparinized to prevent clotting in the pump and its tubing. Although citrate is the preferred anticoagulant for blood storage because it is nontoxic and readily metabolized, sodium citrate alone is not suitable, and pH adjustment is required. This is accomplished by the addition of citric acid and monobasic sodium phosphate to produce a buffer solution that reacts with blood to produce a final mixture of the desired near-neutrality. Improvement of red blood cell viability is effected in storage by the addition of glucose (dextrose) as a source of energy. Recent work indicates that further addition of metabolic intermediates such as adenine, adenosine, or inosine further improves RBC viability in storage. Adenine addition, in particular, has been demonstrated to permit extension of RBC storage life from 21 days in CPD to at least 28 and probably 35 days without clinical complications, while still maintaining cell viability above the 70% survival requirement. Purine nucleosides such as adenosine or inosine have been shown to prevent or restore loss of cellular ATP, thereby prolonging RBC storage life. Inosine also aids in regeneration of 2,3-DPG. Unfortunately, the catabolism of inosine in vivo yields quantities of uric acid that are not clinically acceptable. The advent of cell-washers which are rapid and efficient, may in time obviate this objection. Adenine has also been found to prolong red blood cell viability when added to CPD, but does not prevent depletion of 2,3,-DPG. Obviously, the ideal blood preservative has not been found, but CPD-adenine as recently put into general use is the best compromise currently available. In passing it should be noted that RBC from different donors vary considerably in viability upon storage. The composition of citrate-phosphate-dextrose (CPD) preservative solution is given in Table 23-1. CPD has all but completely replaced the older acid-citrate-dextrose (ACD) solution as a blood preservative. CPD has a slightly higher pH than ACD, preserves red blood cell 2,3-DPG levels better, and is more nearly isotonic with blood than is ACD.

The first 5% to 10% of the RBC collected into preservative are rather severely damaged, with only about half remaining viable. The "collection lesion," i.e., the proportion of RBC irrevocably damaged during phlebotomy, is about 5% of a one pint blood donation. Cell viability then decreases in blood preserved in CPD at 4 C at the rate of 5% to 10% per week. RBC stored as sedimented RBC (hematocrit of 60% to 75%) or as "packed" or centrifuged RBC (hematocrit 80% to 90%) survive as well in storage as do RBC stored as whole blood (hematocrit 35% to 45%). Red blood cells that survive in the circulation of a transfusion recipient for 24 hours can be expected to live out a normal life span. Granulocytes in whole blood deteriorate relatively rapidly under storage conditions, though acceptable survival of WBC concentrates is obtained after 24 hours at 4 C. Lymphocytes may remain viable for many days in blood stored at 4 C and are a theoretical if not actual source of problem, especially in

TABLE 23-1

Composition of CPD Blood Preservative Solution
Volume for use in collection of 450 ± 45 ml of blood is 63 ml.

Sodium citrate	26.3 gm
Citric acid	3.27 gm
Monobasic sodium phosphate monohydrate	2.22 gm
Dextrose	25.5 gm
Water to make	1,000 ml

the immunosuppressed patient being transfused. Platelet survival in whole blood is poor with storage at 4 C, but platelet concentrates may be physiologically effective after up to 72 hours of storage at room temperature.

Today, storage containers for blood are almost wholly plastic bags, which possess numerous advantages. In addition to preserving blood in a sterile system that does not require venting during transfusion, the use of bags with integral attached satellites permits manipulation and transfer of various portions of a unit of blood without entry into the system, which would expose the unit to bacteriologic contamination and reduce its shelf life to 24 hours after entry. A significant advantage of the plastic bag system is its attached tubing with removable segments filled with blood. The use of such segments for compatibility testing precludes the mix-ups possible when detachable pilot tubes were employed. Small amounts of plasticizer leak from storage bags into blood, and although a source of theoretical concern have not caused demonstrable clinical problems. Storage of blood should be carried out at temperatures of 1 C to 6 C, with a variation of no more than 2 C. Refrigeration must be continuous, and units of blood that have been out of refrigeration long enough to warm to 10 C (about 30 minutes under most circumstances) or that have been heated in blood-warmers, are not acceptable for restocking. Refrigerators used for blood storage must be scrupulously clean and used for no other purpose. A recording thermometer, a separate thermometer linked to an audible and visible monitored alarm, and thermometers for checking the reliability of the recording thermometer must be kept in or attached to all refrigerators used for blood storage. Even temporary storage of blood in refrigerators on wards or in operating theaters is unacceptable unless they meet all of the requirements for blood bank refrigerators. The practice of sending blood to floors in advance of its need, i.e., before it is actually to be infused, should be discouraged, as should the attitude of the surgeon who will not operate unless units of blood are physically present in the operating room.

The processing of blood must be a matter of meticulous care. Blood processing is most apt to be inadequate when most of the blood administered is obtained from a central source that also normally does the processing. The laboratory collecting only occasional units of blood needs to be doubly careful in its processing routine. The requirement for routine bacteriologic culturing of units of blood has been waived unless processing occurs in an open system or one that must be entered. All units of blood must have ABO grouping performed, including serum grouping. The D type must be determined, with performance of testing for D^u if the presumptive Rh typing is negative. Testing for other antigens, including other Rh antigens, is not required. A serologic test for syphilis is currently mandated by law on all units, but the requirement may be abandoned in the future. A"third generation" test for HB_SAg (e.g., RIA or RPHA) must be performed. Screening for alloantibodies is required, although the details of the procedure are optional. Any alloantibody present must be identified and preferably removed by washing the RBC before the unit is transfused. If other than ABO group-specific units are issued, testing for hemolytic anti-A and/or anti-B must be carried out. Label requirements are fixed by law. Suitable examples are found in the *Technical Manual of the American Association of Blood Banks*, seventh edition, 1977, or the author's *Blood Bank Policies and Procedures*. Record-keeping requirements are described in Chapters 27 and 28. Processing samples should be retained for seven days.

Testing of units of blood collected and processed at another facility is confined to repetition of the ABO grouping and, in the case of Rh-negative blood, to confirmation of the negative tests for D and D^u on the donor RBC.

RECOMMENDED READING:

Greendyke, R.M. and Banzhaf, J.C.: *Blood Bank Policies and Procedures.* Medical Examination Publishing Co., Garden City, N.Y., 1976

Huestis, D.W. et al: *Practical Blood Transfusion*, 2nd ed. Little, Brown and Co., Boston, 1976

Miller, W.V. (Ed): *Technical Manual of the American Association of Blood Banks.* Am Assn of Blood Banks. Washington, 1977

CHAPTER 24

Blood and Red Blood Cell Transfusion

The blood bank no longer supplies only whole blood, but rather provides a variety of blood components tailored to specific patient needs. Save for large-volume surgical requirements, most blood banks distribute little whole blood. In cases of chronic anemia or moderate acute blood loss, the transfusion of red blood cells should be the rule, and transfusion of whole blood the exception. Chronic shortages make blood too valuable to be used as whole blood when, by separation into components, two or three patients may benefit from a single donation. Moreover, each patient may be better served. If a patient requires added oxygen-carrying capacity, he requires red blood cells. To transfuse him with whole blood is to waste the plasma and unnecessarily burden his cardiovascular system with excess volume. Many anemias are best treated without blood transfusion by diagnosing and rectifying the cause, after which the patient's bone marrow will replace the RBC deficit. As a general rule it may be stated that RBC transfusion should be administered only when the deficiency in the circulating red blood cell mass is too severe to be treated by other means. The indications for transfusion of whole blood are practically confined to cases of massive acute hemorrhage. On the other hand, insistence on separate provision of RBC and plasma in this situation invites ridicule. In the treatment of nonhemorrhagic shock, administration of plasma or other volume expanders alone is frequently sufficient.

The disadvantages of the use of RBC for transfusion as opposed to whole blood are easily dealt with in most situations. Sluggish flow can be corrected by adding saline to the unit through a Y-set. Inadequate volume can be supplemented, at least up to a point, with crystalloid solutions or dextran. Potential deficiencies in coagulation factors are hardly ever a problem unless an abnormal coagulation mechanism antedated the transfusion, transfusion is inadequate and/or massive transfusion has been required, and even then clotting deficiencies are often not clinically significant. The provision of plasma proteins is not a goal of whole blood transfusion. The physiologic advantages of RBC transfusion may be summarized to include: decreases in volume load, citrate load, "waste" load (e.g., potassium, organic acids, ammonia, hemoglobin), and antibody load (including ABO, platelet, and leukocyte antibodies).

The problems, both theoretical and actual, associated with massive transfusion of whole blood have been cited as reasons for giving fresh blood (i.e., blood stored less than 24 hours) to the patient undergoing major surgery. The "storage lesion" found in blood two to three weeks after collection may be reviewed in light of this recommendation:

1) The blood is cold. Routine use of a blood-warming device in massive transfusions is recommended.

2) The blood is acid (pH 6.8 to 6.9), contains lactate (5 to 9 mEq/l), citrate, and other organic acids and is devoid of ionized calcium. Acidosis is rapidly corrected when shock is properly treated. An intact circulatory system and liver can easily cope with the acid load.

3) The blood contains increased amounts of plasma potassium (about 10 mEq/l after seven days, 20 mEq/l after 14 days) and ammonia (about $250\mu g/dl$ after seven days, 700 $\mu g/dl$ after 21 days). The quantities are negligible in comparison to total body stores, though in a patient in renal failure the potassium concentration could be a problem, and in theory the ammonia level might be harmful to patient in hepatic failure.

4) Survival of stored RBC is decreased. About 70% to 80% of RBC are viable after 28 days of storage in CPD-adenine and after 21 days in CPD. The increased plasma hemoglobin levels have no harmful physiologic effects.

5) Stored RBC unload oxygen poorly because of decreased 2,3-DPG concentrations. RBC 2,3-DPG levels are essentially 100% of normal after seven days of storage, and almost 50% of normal after three weeks. Half of the 2,3-DPG deficit is restored after four hours in circulation. Unless compensatory mechanisms in the body have been exhausted, this is primarily a theoretical objection.

6) Microaggregates are present. Even if physiologically signi-

ficant, microaggregates can be removed by appropriate filtration.

7) Labile plasma procoagulants are deficient. Factor VIII levels fall by 20% during the first 24 hours of storage and after a week less than half of the original activity remains. On the other hand, plasma levels of 30% of normal are adequate for surgical hemostasis. Concentrations of Factor V are reduced to two thirds of normal after seven days of storage; half remains after two weeks. Concentrations of 5% of normal are sufficient for control of surgical bleeding. Coagulation problems due to plasma procoagulant deficiency are unusual unless there is a preexisting abnormality.

8) Platelets are deficient. Functional platelet levels in whole blood have fallen to 10% of original values by the time blood has been stored for 24 hours at 4 C, and by 48 hours they are absent. Dilutional thrombocytopenia after rapid administration of twice the patient's blood volume may decrease platelet counts to 40,000 to 70,000/μl. Values under 100,000/μl may persist for up to five days, and normal levels may not be restored for ten or 12 days. Despite this fact, platelet transfusions in this situation are rarely required for hemostasis, although sometimes they are given prophylactically. The administration of whole blood, however fresh, is totally ineffective as therapy for thrombocytopenia.

A routine that has been suggested for use when massive transfusion is given includes regular use of a blood warmer and regular monitoring of blood pH, coagulation status, and serum albumin concentrations. Administration of one ampule of sodium bicarbonate (44.6 mEq) and one unit of fresh frozen plasma after each five units has been proposed if massive transfusion is carried out with aged bank blood.

In the case of total absence of erythropoiesis, the transfusion requirement of a 70-kg subject maintained at a hemoglobin concentration of 10 gm/dl is 24 ml of RBC per day, or allowing for nonviable cells, transfusion of about one unit of blood per week. Shortened survival of transfused RBC may occur in the absence of demonstrable blood group antibodies in patients with diseases such as rheumatoid arthritis or aplastic anemia and with conditions that cause splenomegaly.

The use of autologous blood transfusion is slowly gaining acceptance. The advantages of autologous transfusion from a medical point of view are many: 1) Compatible blood is available for the patient with antibodies to high frequency antigens or combinations of antigens. 2) The recipient does not risk sensitization to RBC, WBC, platelets, or serum protein antigens. 3) No allergic or febrile reactions occur. 4) There is no danger of transfusion-transmitted hepatitis or other infectious disease. 5) If a suitable period of time intervenes between phlebotomy and reinfusion, the bone marrow is stimulated. 6) If only a short period of time intervenes, dilution improves capillary blood flow and diminishes sludging. The disadvantages of the practice revolve about the logistic problems involved in reserving particular units of blood for particular patients, knowing when the patient is admitted to the hospital, knowing when surgery has been canceled, and the like. These problems are at least partly offset by the gain to the blood bank if the autologous unit is not required by its donor.

Many different schemes of exploiting the concept of autologous transfusion can be used. Predeposit plans may use a "leapfrog" technique in which multiple units are collected over a period of weeks and the oldest periodically returned to the donor, although this process is expensive and time-consuming. Frozen storage is preferable for obvious reasons. Intraoperative salvage and reinfusion of shed blood is an appealing notion that has heretofore been hampered by problems such as RBC hemolysis due to mechanical damage, depletion of coagulation factors, and most especially by microembolism and initiation of DIC by particles of fat, tissue debris, and fibrin-WBC-platelet clumps in the salvaged blood. Continuous flow centrifugation technique eliminates much of the problem, but the extra technician required to operate the instrumentation in the operating suite brings the cost-effectiveness of the procedure into question. The technique is not suitable for use in patients with malignancies, sepsis, hepatic or renal failure, or a preoperative coagulopathy. Hemodilution procedures carry substantial benefits by providing intraoperative predeposit of blood for reinfusion at the end of the procedure. This method provides fresh, compatible blood with a normal platelet content when it is most needed, yet it confers the advantages of hemodilution during surgery.

Care must be taken if autologous transfusion is practiced to ensure proper identification of the donor-patient. Signatures and instant photographs have been used for the purpose. It is recommended that blood predeposited for future use be processed in the normal manner to safeguard against problems should the unit be inadvertently selected for administration to another patient or placed in stock after not being used by its donor. No age limits have been set for donation for autologous transfusion: practical considerations and reasonable medical judgment should control the circumstances under which the practice is carried out. A lower limit of hemoglobin concentration of 11 gm/dl has been suggested for predeposit donations. Iron supplements should be prescribed for patients donating multiple units. If frozen storage is contemplated, the patient's RBC should be subjected to a direct antiglobulin test; RBC from patients with a positive direct antiglobulin test, a positive test for S hemoglobin, G-6-PD deficiency, or hereditary spherocytosis preserve poorly by some freezing methods. A positive test for HB_SAg is a contraindication to frozen storage because of the hazard to personnel processing the blood for freezing. Blood from cancer victims or patients with infectious disease can be administered only to the donor and should not be placed in stock. Donors for autologous transfusion should in general be screened in the same fashion as regular blood donors in case their blood is given intentionally or mistakenly to someone else.

The preservation of blood in the frozen state offers many advantages to the blood bank and its patients. Long-term storage (up to five years) of rare blood types and of blood for autologous transfusion is made possible. A frozen blood bank serves as a buffer against excess supply or need. Normal or even augmented concentrations of ATP and 2,3-DPG are maintained during frozen storage. Because of the washing steps required to free frozen RBC of the cryopreservative agent, thawed RBC suspended in saline are almost free from cell debris, granulocytes, platelets, plasma, potassium, ammonia, citrate, lactate, and microaggregates. Hepatitis B virus is markedly reduced in amount, if present. Some 10% to 15% of RBC are lost in the freeze-thaw-wash cycle, and another 10% to 15% do not survive for 24 hours after infusion, but the remainder live out a normal life span in the recipient. Group O frozen RBC suspended in antibody-free fresh frozen group AB plasma approach being "universal donor" blood, save for the recipient with an alloantibody. The major uses of frozen RBC today are in transfusion to potential organ-transplant candidates in whom HLA sensitization by transfused lymphocytes in bank blood is thought undesirable. Other uses include transfusion of patients with potent leukocyte antibodies, transfusion of stockpiled blood of rare types to patients with particular blood group antibodies and autologous transfusion as described above. The principal disadvantages of RBC freezing are its added cost and the current 24-hour limitation on post-thaw storage of frozen RBC because of their potential contamination during the thaw-wash cycle.

The freezing of RBC without the use of a cryoprotective agent results in the formation of ice crystals in the cells separated by tiny pools of fluid in which cell solutes are greatly concentrated. These cause biochemical damage to the cell and hemolysis upon thawing. Glycerol added to red blood cells before freezing rapidly enters their cytoplasm and protects them against osmotic damage. Two basic methods of cryopreservation are in general use, the "low glycerol" method employing 3.8 M glycerol, rapid freezing, and storage at −196 C, and the "high glycerol" methods using 6.2 or 8.6 M glycerol, slow freezing, and storage −65 C to −85 C. The low concentration of glycerol in the first method is permissible because freezing is too rapid for ice crystal formation to occur, and in addition the RBC are first partially dehydrated by suspension in hypertonic solutions of such materials as sugar or albumin. When the RBC are thawed, the glycerol is removed, not because it is toxic (it is not) but to prevent osmotic lysis of the cells. The thawed cells are first washed in hypertonic solution, then in a large volume isotonic wash solution and finally suspended in isotonic saline. The instruments available to deglycerolize thawed RBC include the cytoglomerator, which takes advantage of sedimentation of clumped RBC in fructose solution; the Hemonetics cell washing system, which employs continuous flow centrifugation in a spinning bowl; and the IBM cell washer, which makes use of a round tubular centrifuge bag. Supernatant hemoglobin in the suspending fluid of frozen RBC is less than 300 mg/dl and the osmolality less than 420 mOsm/kg. A proportion of all frozen units of blood should be cultured bacteriologically to ensure that proper sterile technique is being employed.

A substantial part of the frozen RBC transfused in some centers is used simply to secure a product reliably free of most (95% to 99%) of its leukocytes. Leukocyte antibodies are reported to cause recipient reactions in 17% to 67% of transfusions, depending on the patient group and the test methodology used. It appears that tests for granulocyte antibodies are more effective than leukoagglutination or lymphocytotoxicity tests in predicting and elucidating such reactions. The problem of sensitization to HLA antigens in potential organ transplant recipients has been discussed previously. Viable lymphocytes in stored fluid blood may colonize the patient with immunologic deficiency, occasionally leading to the occurrence of graft-versus-host disease. It is necessary to remove over 90% of WBC from blood to prevent transfusion reactions in patients with leukoagglutinins. Various maneuvers have been used to effect this removal, including sedimentation with added high molecular weight polymer solutions, filtration with nylon fiber filters, inverted centrifugation with removal of the buffy coat, saline washing, freeze-thaw-deglycerolization, and various combinations of these approaches. The problems engendered include anaphylactoid reactions to sedimenting agents, failure of nylon fibers to remove lymphocytes, the necessity of heparinizing the blood, red blood cell loss, reduction in shelf life to 24 hours, and cost. Radiation in the amount of 1,500 to 6,000 rads has been used to destroy the capability for DNA synthesis in remaining lymphocytes when the clinical situation demands. Recent reports indicate a beneficial effect of the transfusion of minimal numbers of leukocytes on graft survival in organ transplant recipients. The importance of HLA antigen–containing cell debris and the role of dead lymphocytes in such sensitization is unknown.

RECOMMENDED READING:

Dorner, I.M: Packed cells– now and in the future. In: *A Seminar on Blood Components*. Am Assn of Blood Banks. Washington, 1977, p.17

Greenwalt, T.J., (Ed.): *General Principles of Blood Transfusion*. Am Med Assn Chicago, 1977

Huestis, D.W.: Fresh blood: fact and fancy. In: *A Seminar on Current Technical Topics*. Am Assn of Blood Banks. Washington, 1974, p.117

Huestis, D.W. et al: *Practical Blood Transfusion*, 2nd ed. Little, Brown and Co., Boston, 1976

Huggins, C.: Frozen storage. In: *Autologous Transfusion*. Am Assn of Blood Banks. Washington, 1976. p.27

Kuban, D.J.: Autologous transfusion. In: *Autologous Transfusion*. Am Assn of Blood Banks. Washington, 1976. p.3

Mollison, P.L: *Blood Transfusion in Clinical Medicine,* 5th ed. Blackwell, Oxford, 1972

Polesky, H.F.: Leukocyte poor blood. In: *A Seminar on Blood Components*. Am Assn of Blood Banks. Washington, 1977, p.53

Roberts, S.C.: Cryopreserved RBC: a blood component. In: *A Seminar on Blood Components*. Am Assn of Blood Banks. Washington, 1977, p.37

CHAPTER 25

Platelet and Granulocyte Transfusion

The transfusion of whole blood to treat thrombocytopenia is ineffective and wasteful. The number of platelets contained in two or three units of whole blood, however fresh, cannot make a significant difference in the platelet count of a thrombocytopenic patient. Transfusion of enough fresh blood to supply meaningful numbers of platelets cannot be accomplished without circulatory overload. Practical therapy requires the administration of platelet concentrates, which contain half to three fourths of the viable platelets present in the original unit of blood but in a volume of only about 50 ml. The pooled platelets from 10 units of blood can thus be administered in a volume equivalent to that of one unit of whole blood.

Platelet concentrates are made from platelet-rich plasma prepared within four hours of collection by gentle centrifugation in a controlled temperature centrifuge (nine minutes at 1,000 x G) of unrefrigerated blood collected into double or triple bags. The platelet-rich plasma is expressed into a satellite bag and recentrifuged (20 minutes at 3,000 x G) to produce a cell button. All but 50 ml of the platelet-poor plasma is expressed into a third bag and may be frozen as fresh-frozen plasma or used to prepare cryoprecipitate. The platelet button is left undisturbed for one to two hours at room temperature, then resuspended and stored at 22 ± 2 C with constant gentle agitation. The storage life of platelet concentrates at room temperature is 72 hours. Alternative storage at 4 C without agitation is claimed to yield a product that is more immediately effective in reducing prolonged bleeding times in thrombocytopenic patients, but with reduced viability in vivo (averaging one day as opposed to almost normal survival of viable platelets stored at room temperature). Platelets stored at room temperature have little effect on the bleeding time for the first 24 hours after transfusion. Pooling should not be carried out until immediately before platelets are to be transfused and not more than four hours before administration.

Federal regulations require that 75% of the units of platelet concentrates prepared by a blood bank contain at least 5.5×10^{10} platelets. The yield of platelets from a unit of blood should reach an average value of 86%. Sixty-five percent of autotransfused fresh platelets can be recovered in the circulation; 20% are sequestered in the spleen. After 24 hours of storage at room temperature, recovery is 50%. Platelets stored at room temperature without agitation exhibit survivals averaging only 1.5 days, and their recovery immediately after transfusion may be reduced by half. It should be recalled that in patients with splenomegaly, the platelets trapped in the spleen may number up to seven times the circulating pool. In theory, the transfusion of one unit of platelet concentrate to a 70-kg subject should increase the platelet count by 10,000 per microliter. In practice, the increment is about half of this. The usual dose of platelet concentrates for a bleeding adult is six to ten units repeated every six to 24 hours. The effect of platelet transfusion is markedly reduced in the presence of thrombocytopenia, hemorrhage, fever, sepsis, or splenomegaly and may be totally abolished by antiplatelet antibodies.

Thrombocytopenia is caused by: 1) decreased platelet production (e.g. in acute leukemia, after chemotherapy); 2) increased platelet destruction (e.g. in idiopathic thrombocytopenic purpura, after cardiopulmonary bypass); 3) platelet consumption or dilution (e.g. in DIC, after massive transfusion); or 4) splenic pooling (e.g. in congestive splenomegaly with hypersplenism, in myeloid metaplasia). Congenital and acquired functional defects of platelets also occur, the most common of which follows ingestion of even usual doses of aspirin. The effects of aspirin on the patient's platelets may require four to six days to disappear. Indocin and phenylbutazone have similar effects but these last only a few hours. Transfused platelet preparations from donors with recent aspirin ingestion become normally functional within four to eight hours after administration, but plateletpheresis donors should not have taken aspirin for 48 hours before phlebotomy. Platelet transfusion is much more effective in patients with decreased production of platelets than it is in those with increased destruction or sequestration. General indications for platelet transfusion in patients with leukemia or bone marrow aplasia following chemotherapy are: 1) Platelet counts below $10,000/\mu l$, or 2) hemorrhage with platelet counts of less than $50,000/\mu l$. Platelet transfusions are frequently ineffective in patients with idiopathic thrombocytopenic purpura and are not generally indicated unless surgery is contemplated.

The incidence of formation of antiplatelet (HLA) antibodies reaches 60% to 80% in multitransfused normal volunteers as opposed to about 8% in patients receiving immunosuppressive drugs. However, platelet survival may be decreased in the latter group of subjects, despite the absence of demonstrable antibody. HLA matching may become necessary in patients who have become refractory to random donor platelet transfusions. Matched donor platelets, particularly if from siblings, may survive well in such patients. Sibling donors have a one in four chance of compatibility. ABO compatibility in platelet transfusions is desirable but not mandatory. Platelets from group A or B donors may exhibit shortened survival in group O recipients. The isoantibodies present in platelet preparations from group O donors may cause a positive direct antiglobulin test to appear on the RBC of a non-group O recipient. As described earlier, whenever there is an in vivo reaction between donor antigen and recipient antibody or vice versa, whether the antigen is on platelets, RBC or granulocytes, antigen-antibody complex formation and complement activation can lead to accelerated destruction of donor or recipient "innocent bystander" platelets, RBC, or granulocytes. The transfusion of plasma from patients with idiopathic thrombocytopenia can cause thrombocytopenia in recipients, despite the absence of demonstrable antiplatelet antibodies. Rh compatibility is not required for platelet transfusions except for women who are potential mothers. Recognize that sufficient RBC to cause blood group immunization often contaminate platelet preparations and that a compatibility test between the platelet donor's RBC and the recipient's serum is desirable before transfusion of platelet preparations derived by plateletpheresis from a single donor. Rh immune globulin is occasionally given to D-negative recipients of platelets from D-positive donors.

Platelet transfusions should be administered through a standard blood filter (not a microaggregate filter, which may retain platelets). Febrile reactions are common in recipients of multiple platelet transfusions. The theoretical danger of bacterial growth in platelet preparations stored at room temperature does not present a problem. Monitoring of the in vivo efficacy of platelet transfusions should be carried out routinely by performing platelet counts on recipients one and 24 hours after transfusion and relating the effects of increases in platelet count to body surface area (i.e., change in platelet count per microliter per m² of body surface area).

Plateletpheresis is a very useful technique for obtaining platelet preparations of superior quality: the yield from a typical donation is equivalent to the platelets present in a pool of ten random donor single-unit concentrates, but carries only one tenth the risk of producing post-transfusion hepatitis and decreases the exposure of the recipient to multiple HLA antigens. The volume of a single-donor platelet concentrate prepared by plateletpheresis is about 300 ml. Donor risks from plateletpheresis include the possibilities of hypovolemia, citrate toxicity and chilling. Platelet counts may fall to 40,000 to 90,000/μl and remain depressed for 24 hours. Plasma loss per donation averages 350 ml, RBC loss 25 to 30 ml.

GRANULOCYTE TRANSFUSION

Although still in its infancy, leukapheresis is conducted in many major centers to obtain the large numbers of granulocytes needed to treat neutropenic patients. When the peripheral blood granulocyte count falls below 500 to 1,000/μl the risk of bacterial infection increases substantially, and in the case of patients with aplastic bone marrows unable to produce neutrophilic leukocytes, granulocyte transfusions may be of substantial value in combatting sepsis. At least 10^{10} granulocytes are required to produce any beneficial effect in such recipients. Although granulocytes spend up to four days maturing in the bone marrow, they circulate in the peripheral blood for only about four to six hours before migrating into the tissues, where they survive for an unknown period of time. Granulocyte transfusion, once begun, is usually repeated daily for three to five days. An increase in peripheral blood white count is often not demonstrable as little as an hour after transfusion, even when clinically beneficial, because of margination and migration of the transfused granulocytes. Febrile reactions are common with granulocyte transfusions as a consequence of the liberation of leukocyte pyrogens or alloimmunization. Rigors occur in 20% to 40% of patients treated with granulocytes obtained by filtration leukapheresis (see p. 302). Other complications may include cytomegalovirus infection, graft-versus-host reactions, and the other usual risks of blood transfusion. ABO compatibility between donor and recipient is desirable because of the number of donor RBC contained in granulocyte preparations (up to 1 gm of hemoglobin per dl). A compatibility test should be performed between donor RBC and recipient serum just as in the case of a single-donor platelet transfusion. The value of HLA matching is unclear. The benefits of granulocyte transfusion are difficult to assess in the absence of objective criteria. Those currently employed are comparative increase in patient survival time and demonstration of lysis of fever. The indication for granulocyte transfusion is a peripheral blood granulocyte count of less than $500/\mu l$ in a patient with infection unresponsive to 24 to 48 hours of appropriate antibiotic therapy and in whom there is a potential for bone marrow recovery.

Granulocytes for transfusion may be harvested by either of two general methods: continuous flow centrifugation (CFC) or filtration leukapheresis (FL). In CFC methods, blood is continuously removed from a heparinized donor, passed through a centrifuge bowl with separation and removal of its buffy coat, and returned to the donor. The efficiency of the process is about 25%. At flow rates approximating 40 ml per minute, seven to ten liters of donor blood can be processed at one sitting, with a harvest of 2 to 8 x 10^9 granulocytes. If the donor is pretreated with adrenal corticosteroids or hydroxyethyl starch to raise his peripheral blood white cell count, yields of 1 to 4 x 10^{10} granulocytes can be obtained regularly. FL involves the trapping of granulocytes from donor blood on nylon filters, with their subsequent elution. A continuous flow technique can yield 1 to 4 x 10^{10} granulocytes from seven to 11 liters of blood. FL procedures in comparison to CFC give somewhat better yields of granulocytes with poorer function. Lymphocytes are present in smaller numbers, and platelets are absent. Granulocyte concentrates can be stored up to 24 hours at 4 C with gentle agitation.

Leukapheresis donors must be highly motivated because of the considerable amount of time required for the procedure and because of the slightly greater risks involved as compared to ordinary blood donation. A careful donor history must be taken, with special attention to any bleeding tendency. In addition to the usual hemoglobin requirement, the donor should be demonstrated to have a normal white blood count, a platelet count in excess of $125,000/\mu l$ and a normal partial thromboplastin time. Leukapheresis typically results in a decrease in the donor's hemoglobin concentration of 0.7 to 1.2 gm/dl, no decrease in the white blood cell count, and a fall in platelet count of 30,000 to 50,000/μl. FL may cause a granulocytosis of up to 35%.

The transfusion of viable lymphocytes in a granulocyte preparation (or in RBC or whole blood) to an immunologically deficient patient may result in a graft-versus-host reaction. In this condition transfused foreign lymphocytes colonize the host's tissues and, recognizing them as foreign, mount an immunologic attack, recognizable clinically by the development of bone marrow changes, fever, rash, and diarrhea. The host defenses that would ordinarily destroy viable foreign lymphocytes must be ineffective, or at least impaired, for this phenomenon to occur.

RECOMMENDED READING:

Greenwalt, T.J. et al: *General Principles of Blood Transfusion*, 2nd ed. Am Med Assn Chicago, 1977

Huestis, D.W. et al: *Practical Blood Transfusion*, 2nd ed. Little, Brown and Co., Boston, 1976

MacPherson, J.L.: An overview of granulocyte collection and transfusion. In: *A Seminar on Blood Components*. Am Assn of Blood Banks. Washington, 1977, p. 99

McCullough, J.: Granulocyte transfusion. In: *A Seminar on Current Technical Topics*. Am Assn of Blood Banks. Washington, 1974, p. 95

Mollison, P.L.: *Blood Transfusion in Clinical Medicine*, 5th ed. Blackwell, Oxford, 1972

Morrison, F.S.: The management of disorders of primary hemostasis. In: *Hemostasis for Blood Bankers*. Am Assn of Blood Banks. Washington, 1977, p. 83

Slichter, S.J. and Harker, L.A.: Preparation and storage of platelet concentrates. In: *A Seminar on Current Technical Topics*. Am Assn of Blood Banks. Washington, 1974, p. 87

CHAPTER 26

Plasma Coagulation Factor Deficiencies

The treatment of patients with coagulation defects depends on the diagnosis of the deficiency. The notion that fresh blood contains all coagulation factors and thus is appropriate for the treatment of all coagulation defects is naive, the volume of whole blood required almost always exceeding what the patient's cardiovascular system can tolerate. Even when the patient is bleeding and requires blood transfusion for other reasons, added concentrated preparations of specific factors are usually necessary to permit clotting. The results of transfusion therapy in patients with hemorrhagic diseases are dependent upon the original concentration and the amount of the missing factor administered, the space in which it is distributed and the presence or absence of inhibitors. The time interval between transfusions is governed by the normal rate of catabolism of the factor administered and the presence of conditions that may affect its turnover time. Appropriate treatment of the patient with a clotting disorder is directed at removing the cause if possible and temporarily rectifying the deficiency. Thus, therapy depends on a knowledge of what is deficient, what appropriate products are available for treatment, the concentration of the desired factor in the material available, its half-life on transfusion, and the levels necessary to effect, for example, surgical hemostasis. Table 26-1 summarizes some of the pertinent data relating to congenital deficiencies of plasma procoagulants.

Of the congenital clotting factor deficiency diseases, Factor VIII deficiency, or hemophilia, is the most common, comprising about 85% of cases. Factor IX deficiency (PTC deficiency or Christmas disease) accounts for about 14%, and Factor XI deficiency (PTA

TABLE 26-1
Plasma Coagulation Factors

Factor	Common Name	Normal Concentration (in vivo)	Half-life (in vivo)	Requirement for Surgical Hemostasis	Available Therapeutic Materials
I	Fibrinogen	150–400 mg/dl	4–6 days	70 mg/dl	Cryo., Plasma
II	Prothrombin	60–120%	2–5 days	20%	Plasma, Commercial conc.
V	Proaccelerin (Labile factor)	70–130%	12 hr	5%	FFP
VII	Proconvertin (Stable factor)	75–150%	1–7 hr	20%	Plasma, Commercial conc.
VIII	Antihemophiliac factor	50–200%	8–16 hr	30%	FFP, Cryo., Commercial conc.
IX	Christmas factor (PTC)	70–130%	18–36 hr	20%	Plasma, Commercial conc.
X	Stuart factor	70–130%	20–40 hr	10%	Plasma, Commercial conc.
XI	PTA	70–130%	40–80 hr	20%	FFP
XII	Hageman factor	40–150%	?	0	Not required
XIII	Fibrin stabilizing factor	50–200%	6–12 days	1%	Plasma

Cryo. = cryoprecipitate; Plasma = stored bank plasma; FFP = fresh frozen plasma.
All are stable in storage at 4 C except for Factors V and VIII. All retain full activity in fresh frozen plasma.

TABLE 26-2

Inherited Disorders of Plasma Coagulation

Factor Deficiency	Frequency	Usual Clinical Severity	Inheritance
I, II, V, VII, X, XI, XIII	< 1 per 10^4	Mild	Autosomal recessive
VIII	1 per 2×10^4 (males)	Mild to severe	Sex-linked recessive
von Willebrand's	5–10 per 10^4	Mild to moderate	Autosomal dominant
IX	5 per 10^5 (males)	Mild to moderate	Sex-linked recessive
XII	< 1 per 10^4	None	Autosomal recessive

deficiency) for about 1%. The remainder are extremely rare (Table 26-2). Hemophilia is an hereditary syndrome due to the presence of sex-linked recessive gene(s) that determine the formation of defective Factor VIII (A+ type) or its underproduction (A− type), the latter comprising some 85% to 90% of cases. Hemophilia is transmitted by carrier mothers, but expressed only in their sons. Factor VIII has been shown to be a molecular complex, the functional components of which are designated VIII_C (the procoagulant), VIII_{ag} (the antigenic portion), and VIII_{vw} (the von Willebrand factor). The VIII_{ag} and VIII_{vw} activities are found on the same molecule, while VIII_C activity is separable. In classic hemophilia, Factor VIII_C activity in plasma is deficient, while the concentrations of the other components are normal. Normal concentrations of Factor VIII procoagulant activity range from 50% to 250% of the mean value of 100 units/dl: 1 ml of normal plasma contains an average of one unit of Factor VIII procoagulant activity. As summarized in Table 26-3, spontaneous bleeding may occur in the moderately affected hemophiliac with Factor VIII_C levels of 1% to 5% of normal. Patients with higher concentrations usually experience little difficulty unless subjected to trauma or surgery (including tooth extraction). The amount of Factor VIII_C necessary to limit hemorrhage depends on the nature and site of the bleeding: levels of 5% prevent spontaneous

TABLE 26-3

Relationship of Plasma Content of Factors VIII and IX to
Clinical Manifestations

Clinical Severity	Plasma Content of Factor (%)	Symptoms and Signs
Carrier	30–60	May bleed excessively with tooth extraction or major surgery
Mild	10–30	Excessive bleeding with surgery, no spontaneous hemorrhage
Moderate	2–10	Excessive bleeding with minor trauma, occasional spontaneous hemorrhage
Severe	< 2	Spontaneous hemorrhage, especially into joints

hemorrhage, but concentrations of 15% to 20% are required to stop hemarthrosis, and levels of 30% are considered necessary for surgical hemostasis.

Factor VIII_C is labile. Plasma stored at 4 C loses on the average about 20% of its VIII_C activity in 24 hours, 40% in 48 hours, and 55% in a week. Although the content of Factor VIII_C in normal plasma varies widely, only 15% of samples have levels initially less than 90% of the mean value of 100 units/dl. Factor VIII_C levels in fresh frozen plasma show only 60% to 70% of the original activity because of dilution by anticoagulant solution and losses in processing. The patient with hemophilia is most effectively treated with concentrates of Factor VIII or, less effectively, with cryoprecipitate. Cryoprecipitate is prepared by harvesting the sediment remaining after fresh frozen plasma is thawed. Because Factor VIII_C is heat labile, continuous refrigeration is required before and during its preparation, and units of blood intended for fractionation into cryoprecipitate must be processed within four hours of collection. Cryoprecipitates contain an average of half of the Factor VIII_C activity present in the plasma from which they were prepared; because they are unassayed, rather more material than theoretically required should be given. Anti-A and anti-B blood group antibodies are present in Factor VIII preparations, and although rare complications do occur, their presence is usually ignored. The risk of transfusion-transmitted hepatitis is present in Factor VIII preparations, especially the concentrates prepared from pooled plasma, despite negative radioimmunoassays for HB_SAg. Essentially 100% of patients with hemophilia treated with commercial Factor VIII concentrates develop positive tests for HB_SAg or anti-HB_S. About 20% of patients develop clinical hepatitis B after their first treatment with commercial concentrate. Up to 80% of patients treated with commercial concentrates display intermittently abnormal liver function tests, and 40% have chronic abnormalities.

Cryoprecipitate generally contains 50 to 150 units of Factor VIII_C activity per bag, plus about 250 mg of fibrinogen and 75 to 100 units of Factor XIII. Commercial lyophilized concentrates of Factor VIII are available in assayed vials containing 250 to 1000 units, giving a concentration factor of 10 to 20 times over plasma. The advantages of the commercial concentrates are their low volume (advantageous in children) and assayed potency; their disadvantages are their risk of transmitting hepatitis B and their cost. Various dosage schemes for treatment of plasma procoagulant deficiencies have been proposed:

Dose of Factor required (units) =

$$\frac{\text{Desired increase in concentration (\%)} \times \text{plasma volume (ml)}}{100}$$

Plasma volume may be calculated from the formula:

$$\text{Plasma volume (ml)} = 0.08 \times \text{body weight (kg)} \times 1000 \times \frac{100 - \text{Hematocrit}}{\text{Hematocrit}}$$

As a rule of thumb, administration of one unit of Factor VIII per kg of body weight increases the plasma Factor VIII concentration by 2%. For treatment of a severe hemophiliac with hemarthrosis or a soft tissue hematoma, Factor VIII_C levels should be maintained above 25% for at least one day. If tooth extraction is contemplated levels of 30% to 50% are optimally required for one to two days, and in the case of surgery or trauma, even higher levels are ideally maintained for seven to ten days. Factor VIII preparations must be administered every 12 hours because of their short half-life (eight to 16 hours); Factor IX concentrates (see p. 309) on the other hand are more slowly catabolized (half-life of 18 to 36 hours) and can be administered once daily. It must be recalled, however, that Factor IX, being a small molecule, is distributed in the extravascular space as well as the plasma, while transfused Factor VIII is largely (60% to 80%) retained in the plasma. To maintain Factor VIII concentrations above 30%, levels of 60% must be attained every 12 hours. While severe treated hemophiliacs probably have acquired hepatitis B immunity (or chronic hepatitis,) the mild, little-treated case of hemophilia should receive only cryoprecipitates. Up to 8% of treated patients with severe hemophilia produce an IgG anti-Factor VIII inhibitor. If the antibody is of low potency, it may sometimes be overcome with massive Factor VIII administration. Plasmapheresis and immunosuppression have been tried in the treatment of such cases. More recently, success has been achieved in halting hemorrhage in patients with refractory Factor VIII$_C$ deficiency by administering Factor IX concentrates: the activated coagulation factors in some lots of some brands are thrombogenic.

Von Willebrand's disease is an hereditary mild-to-moderate coagulation disorder characterized by ecchymosis and mucous membrane bleeding, occurring in both sexes and constituting the most common inherited bleeding disorder in women. All portions of the Factor VIII complex are deficient, resulting in both decreased plasma procoagulant activity in tests for Factor VIII$_C$ and in defective platelet function due to deficiency of Factor VIII$_{VW}$ and manifested by prolonged bleeding times and defective platelet aggregation by ristocetin. The von Willebrand component of Factor VIII plays an essential but unelucidated role in normal platelet function, and its absence results in qualitative platelet abnormality. Transfusion with normal fresh frozen plasma or cryoprecipitate results in a greater increase in plasma Factor VIII$_C$ concentrations in patients with von Willebrand's disease than can be accounted for by the amount of Factor VIII administered, suggesting the absence of a precursor or regulator substance in their plasma. This material is deficient in commercial Factor VIII concentrates, making cryoprecipitate the agent of choice for treatment.

Factor IX deficiency, or Christmas disease (also called hemophilia B, as distinguished from hemophilia A, or Factor VIII deficiency), is a sex-linked recessive coagulation disorder occurring about one tenth as commonly as classic hemophilia and usually as a less crippling disorder. The significance of a given concentration of Factor IX parallels that of a similar level of Factor VIII. As in hemophilia, both quantitative and qualitative abnormalities of Factor IX have been identified. Factor IX is stable in plasma stored at 4 C, with 80% remaining after 21 days. There is no advantage to the use of fresh rather than stored plasma for transfusion. Because Factor IX is widely distributed in extravascular body water, the amount found in the plasma at the conclusion of transfusion is only 20% of the amount infused. A concentrated preparation of the vitamin K–dependent coagulation factors produced in the liver (Factors II, VII, IX and X) is available commercially. The product contains about equal amounts of each factor, but is assayed only for Factor IX. The hepatitis B risk from this concentrate is high. A further risk is associated with its use in that partially activated coagulation factors are present in some lots and may induce thrombosis in the recipient, especially in the presence of chronic liver disease. Concomitant heparin administration in the amount of five units per ml of reconstituted volume has been recommended.

Hypofibrinogenemia is rare as a primary cause of bleeding and is usually secondary to DIC. Concentrations of fibrinogen must fall below 50 mg/dl to result in a coagulation deficit. Replacement therapy is rarely, if ever, indicated. Commercial fibrinogen preparations are no longer available because of the high hepatitis risk to the recipient. It should be recalled that each unit of cryoprecipitate supplies about 250 mg of fibrinogen.

Congenital Factor XIII deficiency has been recognized only recently. Affected infants may be suspected when excessive bleeding occurs from the cut end of the umbilical cord. Poor wound healing also has been described in this condition. Other congenital coagulation factor deficiencies are extremely rare and are usually manifested by clinically mild disease.

ACQUIRED PLASMA COAGULATION DEFECTS

Acquired abnormalities of the plasma coagulation system can be categorized under the headings of decreased procoagulant production, increased consumption or inhibition. Decreased production of plasma coagulation Factors II, VII, IX, and X occurs in patients with chronic liver disease (primarily cirrhosis) and in those treated with coumadin anticoagulants such as warfarin or dicumarol. The liver synthesizes all of the plasma procoagulants save for Factor VIII_{ag} and Factor VIII_{vw}. Coumadin anticoagulants act as vitamin K analogs and prevent completion of the synthesis of the vitamin-K dependent factors. Vitamin K causes carboxylation in the liver of a prothrombin precursor (and probably of the precursors of Factors VII, IX, and X) to form a calcium-binding site that is essential to activation by Factor Xa. Oral anticoagulants depress the formation of Factor VII first, followed by interference with the synthesis of Factors IX, X, and II. Certain drugs may inhibit the action of oral anticoagulants (e.g., phenobarbital) or potentiate them (e.g., phenylbutazone). In patients with cirrhosis the decrease in production of Factors II, VII, IX, and X is reflected in abnormalities in the prothrombin time and parallels abnormalities in other tests of hepatic function. In addition, there may occur varying amounts of low-grade DIC, impaired clearance of plasminogen activator, increased fibrinolysis, and thrombocytopenia caused both by DIC and congestive splenomegaly secondary to the cirrhosis.

Inhibitors of coagulation factors are encountered in the form of anti-Factor VIII_C antibodies in 5% to 10% of treated hemophiliacs with severe forms of the disorder, and in rare cases of drug reaction, immunologic disease, pregnancy, and in otherwise healthy elderly patients. Anti-Factor VIII_C antibodies are characterized by the slowness of their neutralizing reactions. Antibodies that inhibit the Factor Xa-Factor V-platelet factor 3-calcium complex are occasionally found in the sera of patients with systemic lupus erythematosus, especially those giving biologic false-positive serologic tests for syphilis. Tests of partial thromboplastin time or recalcification time using mixtures of patient and normal plasma are used to detect circulating anticoagulants. Prolonged thrombin times (as well as prothrombin times and partial thromboplastin times), which falsely suggest the presence of a circulating anticoagulant, may be seen as a result of interference with fibrin polymerization in patients with dysproteinemias.

Consumption of coagulation factors may be excessive in patients with acute DIC occurring as a consequence of obstetric accidents, shock, liberation of thromboplastic substances into the bloodstream (e.g., after surgery, intravascular hemolysis, or venomous snakebite, sepsis, antigen-antibody reactions, severe trauma, heatstroke, or extracorporeal circulation). Any of these conditions may activate both the coagulation mechanism and reactive fibrinolysis. Chronic, low-grade forms of DIC occur commonly in patients with chronic liver disease, malignancy, leukemia, and vascular malformations. Neonatal DIC may occur as a complication of HDN, maternal toxemia, or abruptio placentae. In DIC, several factors are operative simultaneously: 1) Clotting leads to consumption of coagulation factors. 2) Reactive fibrinolysis produces fibrin split products that interfere with platelet function and fibrin polymerization. 3) Plasmin also destroys certain plasma procoagulants. 4) Thrombosis and microembolism take place. RBC destruction (microangiopathic hemolysis) is a result of red blood cell injury by fibrin threads. 5) Shock occurs, with obstruction of pulmonary capillaries. There is some question as to whether shock is cause or effect in DIC. 6) Complement is activated, a process, as described previously, that is linked to plasmin release.

Laboratory testing of patients with DIC classically demonstrates an abnormal peripheral blood smear, with schistocytes, nucleated RBC, and polychromatophilia. Also present are thrombocytopenia, prolonged partial thromboplastin, prothrombin, and thrombin times, decreased plasma levels of fibrinogen, and increased concentrations of fibrin split products. The partial thromboplastin time is sensitive to a 30% plasma level of Factor VIII and discloses abnormalities of all of the consituents of the intrinsic coagulation scheme except for phospholipid. The prothrombin time assesses the extrinsic system and detects abnormalities in the concentrations of Factors II, VII, X, and fibrinogen. The thrombin time is used to discover abnormalities in the late stages of coagulation and is sensitive to reduced plasma concentrations of fibrinogen, to fibrin split products and to paraproteins. Treatment of DIC varies with the cause of the disease. Frequently, if the exciting cause is controlled (e.g. the removal of a dead fetus), DIC will subside spontaneously. In cases where fibrinolysis is excessive (e.g. after cardiopulmonary bypass or in chronic liver disease), administration of epsilon aminocaproic acid may be beneficial. In situations in which thromboplastic substances have been liberated in excess (e.g. after amniotic fluid embolism or in hemolytic transfusion reactions), heparinization is indicated. Simultaneous replacement therapy is also administered.

Coagulation problems are occasionally encountered in patients undergoing extracorporeal circulation. Causes include incomplete or excessive neutralization of the heparin used to anticoagulate the patient's blood during the bypass, thrombocytopenia as a consequence of platelet adherence to the pump and tubing surfaces, activation of

DIC, dilutional procoagulant deficiency, and incomplete surgical hemostasis.

Although not concerned in the production of blood clots, albumin and gamma globulin comprise two other plasma constituents administered as blood components and may be conveniently considered at this time. The plasma of a 70-kg adult contains about 125 gm of albumin and the extravascular space an additional 190 gm. Daily turnover is of the order of 10 to 16 gm, most of which occurs in the plasma compartment, so that about 10% of the plasma albumin is replaced daily. Human serum albumin as a 5% or 25% solution is prepared from plasma for use as a volume expander. Its advantages include freedom from blood group antibody and hepatitis virus, plus stability on storage; its disadvantage is its high cost. The indications for the transfusion of albumin are 1) to restore rapidly the plasma volume, and 2) to increase intravascular binding of bilirubin in babies with HDN. There is no place for transfusion of albumin in the management of chronic hypoalbuminemia, such as occurs in cirrhosis, nephrosis, or malignancies. The half-life of transfused albumin is about 15 days.

Gamma globulin for intramuscular injection is another plasma byproduct and like albumin is free from hepatitis virus. Because it is made from a pool of plasma from many persons, such gamma globulin contains a variety of antibodies and is therefore useful for prophylaxis against a number of infections in susceptible exposed people and in patients deficient in gamma globulin. Both albumin and gamma globulin are prepared commercially or at a national center. Specific immune globulin preparations are now also available for use in high-risk patients. These are prepared from the plasma of convalescent patients or donors with antibodies to the agents of specific diseases (e.g., mumps, herpes zoster, hepatitis B).

Immunoglobulin injected intravenously equilibrates between the intravascular and extravascular compartments in about five days, and disappears with a half-life of about 23 days. Seven percent to 8% of the intravascular pool of immunoglobulin is turned over per day, independently of concentration. IgG injected intramuscularly is cleared into the plasma at the rate of about 40% per day. Plasma levels after intramuscular injection are maximal at two days and reach about 40% of the total dose. Absorption of subcutaneously injected IgG is slower, with maximal plasma concentrations not reached for five days.

CHAPTER 27

Administrative Regulations and Practices

A detailed discussion of the operational aspects of blood banking is beyond the scope of this volume. Recommended regulations and practices will only be summarized in this chapter. It is emphasized that a procedure manual that details all of the areas touched upon below must exist in the blood bank. For an example of such a manual that is adaptable to the needs of most blood banks, the reader is referred to the author's companion volume *Blood Bank Policies and Procedures.*

Proper physical facilities and their appropriate maintenance are essential to quality work. Subject to the size of the hospital and the range of services offered, space is required for the following activities: reception, donor interviewing, blood collection, blood processing, component preparation, antibody identification, special testing, sterile procedures, patient typing and compatibility testing, developmental and evaluation studies, quality control activities, secretarial services and record keeping, supply storage, office space for the director and supervisory staff, and a library-teaching area. Illumination must be adequate for close work. Temperatures and humidity should be controlled within comfortable working limits. Floors, benches, walls, and ceilings should be finished to permit scrubbing. Clutter should be minimized; aisles must be kept clear. Reagents and supplies not in immediate use should be returned to their proper place of storage at once. Only one day's supplies should be kept at work station at one time. Personal items and decorations should be minimized.

Communications facilities should include adequate telephone

lines, including, at least in larger facilities, an unlisted direct outside line for use in emergency situations. Telephone extensions without bells should be located at appropriate locations, as should intercom connections. The blood bank should be quiet and serene: harassed technologists make mistakes. Non-blood bank personnel should be politely but firmly excluded from the premises. Confusion, blaring radios, funny stories, and vivid accounts of a new girlfriend may distract the technologist at the next bench who holds someone's life in his hands.

Emergency power must be available to the blood bank in the event of a disaster. Housekeeping must be immaculate. Floors, sinks, and benches must be spotlessly clean and free from spills. Instrument and equipment surfaces and interiors must be immaculate. The technical staff should be responsible for maintenance of work areas and instruments. Daily disinfection of work surfaces is recommended. A posted protocol should exist for dealing with spilled biologic products, in light of their potential contamination with hepatitis B virus. Disposal of potentially contaminated wastes, including biologics, tubes, bags, gauzes, and needles should be conducted according to written policy designed to minimize the risk of infection. Radioactive wastes must be accorded special treatment, again per a written protocol.

An organized file of equipment items should be maintained, listing such items as manufacturer, model, serial number, supplier, date of purchase, cost, service records, records of preventive maintenance, and the source of routine and emergency service. A similar file is recommended for supply items including specifications, source, catalogue number, price, an alternative source of emergency supply, the usual inventory, the procedure for putting a supply into use (with attention to expiration dates), special storage conditions required, the procedure for clearing an item for use (e.g., completion of quality assurance testing on a new reagent) and the procedure for rejection of faulty items.

Blood inventory control should be exacting, both to ensure against unexpected shortages and to minimize outdating. Every effort should be made to minimize holding blood "on call" for protracted intervals. Except under unusual circumstances it is suggested that blood crossmatched for a patient not be reserved for more than 24 hours after the time of anticipated use indicated on the requisition. Minimum desirable blood inventory levels will be established by experience, but rarely need exceed a 48-hour supply if blood is obtained from a readily accessible central depot. Larger stocks may be warranted if a hospital has an active emergency service or if considerable delays can occur in securing new blood supplies. An ongoing effort should be made to minimize outdating of blood and its products. This should include an inventory system that alerts the blood bank to impending outdating so that special efforts can be made to transfuse the product to a patient who requires it.

Blood shortages require a variety of maneuvers. The attending physicians of patients with blood on reserve can be called to request its release for emergency use. A given unit of blood may be cross-matched for two potential recipients. Frozen blood reserves may be used. Group O RBC, preferably washed, may be supplied to non-group O recipients. Under documented urgent circumstances, with the authorization of the blood bank director and the written consent of the attending physician, incompletely processed units of blood (e.g. those lacking serologic testing for syphilis) or blood tested by an abbreviated or alternate method, may be issued. Under documented life-threatening circumstances with the same conditions as above, D-positive blood has been issued for administration to D-negative recipients whose serum has been shown by sensitive (enzyme plus antiglobulin) testing to lack anti-D. Before such desperation measures are employed, if time permits, a broadcast appeal for blood donors over the hospital's public address system or by radio, or telephone solicitation of an immediately available group such as a college class, will generally bring donors quickly.

A table of organization should be drawn for the blood bank staff, detailing the chain of responsibility. Written personnel rules should exist, together with job description and position requirements including licensing requirements of governmental agencies. Personnel records should include references, a resume of training, experience and certification with dates, annual performance evaluations, records of advancement, salary data, health records, and disciplinary and commendation records. Incident reports must be filed in the case of any accident or occurrence that involves personal injury or that could eventuate in legal action. Specific blood bank personnel rules should be posted. Schedules of work, arrangements for staggering coffee breaks and lunch hours, assignments for "on-call," weekend and holiday work, the dress code, and regulations concerning eating, smoking, personal visitors, and telephone calls are all potential areas for friction unless clearly specified and fairly administered. Every effort should be made to avoid technologist fatigue and boredom: accuracy and productivity fall off alarmingly in tired or disinterested people. An occasional change in responsibilities often engenders renewed enthusiasm and interest.

Quality blood banking begins with informed, enthusiastic, concerned people. An on-going educational program can contribute in a major way, and should be regarded by the blood bank director and hospital administration as an integral part of the provision of high-quality patient care. As parts of such an effort, the following are recommended: 1) a familiarization program for all new blood bank technologists. This should be more than a "where to find it" and "this is how we do it here" orientation, but a review of fundamental principles of blood banking, an introduction to new techniques with which the technologist may not be familiar, a chance for the technologist to fill out gaps in his background, and an opportunity for the blood bank supervisory staff to assess the knowledge, skill, and personal factors that must be known before proper assignment of duties and level of responsibility can be made. 2) An in-service, regularly scheduled program of continuing education for the blood bank staff. 3) Attendance by the blood bank staff at selected appropriate medical staff conferences, rounds, or special lectures. 4) Membership and participation in local and professional societies, including the American Association of Blood Banks. 5) Ready availability of current reference materials and pertinent professional journals.

Major efforts should be made to ensure the health and safety of the blood bank staff. The possibility of viral hepatitis represents the major hazard. All blood samples should be handled as if they were infectious, and the same precautions should be taken with reagents of human origin and samples received for proficiency testing. Shipments of blood and packages of sera should be examined for leakage when received. If containers are damaged, the product should be discarded and the contaminated area disinfected. Contaminated packing materials should be treated as infectious. Frozen blood products should be enclosed in a leakproof overwrap before being thawed in a waterbath to guard against contamination of the bath if the bag has cracked while frozen. Bags of blood subjected to centrifugation must be similarly enclosed in an overwrap in case of breakage. Special care must be taken to prevent soiling of records, worksheets, and labels by spilled blood or reagents. Testing materials, positive control sera, and positive specimens from HB$_S$Ag testing should be autoclaved before disposal. Protective clothing must be worn in the hepatitis testing area, and the work should be carried out in a separate, isolated and properly identified area. No mouth-pipetting should be allowed, and disposable pipettes should be used. The staff should be cautioned against the possibility of aerosols when opening capped tubes of blood or centrifuging uncapped specimens. Serum from donors of reagent test cells prepared in the blood bank should be tested for HB$_S$Ag every six months. It is recommended that all blood bank staff have a blood specimen tested for HB$_S$Ag upon employment and yearly thereafter.

Fire safety needs regular emphasis, with periodic drills, posted escape routes and procedures for reporting a fire, and instruction in use of fire extinguishers. Electrical safety should be ensured by periodic inspection and testing of blood bank equipment by a competent service representative.

RECOMMENDED READING:

Abelson, N.M.: *Topics in Blood Banking.* Lea & Febiger, Philadelphia, 1974

Greendyke, R.M. and Banzhaf, J.C.: *Blood Bank Policies and Procedures.* Medical Examination Publishing Co., Garden City, N.Y., 1976

Huestis, D.W. et al: *Practical Blood Transfusion,* 2nd ed., Little, Brown and Co., Boston, 1976

Kammerer, R.C. (Ed.): *Administrative Procedures and Practices,* 2nd ed. Am Assn of Blood Banks. Washington, 1974

Miller, W.V. (Ed.): *Technical Manual of the American Association of Blood Banks.* Am Assn of Blood Banks. Washington, 1977

Myhre, B.A.: *Quality Control in Blood Banking.* John Wiley & Sons, New York, 1974

Oberman, H.A. (Ed.): *Standards for Blood Banks and Transfusion Services,* 8th ed. Am Assn of Blood Banks, Washington, 1976.

CHAPTER 28

Quality Assurance

A functioning quality control program is essential to the proper, safe operation of a blood bank. It is not safe to assume that a person, a reagent, a supply, a process, a product, or a piece of equipment performs the way you want it to or the way the manufacturer says it does without proving so. Errors of both omission and commission may be perpetuated almost indefinitely unless detected by routine monitoring or by the occurrence of a problem. Other people's quality assurance programs may leave something to be desired, and the inspection programs on industrial production lines miss defects with regularity. Even the best of products may be damaged in shipment or deteriorate in storage.

The major thrust of the quality assurance program in the blood bank, however, should, in the author's judgement, be directed at people, not things. This is not to minimize the importance of quality control procedures on supplies, reagents, and instruments, but to insist that the problem be viewed in perspective: How much patient morbidity and mortality result each year from material defects and how much from human error? Both sets of problems should be attacked but it is apparent that in most quality assurance programs emphasis is laid on those aspects that are concrete and susceptible to testing, quantitation, documentation, and statistical analysis, and that the more nebulous area of trying to get people to understand and to perform their work properly is usually dismissed, albeit uneasily.

The following discussion is divided into sections dealing with:
1. Assurance of personnel competence
2. Control of incoming material (reagents and supplies)
3. Process control (equipment and procedures)

4. Control of outgoing material (products and reports)
5. Exercise of supervisory controls

PERSONNEL COMPETENCE

Education and experience are most desirable in the blood bank staff but do not guarantee superior work. On the other hand, the motivation that has led the technologist to secure a sound educational background seems to correlate with job performance. The pursuit of additional education should be encouraged in all staff members. The enthusiasm and interest of people who are involved almost guarantees superior performance and tends to be infectious.

The necessity for technical orientation of new staff members was discussed in Chapter 27. Such a program must emphasize the necessity of doing things as prescribed in the procedure manual, irrespective of how the technologist may have performed the test elsewhere. The prohibition of short-cuts or personal modifications of procedures must be made very clear. At the same time, the technologist must be encouraged to offer constructive suggestions and to participate if studies are undertaken to evaluate the feasibility or utility of his ideas. All staff members must read the procedure manual during their orientation period, and it is suggested that they review it yearly, as documented by their signature in the manual.

Continuing educational programs were mentioned in Chapter 27 and have been discussed in detail in the companion book to this volume, *Blood Bank Policies and Procedures.* Participation by the blood bank in proficiency testing programs such as those sponsored by the College of American Pathologists or various governmental regulatory agencies is desirable. Communication is vitally important in the area of quality assurance: procedure and policy changes must be disseminated to all staff members on all shifts, and care must be taken to include part-time staff, those who rotate through the blood bank but may currently be working elsewhere, and those on vacation, or absent because of illness or other reason. It is not sufficient with professional blood bank technologists to say "Do it this way." Reasons for changes and data that show why the new way is better must be given to enlist support for change. The staff must be encouraged to participate in decisions and their objections or recommendations evaluated seriously. With regard to the quality assurance program particularly, its purpose and means of implementation must be explained.

Procedural uniformity should be tested at regular intervals to ensure that the results are similar and reproducible. Examples of such testing include exercises in the reading of agglutination, the preparation of RBC suspensions of a given strength, titering, eluate, preparation, and taking of blood pressures. A regular schedule should be used for this testing, and all results should be kept as permanent records. Emphasis should be laid on the fact that the purpose of the testing is constructive, not punitive; assistance, not criticism should be provided when indicated.

REAGENTS

Most blood bank reagents are of animal or human origin and as such have the undesirable characteristics common to biologic materials: impurity, variability, and instability. Impurity is imparted to antisera by various additives and by the presence of reactivities other than that desired, e.g., anti-A and anti-B typing sera usually also contain anti-T, anti-Tn, and occasionally anti-Sd^a, plus even anti-Bg and anti-Gm activity. Antibodies to dyes such as acriflavine or yellow #5 tartrazine added to color anti-B typing sera may cause false-positive cell grouping reactions when slide technics are used. Antibodies to caprylate-stabilized bovine albumin are responsible for albumin autoagglutination. Rare typing sera often contain additional antibodies not reactive if the recommended technique is employed but which may cause error if the supplier's directions are not followed. Antibodies to white blood cell antigens shared by RBC (e.g., anti-Bg) are present in up to one third of typing sera. It is desirable to have antisera of a given specificity from more than one manufacturer available for use in checking suspicious results. Anti-A or anti-B antibodies or antihuman antibodies may reappear in sera thought to be completely absorbed or neutralized, the latter occurring as the result of dissociation of antigen-antibody complexes on storage. Although the manufacturers of blood bank reagents exert every effort to ensure uniformity in their products, no two patients or animals produce identical antisera, and the antibodies produced by a single subject may vary with time. Two antisera may react identically in one situation but quite differently in another (e.g., two antiglobulin sera may detect RBC sensitization with anti-D equally well, but vary in their ability to react with anti-c or anti-Jk^a). Manufacturers overcome part of the difficulty by pooling materials from several sources, but in the case of rare antisera this may not always be possible, and considerable variability may be found among lots or among the products of different suppliers, especially for the many items for which no federal regulation on potency exists.

Biologic reagents are prone to denaturation and may deteriorate readily if improperly handled. Continuous refrigeration and the exercise of care to prevent bacterial or other contamination are required. Frequent warming and cooling of antisera are undesirable. The presence of sodium azide in a serum does not guarantee its sterility. On receipt of reagents, examination for breakage, expiration dates, and evidence of deterioration as manifested by turbidity or a precipitate should be made. The package insert should be checked for changes; if found, the procedure manual should be appropriately modified and the staff informed. Antisera for routine use should be stored at 2 C to 8 C, not frozen. Freezing and thawing may denature proteins and unpredictably affect antisera containing additives such as bovine albumin. Especial care should be taken when supply sources for blood bank reagents are changed. One manufacturer's directions must never be used with another's product. Each shipment and each lot number of reagent should be completely tested upon receipt. Thereafter retesting by a less elaborate protocol should be carried out daily, or for less commonly used reagents, whenever employed.

Quality control of saline requires that the water used be distilled, with resistance greater than 0.1 meg-ohms (conductance less than 4 ppm of NaCl), sterile, and of pH 6.0 to 7.0. The sodium chloride used should be USP grade. Concentration should be 0.15 M ± .005 M (300 ± 10 mOsm per liter). Each batch of saline should be tested to ensure that it does not crenate, lyse, or produce a positive direct antiglobulin test with normal RBC. ABO grouping sera must cause 1+ agglutination of A$_1$ or B RBC at a dilution of 256. Weakly reactive (cord) red blood cells should be readily agglutinated by undiluted grouping sera. There should be no nonspecific agglutination. Avidity tests must meet federal requirements (see *Blood Bank Policies and Procedures*). Daily testing should demonstrate appropriate reactivity with group A$_1$, A$_2$, B, and O RBC.

Anti-D typing sera must yield 1+ agglutination in tube tests at a dilution of 32 in 22% albumin. D^u cells should react with the undiluted typing serum upon antiglobulin testing. All reactions must be specific. Appropriate avidity must be present. Daily testing should include the use of positive and negative controls. Tests with other typing sera, not subject to federal standards, should be routinely monitored with negative and heterozygous positive controls. It should be noted that if Bureau of Biologics reference sera are available for comparison, titering is not necessary with anti-A, anti-B, or anti-D typing sera.

Antiglobulin sera must be tested on receipt for anti-IgG and anti-C3b activity, using appropriately sensitized RBC. The potency and specificity of the anti-IgG must be demonstrated by a technique such as that described in *Blood Bank Policies and Procedures*. Daily testing should include demonstrable reactivity with the antiglobulin check cells employed at the end of compatibility testing. Anti-C3d activity must be demonstrable in sera employed for direct antiglobulin tests.

Reagent RBC for ABO serum grouping must show 1+ agglutination by a 1:250 dilution of ABO cell grouping serum. A_1 RBC must react with anti-A_1 lectin. Reagent RBC for antibody screening and identification tests should be tested upon receipt for reactivity of those antigens that deteriorate readily – Lewis, MN, and P.

Albumin should be tested upon receipt for the presence of agglutinating or hemolytic activity. Enhancement of agglutination by anti-D should be demonstrated with the albumin. Lectins should be checked for reactivity and specificity.

EQUIPMENT

Scheduled preventive maintenance of instrumentation should be performed regularly and detailed records kept including the nature of any repairs made. A 12-month calendar is recommended, listing the dates and nature of all scheduled quality control activities. Instrument maintenance is conveniently scheduled on this calendar.

Function checks of all equipment used in the blood bank should be carried out regularly. This monitoring is also easily scheduled on the quality control calendar and recorded on the daily quality control log. In general, equipment should be tested with the frequency with which malfunction is expected to occur, as modified by how vital the device is. A blood bank refrigerator, for example, is not expected to break down daily, yet its perfect performance is so essential that it is monitored continuously and additionally inspected every 24 hours.

Thermometers must be checked against a reference thermometer, preferably one calibrated by the National Bureau of Standards. Daily recording of temperatures of water baths, heat blocks, warming stages, refrigerated centrifuges, freezers, and refrigerators is required. The adequacy of glassware washing should be checked routinely. Wash bottles require regular cleaning and appropriate labeling. Centrifuges should be calibrated for both speed and timing. Maintenance of refrigerators and freezers used for blood storage must include checks of the temperature recorder, actual inside temperature, lighting, air circulation fans, cleanliness, and the alarm system. Appropriate function checks must be performed on serologic rotators, blood pressure cuffs, trip balances used in blood collection, and blood warmers. Voltages of electrical circuits should be tested periodically. Microscopes require regular professional maintenance.

PROCEDURES AND TECHNIQUES

The most simple of techniques is subject to disarmingly numerous variations and procedural faults. All procedures should be periodically reviewed for uniformity of performance and suitability. Among the many procedures and techniques requiring monitoring may be listed the preparation of the venipuncture site, the microhematocrit method, the amount of blood drawn, the testing procedures for syphilis and HB_SAg, the preparation of red blood cell suspensions, the adequacy of the cell washing technique, the techniques of saline addition, RBC suspension, decanting, and reagent addition, the centrifugation procedure, the reading of agglutination reactions, the performance of enzyme tests, and the detection and identification procedures used in testing for alloantibodies.

BLOOD COMPONENTS

Quality control of blood components requires an assessment of their functional capacity, i.e., an in vivo performance evaluation. The effectiveness of a blood component in vivo is influenced by the amount of loss and damage sustained before and during manufacture, the amount of deterioration during storage, the clinical state of the recipient, and the infusion technique. Frozen RBC may be evaluated by determining their efficiency in raising the hematocrit of the recipient: one unit of frozen RBC should increase the hematocrit of a 70-kg recipient by about 4 volumes per dl. Studies of frozen RBC should be conducted regularly to ascertain the percentage of red blood cell recovery. The efficiency of the post-thaw deglycerolization may be assessed by determining the osmolality of the suspending fluid. Periodic bacteriologic study of frozen RBC should be conducted to ensure that breaks in sterile technique are not occurring.

Regular studies on platelet concentrates are required to determine the percentage yield of platelets from a pint of whole blood and the total number of platelets present in each unit. Recovery in vitro should ideally be greater than 60% of the original platelets present. Platelet concentrates should contain 5.5×10^{10} platelets in 75% of units tested. The red blood cell counts should be less than $20,000/\mu l$. Platelet concentrates should be free from visible clumping. The pH of a platelet concentrate after 72 hours of storage should be not less than 6.0 as measured at the storage temperature. The plasma volume should be determined by weight to be 30 to 50 ml. The in vivo effectiveness of platelet transfusion in raising the platelet count of the recipient should also be determined regularly by performing platelet counts before and at one and 24 hours after platelet infusion. The effective in vivo yield of platelets rarely exceeds half of the calculated number of platelets administered, and in patients with platelet antibodies or the conditions listed in Chapter 25 will be substantially less.

If cryoprecipitate is prepared in the blood bank, Factor VIII activity must be assayed on at least four bags per month. Cryoprecipitate preparations should exhibit 40 units of Factor VIII activity for each 100 ml of source plasma. An in vivo assay should also be performed regularly to determine the potency of the preparations. Active bleeding in a hemophiliac or the presence of anti-Factor VIII in his serum will markedly reduce the in vivo effectiveness of transfused cryoprecipitate.

RECORD KEEPING

Complete and detailed records of every aspect of the blood bank quality control program are essential. Inspectors and regulatory agencies take the approach "If it wasn't documented, it wasn't done" with reasonable justification. Every piece of data generated by the quality control program must be recorded as the work is done (not later from memory) on a permanent, signed record (not on a slip of paper to be copied later). Criteria for normalcy must be established, together with the action to be taken if limits are exceeded. All variations from normal or expected results must be explained on the record, and there must be a notation of what corrective measures were employed. Quality control records are permanent documents to be preserved with other blood bank records for at least five years.

A 12-month calendar should be prepared yearly listing the dates for performance of each part of the quality control program save for those checks performed daily. Items or areas of testing susceptible to periodic review may be scheduled according to Table 28-1. A daily quality control log is useful for recording the results of all quality assurance procedures performed that day. All testing performed on a daily basis is recorded, including a general inspection of the facilities, testing of antisera and reagent RBC, visual inspection of all units of blood in stock, and temperatures of water baths, heat blocks, refrigerators, and freezers. The form is also used to note the results of testing performed as scheduled on the calendar described above or on an irregular basis.

At intervals, clerical errors known only to the quality control officer should be introduced into the blood bank system. The staff should be made aware of what is being done, but the timing should not be predictable. Such a program almost always detects more errors than were introduced.

The list of records required of a blood bank comprises a discouraging array, yet compelling medical, logistic, and legal arguments exist for their maintenance. Sample forms and discussion of their use are found in *Blood Bank Policies and Procedures* and in the *Technical Manual of the American Association of Blood Banks*. Only a listing will be presented here of the necessary records: Blood donor record (history, physical examination, release form), record of emergency treatment of donor reactions, blood-processing record, blood receipt and retesting record, blood transfusion requisitions, daily technologist worksheets (including quality assurance testing by individual technologists), blood issue records, transfusion records (in patient's clinical charts), reports of transfusion reactions, transfusion reaction investigation record (including investigation of cases of

TABLE 28-1

Checklist of Quality Control Procedures

Daily or Whenever Used:

Typing sera
Antiglobulin sera
Reagent RBC
Lectins
Enzyme solutions
Water baths (refill, temp)
Heat blocks
Refrigerators, freezers (temp, general)
Blood units and products (inspection)
Weights of donor units
Serologic tests for syphilis
Tests for HB_SAg and anti-HB_S
Frozen RBC (sterility)
Cryoprecipitate pools (in vivo)
Bench tops (clean)
Microscopes (clean)
Refrigerated centrifuges (temp)
Hematocrit determination (controls)

Weekly:

Glassware washing
Forceps containers
Wash bottles
Refrigerator and freezer temperature
   records
Stock enzyme reactivity
Shipments from central blood
   depot (temp)
Water baths (drain, clean)
Centrifuges, refrigerators (clean)
Staff meeting

Monthly:

Temp alarms (refrigerators, freezers)
Phlebotomy site preparation (culture)
Frozen RBC (Hct, % recovery, WBC)
Platelet concentrates
RBC suspensions (2%)
Technologist unknowns
Clerical error introduction
Housekeeping inspection

Quarterly:

Centrifuges
RPR rotator
Blood pressure cuffs
Trip balance (donor phlebotomy)
Blood warmers
Line voltage

Yearly:

Hematocrit centrifugation procedure
Technologist techniques
Microscopes
Record forms
Procedure manual
Water purity

On Receipt or as Changed:

Thermometers
Water baths
Heat blocks
Saline
Typing sera
Antiglobulin sera
Reagent RBC
Albumin
Lectins
Sterile supplies
New technologists (orientation,
   procedure manual)
Staff notification, changes in procedure
Shipments of blood (irregular suppliers)

possible posttransfusion hepatitis), antibody identification records, equipment and maintenance records, personnel records, and quality assurance records. A daily log in which notations of problems, special action, and incidents are recorded is useful, though not required.

SUPERVISION

There must be documentation of constant surveillance of the blood bank by the supervisor or chief techologist. A supervisor two corridors away buried in paperwork is not effective; neither is one who spends the day performing crossmatches. The professional functions of the supervisor are, among others, to coordinate, solve problems, provide guidance and assistance, and serve as liason between the technical staff and the blood bank director. These responsibilities must not be subordinated to those of being the schedule maker, father confessor, order clerk, committee and fund-drive representative and general factotum in the laboratory. The minute-to-minute operation of the blood bank is the first priority of business for its supervisor; other responsibilities can be delegated if necessary.

RECOMMENDED READING

Greendyke, R.M. and Banzhaf, J.C.: *Blood Bank Policies and Procedures.* Medical Examination Publishing Co., Garden City, N.Y., 1976

Hoppe, P.A.H.: Performance criteria for blood grouping sera. In: *A Seminar on Performance Evaluation.* Am Assn of Blood Banks. Washington, 1976, p. 1

Issitt, P.D.: The antiglobulin test and the evaluation of antiglobulin reagents. In: *Advances in Immunohematology.* Vol. 4, Nos. 5 & 6. Spectra. Oxnard, Calif., N.D.

Issitt, P.D. and Smith, T.R.: Evaluation of antiglobulin reagents. In: *A Seminar on Performance Evaluation.* Am Assn of Blood Banks. Washington, 1976, p. 25

Miller, W.V., (Ed.): *Technical Manual of the American Association of Blood Banks.* Am Assn of Blood Banks. Washington, 1977

Zuck, T.F.: In vivo performance evaluation of blood bank components. In: *A Seminar on Blood Components.* Am Assn of Blood Banks. Washington, 1977, p. 1

Index

ABH antigens
  acquired B antigens, 107
  Bombay types, 104
  chemical nature of, 114, 115
  cis-AB, 107, 108
  combining sites, numbers of, 99
  distribution of
    genotypes, 102
    phenotypes, 101
  modification in disease, 107
  para-Bombay types, 106
  relationship to
    disease, 100
    Lewis and I antigens, 107
  scheme of development, 105, 106
  weak variants, 102-104
ABO
  antibodies
    anti-H, 110
    cross-reacting anti-A,B, 109
    immune isoantibodies, 109
    in infants, 108
    reciprocal relationship with ABO
      antigens, 98, 99, 108
    serologic properties, 108, 109
  genotypes, frequency distribution, 102
  grouping
    false-negative reactions
      RBC, 202
      serum, 203
    false-positive reactions
      RBC, 202
      serum, 203
    in infants, 201
  investigation of problems in, 204
    principle of, 201
    technics, 201
  -HDN, 267
    clinical occurrence, 267
    laboratory diagnosis, 268
  phenotypes, frequency distribution,
    101
Absorption tests, 190
Acid-base balance, 248
Acquired B antigens, 107, 164

Acriflavine, 185
Adenine, 287
ADP, 12
Agglutination of RBC
  causes of anomalous results, 185
  centrifugation, 189
  effect of
    cell concentration, 183
    cell storage, 65, 182
    LISS, 184
    time, 184
  first stage
    effect of
      albumin, 68
      enzymes, 68
      ionic strength, 68
      pH, 68
      temperature, 68
    size relationships, 69
  grading of, 192
  second stage
    effect of
      albumin and ionic strength, 69
      enzymes, 69
      temperature, 69
Agglutinins
  in albumin, 218
  in saline, 218
Agranulocytosis, 25
Albumin autoagglutinins, 185
Albumin
  bovine, 185
  human serum, 313
Alloantibodies
  criteria for identification, 218-223
  definition of, 119
  determination of specificity, 215
  level of confidence of identification,
    217
  occurrence of, 129
  reasons for detecting, 213, 214
  screening cells to detect, 214
  screening technics, 214
Alpha-methyldopa, and positive direct
  antiglobulin tests, 177

Ammonia, 250
Amniocentesis, 266
Anamnestic response, 52, 53
Anaphylotoxins, 84, 85
Anemia
  classification, 21
  physiologic compensations, 34
Anti-A$_1$ lectin, 102
Anti-A,B, 109
Anti-C, 131
Anti-C^w, 131
Anti-C^x, 131
Anti-D
  amount of D antigen required to elicit,
    128, 129
  appearance postpartum, 263
  IgG subclasses of, 128
  maternal immunization, 130
  serologic properties, 127, 128
Anti-E, 131
Anti-Factor VIII$_c$, 311
Anti-Fy^a, 140, 141
Anti-Fy^b, 140, 141
Anti-Fy3, 141
Anti-Fy4, 141
Anti-Fy5, 141
Anti-H, 110
Anti-HB$_c$, 254
Anti-HB$_s$, 256
Anti-Hr, 133
Anti-Hr$_0$, 133
Anti-I
  clinical significance, 157
  occurrence, 156
  serologic properties, 157
Anti-i, occurrence in infectious
  mononucleosis, 157
Anti-Jk^a, 142
Anti-Jk^b, 142
Anti-K, 134, 139, 140
Anti-leukocyte antibodies reactive with
  RBC, 160, 161
Anti-Lu^a, 152, 154
Anti-Lu^b, 152, 154
Anti-Lu3, 152
Anti-M, 147, 148
  lectin, 147
Anti-M$_1$, 148
Anti-M^g, 148
Anti-N, 147, 148
Anti-P, 150
Anti-P$_1$, 148, 150
  clinical significance, 150

Anti-P+P$_1$+P^k, 150
Antiplatelet antibodies, 300
Anti-S, 147, 148
Anti-s, 147, 148
Anti-Tj^a, 150
Anti-U, 147
Anti-Wr^a, 159
Antibody
  affinity, 63
  avidity, 63
  cellular, 42
  classification, 42
  definition of, 39
  elution, 69
  enhancing, 276
  humoral, 42
  Ig class vs. pattern of RBC
    destruction, 229, 230
  naturally occurring, 39, 55
  to platelet antigens, 278
  production, 55, 57
  specificity, definition of, 40
  types of serologic reactivity, 44
Anticoagulants, 19
Anticomplement antiglobulin test, 88
Anticomplementary sera, 188
Antigen
  -antibody reactions
    binding forces, 66, 67
    characteristics, 61
    complementarity of structure, 47
    conformational shifts, 67
    effect of
      time, 73
      relative concentrations, 66
    -lattice formation, 67
  definition of, 39
  specificity, 40
  system, 92
Antigenic
  determinant, 40
  sites, 64
    definition of, 40
Antigenicity, 40
  factors affecting, 50
  of RBC antigens, 199, 200
Antigens
  RBC
    at birth, 42
    chemical properties, 41
    damaged by enzymes, 78, 186
    immunogenicity of various RBC,
      199

racial variation, 51
platelet
   frequency distribution, 278
   stimulus to formation, 278
   types, 278
related to RBC membrane
   abnormalities, 163
Antiglobulin
   sera
      anti-C3b, 88
      anti-C3d, 89
      anti-C4b, 89
      anticomplement, 88
      anti-IgG, 88
      broad spectrum, 88
   test
      anticomplement, 88
      direct, 75, 89
      indirect, 75
      methodological considerations
         false-negative results, 186, 188
         false-positive results, 187
         two-stage test, 188
         use of check cells, 187
      sensitivity, 77
      washing step, 77
Antisera
   quality control of, 322-324
   potency, 62
Antithrombin III, 19
ATP, 246
Autoanalyzer applications, 193, 194
Autoantibodies
   factors influencing biologic activity,
      169, 173
   mechanisms of RBC destruction
      mediated by, 169
   production of, 167
   serologic properties, 168, 170, 171
   significance, 167, 168
   specificity of cold-reacting, 171
   specificity of warm-reacting, 170
   transfusion of patients with, 171
Autoimmune acquired hemolytic
   disease, 167
   drug-induced, 175
   in infectious mononucleosis, 173
   laboratory testing in, 174, 175
   with negative direct antiglobulin test,
      168
   occurrence of, 167
   occurrence of alloantibodies in, 132,
      160

in paroxysmal cold hemoglobinuria,
   173
Autologous transfusion, 293-295

B-lymphocytes, 9, 58
   antibody production by, 57, 58
   differentiation of, 58, 59
Bacterial contamination of stored blood,
   257
Bg antigens, 161
Bilirubin, estimation in amniotic fluid,
   266, 267
Binding constant, 52, 64
Blood
   bank
      administrative rules, 317
      inventory control, 316
      education program, 318
      equipment file, 316
      physical facilities, 315
      safety precautions, 318, 319
   components, quality control of, 325,
      326
   compositon of, 3
   donors
      medical history, 283-285
      physical examination, 285
      public relations, 281, 282
      reactions, 285, 286
      records, 282
   group antibodies, classification by
      serologic reactivity, 61
   preservative solutions, 287
   processing, 290
   shortages, 317
   sludging, 252, 253
   storage conditions, 289
   transfusion
      facilitation of, 35
      indications for, 33
      rate of administration, 35
   transfusion, pediatric
      syringe transfusion, 38
      volume to be administered, 37
Bombay RBC, 103

C antigen, 132
C3b inactivator, 84
C3INA, 89
Cad-positive RBC, 159, 164
Calcium, 19
Cartwright system, 159
Cell panel
   further testing, 222

interpretation of reactions, 217, 222
Cellular immunity, 8
Centrifugation, 73, 189
Cephalosporins and positive direct
  antiglobulin tests, 177
Chemotaxins, 85
Chido antigen, 161
Chimeras, 54
Christmas disease (see Factor IX
  deficiency)
Chromosomes, 91
Chronic granulomatous disease, 137
Chronic hepatitis, 254
Circulatory overload, 245
Cis-AB antigens, 107
  -differentiation from acquired B, 108
Citrate load, 249
Coagulation
  blood
    acquired defects of, 27
    congenital defects of, 27
    disseminated intravascular
      coagulation, 28
    extrinsic system, 16
    fibrinolysis, 16
    inhibitors, 16, 19
    intrinsic system, 16
    in open-heart surgery, 28
    plasma factors, 18
    scheme, 10
  defects after surgery, 250
  factor deficiencies, acquired, 310
    caused by
      anticoagulants, 310, 311
      inhibitors, 311
      DIC, 311
    in extracorporeal circulation, 312
    in hepatic disease, 310
  factor deficiencies, congenital, 304-
    310
Cold autoantibodies, specificity of, 223,
  224
Collection lesion, 288
Compatibility testing
  antiglobulin serum, requirements, 210
  cold autoantibodies and, 223
  crossmatches when various
    alloantibodies are present,
    frequency, 219
  issue procedure, 208
  limitations of, 205, 206
  minor crossmatch, 207
  patient samples, age of, 207

procedure, 206
rationale for, 205
review of old records, 206
sample identification, 207
selection of blood for, 196, 201
Complement
  activation in transfusion reactions, 233
  alternate pathway, 85
  anticomplementary effects, 88
  antigen-antibody activation of, 80
  biologic role, 78, 85
  classic activation sequence, 80-84
  complement and coagulation schemes,
    similarities, 79
  components of, 79
  effect of disease on, 87
  fixation by IgM vs. IgG antibodies,
    230
  hemolysis, cause of, 78
  inhibition, 79
  lability, 87
  notation, 80
  role in antibody-mediated RBC
    destruction, 228
Component therapy, 291
Compound Rh antigens, 132
Conformational shift, 41
Coumadin, 310, 311
CPD, 287
Cryoprecipitate, 307, 308
C^W antigen, 131
C^X antigen, 131
Cytomegalovirus, 256

D antigen
  antigenicity, 128, 129
  factors influencing sensitization to,
    130
  increased reactivity, 126
  mosaic, 124
  RBC, number of D sites, 126, 127
  replacement antigens, 124
  variant D (D^u), 122
Delayed transfusion reactions, 143
DIC, 28, 311
  laboratory evaluation, 312
  in transfusion reactions, 223
  treatment, 312
Diego system, 158
Dielectric constant, 72
2,3-diphosphoglycerate, 34, 246, 247
Disseminated intravascular coagulation
  (see DIC)

Dithiothreitol, 46
Domains, antibody, 48
  biologic activity, 49
Donath-Landsteiner antibody, 173
Dosage effects, 94
  certain specificities, with antisera, 132
2,3-DPG (see 2,3-diphosphoglycerate)
Drug-induced positive direct antiglobulin
  tests, 175
  due to
    drug adsorption, 176
    drug modification of RBC, 177
    immune complex adsorption, 176
  laboratory investigation of, 178
  due to unknown mechanism, 177
Duffy antigens
  antigenicity, 140
  biosynthetic pathway, 141, 142
  Fy(a–b–), 141
  Fy^X, 141
  Fy3, 141
  Fy4, 141
  Fy5, 141
  inactivation by enzymes, 141, 142
  phenotypes, frequency distribution,
    140
  receptor for *Plasmodium vivax*, 142
D^W antigen, 124

E antigen, 132
  of hepatitis B, 254
Electrophoresis, 12
Elution procedures, 191
Enzyme testing, 78, 186
Epstein-Barr virus, 256
Erythroblastosis fetalis (see Hemolytic
  disease of the newborn)
Erythrocytes (see RBC)
Erythropoietin, 22
E^T antigen, 132
E^W antigen, 132
Exchange transfusion, 269
  choice of blood for, 270, 271
  efficiency of, 270
  indications for, 270

F antigen, 132
Factor VIII, 306
  components, 306
  deficiency, 304
    clinical severity, 306, 307
    complications of treatment, 307
    dosage for treatment, 308, 309

preparations, 307, 308
  storage, 307
  treatment, 307, 309
  types, 306
Factor IX
  clinical disease, 309
  concentrates, 308-310
  deficiency, 304
  treatment, 310
Factor XI deficiency, 304
Factor XIII deficiency, 310
Fetal-maternal hemorrhage, 263, 273
Fibrinolysin (see Plasmin)
Fresh blood, 304
Frozen RBC, 295, 296

G antigen, 132
Gamma globulin, 313
Genetic
  disequilibrium, 274
  polymorphism, 48
Genes, 91
  allelic, 91
  amorphic, 92
  codominant, 92
  deletion, 94
  dominant, 92
  expressed, 92
  frequency, 95
  heterozygous, 91
  homozygous, 91
  interaction of, 94
  linked, 91
  mode of action, 92-94
  operator, 94
  recessive, 92
  regulator, 94
  structural, 92
Genotype, 92
Glycophorin A, 6
Glycosyltransferases, 114
Go^a antigen, 124
Graft vs. host reaction, 303
Grafting, organ, 275
Granulocyte
  concentrates, 302
  transfusion reactions, 237

H-chains, 44
H substance
  on RBC, 100
  in secretions, 100
Hapten, 40

Hardy-Weinberg equation, 95
HB$_S$Ag, 254
  radioimmunoassay for, 255
Hemodilution, 253
Hemoglobin
  catabolism after hemolysis, 234, 235
  functions of, 5
Hemolysis, factors affecting, 184
Hemolytic disease of the newborn, 259
  due to ABO incompatibility, 267
  amniocentesis, 266
  causative antibodies, 261
  criteria of severity, 260
  effect of ABO incompatibility, 262, 263
  factors determining development of, 261
  fetal-maternal hemorrhage, 262
  laboratory testing, 268
  natural history, 261
  pathogenesis, 259, 262
  placental transport of antibody, 263
  prenatal prediction of severity, 263, 264
  prophylaxis, 272
  protocol for prenatal testing, 264, 265
  titers in, 266
  transfusion in, 269-271
Hemophilia (see Factor VIII deficiency)
Hemorrhage
  causes, 29
  consequences, 30
  estimation of extent, 31
  repair of, 31
Hemosiderosis, 251
Hemostasis
  platelet factors participating in, 11
  sequence of events in, 12
HEMPAS, 165
Heparin, 19
Hepatitis B, 253-255
  prophylaxis, 255
HLA
  antibodies, 274, 275
    and febrile transfusion reactions, 277
  system
    disease associations, 277
    genetics, 274
    testing, 276, 277
HTLA antibodies, 161, 162
Humoral immunity, 8
Hydrops fetalis, 259

Hyperglobulinemia, 26
Hypocalcemia, 249
Hypofibrinogenemia, 310
Hypogammaglobulinemia, 26
Hypothermia with transfusion, 251

I antigen
  development of, 155
  effect of ABO and P groups, 156, 157
  I$_{int}$, 155
  mosaic character, 156
  number of combining sites, 156
  soluble forms, 156
i antigen
  on cord RBC, 156
  i$_{adult}$, 155
  and RBC marrow transit time, 156
  soluble forms, 156
Icterus gravis, 259
IgA
  structure of, 45
  transfusion reactions to, 238
IgG
  structure of, 44, 48
  subclasses, 46, 47
IgM, structure of, 44
Immune
  adherence, 85
  paralysis, 55
  response, 50-52
Immunoconglutinin, 89
Immunoelectrophoresis, 13
Immunoglobulins
  classes, 42
  properties, 42
  structure of, 44
Immunologic
  competence, 39
  enhancement, 54
  tolerance, 54
Incompatible crossmatch
  common causes of, 209
  falsely compatible, 209
Index of heterogeneity, 53
Infectious mononucleosis, 24
Inhibition tests, 190
Inosine, 287
Intrauterine transfusion, 267

Jaundice, neonatal, 268
  albumin, effect of, 269
  phototherapy, 271

Kell antigens, 134-140
  alleles, 136
  antigen frequency, 136
  biosynthetic pathway, 139
  frequency distribution of phenotypes,
    135
  gene complexes, 137
  importance to RBC membrane, 139
  K_O, 136
  K_X, 139
  McLeod phenotype, 139
  nomenclature, 136
  number of combining sites, 135
  relationship to chronic granulomatous
    disease, 137
Kidd antigens, frequency distribution of
  phenotypes, 143
Kleihauer—Betke test, 272

L-chains, 44
Law of mass action, 63, 64
Leukapheresis, 302
Leukemia, 23
Leukoagglutinins, 237
Leukocyte-poor blood, 296, 297
Leukocyte transfusion reactions, 236,
  237
Leukocytes (see WBC)
Lewis antibodies
  blood transfusion to patients with,
    118, 231
  production of, 117
  serologic properties, 117, 118
  spectrum of specificity, 117
Lewis antigens
  chemical nature of, 114, 115
  in infancy, 116
  interference by A_1, 116
  Le^X, 116
  phenotypes, distribution, 117
  scheme of development, 112, 113
Locus, 91
  syngeneic, 92
Lutheran antigens
  alleles, 152
  amorphs, 151
  biosynthetic pathway, 153
  dosage effects, 152
  phenotypes, frequency distribution,
    151
  on RBC of newborn, 151
LW antigen, 125
Lymphocytes, 8 (also see T-lymphocytes,

  B-lymphocytes)
  committed, 57
Lymphocytotoxins, 237
Lymphoma, 23
Lyonization, 139

Macroglobulin, alpha-2, 19
Macrophages, 10
  role in antibody production, 58
Malaria, 257
Matuhasi-Ogata phenomenon, 191
McLeod type RBC, 139
Memory cells, 57
2-mercaptoethanol, 46
Microemboli, 252
Mixed-field agglutination, 152, 192
MNSs antigens
  aberrant and satellite antigens, 146
  biochemical nature, 146
  M_1, 147
  M_2, N_2, 147
  M^c, 147
  M^g, 147
  M^k, 147
  M^v, 147
  phenotypes, frequency distribution,
    146
  U, 145
Monoclonal gammopathy, 26
Monocytes, 10 (Also see Macrophages)
Mosaicism, 54
Multiple myeloma, 26

Nephelometry, 15
Neutropenia, 25
Neutrophils, 8
Non-A, non-B hepatitis, 256
"Null" lymphocytes, 10

Operon, 94
Opsonization, 85
Oxygen dissociation curve, 34

P antigens
  biochemical nature, 150
  biosynthetic pathway, 148
  at birth, 150
  effect of In(Lu), 150
  phenotypes, frequency distribution,
    149
  parallels with A and O blood groups,
    148, 150
  storage characteristics, 150

Pancytopenia, 25
Para-Bombay RBC, 106
Paraproteins, 126
Paroxysmal cold hemoglobinuria, 151
Paternity testing, 95, 96
Penicillin, and positive direct
  antiglobulin tests, 176
pH of blood, 248
Phagocytosis, 85
Phenotype, 92
Plasma, composition of, 12
Plasma proteins
  electrophoretic separation, 12
  immunoelectrophoretic separation, 13
  major fractions, 13
  quantitation of fractions, 15
  ultracentrifugation, 15
Plasmin, 16
Plastic bags, blood storage in, 239
Platelet
  concentrates, 298
  preparation, 298
  storage, 298
  yields, 299
  transfusion reactions, 237
Plateletpheresis, 301
Platelets
  acquired abnormalities, 24
  functions, 11
  hereditary diseases of, 12
  properties, 10
Polyagglutinins, 163
  differentiation, 165
  serologic properties of, 165
Polycythemia, 23
Position effects, 122
Post-perfusion syndrome, 256
Potassium load, 249
Practical considerations, serological
  avoidance of contamination, 181
  effect of RBC concentration, 183
  loss of RBC agglutinability, 182
  procedural errors, 182, 183
  rouleaux formation, 182
  serum vs. plasma, 181
  use of
    clotted specimens, 182
    hemolyzed specimens, 182
    thrombin, 181
Procoagulant deficiences (see
  Coagulation factor deficiencies)
Properdin, 85
Prostaglandins, 12

Prozone phenomenon, 62

Quality assurance
  blood components, 325, 326
  checklist, 328
  equipment, 324, 325
  personnel competency, 321
  procedures and technics, 325
  reagents, 322-324
  records, 326, 327
  supervision, 329

RBC
  destruction of antibody, mechanisms
    of, 227
  membrane composition, 5, 7
  properties, 4
  survival after storage, 246
  viability in storage, 288
Renal failure, in transfusion reactions,
  233
Reticulocytosis, and positive direct
  antiglobulin tests, 179
Rh antigens
  antigenicity of, 128, 129
  compound, 132
  deleted phenotypes, 126
  distribution of genotypes, 123
  frequency of common gene complexes,
    124
  major components, 119
  most probable genotypes, 123
  nomenclature and genetics, 119-121
  and RBC membrane integrity, 126
Rh
  control solutions, 185
  immune globulin, 272
    dosage, 272
    failure, 273
    indications for administration, 272
    pre-administration laboratory
      workup, 272
    use in Rh-incompatible transfusion,
      272
  typing
    D^u testing, 205
    technical considerations, 204, 205
Rh_{null}, 124-126
Rogers antigen, 161
Rouleaux formation, 182

Saline, 188
Scoring, 63

Screening cells, 214
Sd^a antigen, 159, 160
Secretors, 98
Sensitization, 75
Shock, 29
  management of, 36
Sid system, 159
Soluble blood group antigens, 163
  adsorption on lymphocytes, 161
Specific mixed agglutination, 190
Spectrin, 6
Storage containers, blood, 289
Storage lesion, RBC, 246, 247
Syphilis, 256, 257

T-activation, 163
T-lymphocytes, 8, 58
  role in production of humoral
    antibody, 57
Thrombocytopenia
  causes, 299
  drug-induced immune, 279
  during quinidine treatment, 176
  neonatal, 279
  post-transfusion, 279
Thrombocytosis, 24
Thymosin, 8
Tissue typing, 275
Titer, 62, 63
  factors affecting, 184
Tn-activation, 164
Transfusion
  blood
    ABO compatibility, 198
    administration of blood of types
      other than the recipient's, 210,
      211
    autologous, 293-295
    chronic, 200
    component therapy, 291
    D-compatibility, 198
    emergency procedures, 196, 197
    fresh blood, 304
    frozen RBC, 295, 296
    leukocyte poor, 296, 297
    massive, 293
    RBC transfusion, 291-293
    selection of blood for, 196-198, 210
    statistical considerations in, 198,
      199
  granulocyte, 280, 301
    ABO compatibility, 300

effects, 300
  indications for, 301
  reactions to, 301
platelet, 278, 279, 298-301
  ABO compatibility, 300
  administration, 300
  effects of antiplatelet antibodies,
    300
  indications for, 299, 300
reaction
  allergic
    cause, 237
    signs and symptoms, 237, 238
  due to transfused Ig
    anaphylactoid, due to IgA, 238
    resembling serum sickness, 238
  febrile, 217
    causes, 236
    signs and symptoms, 236, 237
  hemolytic
    in absence of antibody, 231
    definition, 232
    due to plasma transfusion, 232
    factors influencing severity of,
      226, 227
    laboratory findings, 236
    and Lewis antibodies, 231
    mechanisms of RBC destruction,
      227-229
    rate of RBC destruction, 230
    renal failure in, 233
    role of complement, 228
    signs and symptoms, 232
    treatment of, 234
  laboratory investigation of, 239-243

U antigen, 145
Ultracentrifugation, 15

Valence, antibody, 40
Von Willebrand's disease, 309

Waldenström's macroglobulinemia, 26
Water of hydration theory, 72
WBC, properties of, 6 (Also see specific
  WBC types)
Wright system, 159

Xg^a antigen, 158

Yt^a antigen, 159

Zeta potential, 70